Biliary Tract Surgery

Editor

JESSICA A. WERNBERG

SURGICAL CLINICS
OF NORTH AMERICA

www.surgical.theclinics.com

Consulting Editor
RONALD F. MARTIN

April 2014 • Volume 94 • Number 2

ELSEVIER

1600 John F. Kennedy Boulevard • Suite 1800 • Philadelphia, Pennsylvania, 19103-2899

http://www.surgical.theclinics.com

SURGICAL CLINICS OF NORTH AMERICA Volume 94, Number 2
April 2014 ISSN 0039–6109, ISBN-13: 978-0-323-29016-6

Editor: John Vassallo, j.vassallo@elsevier.com
Developmental Editor: Yonah Korngold

Surgical Clinics of North America (ISSN 0039–6109) is published bimonthly by Elsevier Inc., 360 Park Avenue South, New York, NY 10010-1710. Months of publication are February, April, June, August, October, and December. Business and Editorial Offices: 1600 John F. Kennedy Blvd., Suite 1800, Philadelphia, PA 19103-2899. Periodicals postage paid at New York, NY and additional mailing offices. Subscription prices are $370.00 per year for US individuals, $627.00 per year for US institutions, $180.00 per year for US students and residents, $455.00 per year for Canadian individuals, $793.00 per year for Canadian institutions, $510.00 for international individuals, $793.00 per year for international institutions and $250.00 per year for Canadian and foreign students/residents. To receive student/resident rate, orders must be accompanied by name of affiliated institution, date of term, and the *signature* of program/residency coordinator on institution letterhead. Orders will be billed at individual rate until proof of status is received. Foreign air speed delivery is included in all *Clinics* subscription prices. All prices are subject to change without notice. POSTMASTER: Send address changes to *Surgical Clinics*, Elsevier Health Sciences Division, Subscription Customer Service, 3251 Riverport Lane, Maryland Heights, MO 63043. **Customer Service (orders, claims, online, change of address): Telephone: 1-800-654-2452 (U.S. and Canada); 314-447-8871 (outside U.S. and Canada). Fax: 314-447-8029. E-mail: journalscustomerservice-usa@elsevier.com (for print support); journalsonline support-usa@elsevier.com (for online support).**

Reprints. For copies of 100 or more, of articles in this publication, please contact the Commercial Reprints Department, Elsevier Inc., 360 Park Avenue South, New York, New York 10010-1710. Tel. 212-633-3874, Fax: 212-633-3820, E-mail: reprints@elsevier.com.

The Surgical Clinics of North America is also published in Spanish by McGraw-Hill Interamericana Editores S.A., P.O. Box 5-237 06500 Mexico D.F. Mexico; and in Portuguese by Interlivros Edicoes Ltda., Rua Comandante Coelho 1085, CEP 21250, Rio de Janeiro, Brazil; and in Greek by Paschalidis Medical Publications, Athens Greece.

The Surgical Clinics of North America is covered in *MEDLINE/PubMed (Index Medicus), EMBASE/Excerpta Medica, Current Contents/Clinical Medicine, Current Contents/Life Sciences, Science Citation Index,* and *ISI/BIOMED.*

Contributors

CONSULTING EDITOR

RONALD F. MARTIN, MD, FACS
Staff Surgeon, Department of Surgery, Marshfield Clinic, Marshfield; Clinical Associate
Professor, University of Wisconsin School of Medicine and Public Health, Madison,
Wisconsin; Colonel, Medical Corps, United States Army Reserve

EDITOR

JESSICA A. WERNBERG, MD, FACS
Adjunct Clinical Assistant Professor, Department of Surgery, University of Wisconsin,
Madison; Department of General Surgery, Marshfield Clinic, Marshfield, Wisconsin

AUTHORS

HORACIO J. ASBUN, MD, FACS
Director, Hepatobiliary and Pancreas Program, Chair, General Surgery, Professor of
Surgery, Mayo College of Medicine, Mayo Clinic, Jacksonville, Florida

TODD H. BARON, MD
Professor of Medicine, Division of Gastroenterology and Hepatology, University of North
Carolina School of Medicine, Chapel Hill, North Carolina

STEPHEN W. BEHRMAN, MD, FACS
Professor, Division of Surgical Oncology, Department of Surgery, University of Tennessee
Health Science Center, Memphis, Tennessee

MARK BLOOMSTON, MD, FACS
Associate Professor of Surgery, Director, Surgical Oncology Fellowship, Division of
Surgical Oncology, Department of Surgery, Wexner Medical Center, The Ohio State
University, Columbus, Ohio

ANNE-MARIE BOLLER, MD
Assistant Professor, Department of Surgery, Northwestern University Feinberg School
of Medicine, Chicago, Illinois

KAREN BRASEL, MD, MPH
Professor, Surgery, Bioethics and Medical Humanities, Medical College of Wisconsin,
Milwaukee, Wisconsin

CARLOS V.R. BROWN, MD
Associate Professor and Vice-Chairman of Surgery, University of Texas Southwestern -
Austin; Trauma Medical Director, University Medical Center Brackenridge, Austin, Texas

KIMBERLY M. BROWN, MD, FACS
Assistant Professor, Department of Surgery, University of Texas Medical Branch, Galveston, Texas

DANIELLE E. CAFASSO, DO, MPH
Department of Surgery, Tripler Army Medical Center, Honolulu, Hawaii

DANIEL CUCHER, MD
Department of Surgery, College of Medicine, University of Arizona, Tucson, Arizona

DANIEL J. DEZIEL, MD
Helen Shedd Keith Professor and Chair, Department of General Surgery, Rush Medical College, Rush University Medical Center, Chicago, Illinois

PAXTON V. DICKSON, MD
Assistant Professor, Division of Surgical Oncology, Department of Surgery, University of Tennessee Health Science Center, Memphis, Tennessee

ALBERTO R. FERRERES, MD, PhD, FACS
Professor of Surgery and Chair, Division of Gastrointestinal Surgery, University of Buenos Aires, Buenos Aires, Argentina

DAVID A. GELLER, MD, FACS
Richard L. Simmons Professor of Surgery, Chief, Division of Hepatobiliary and Transplant Surgery; Co-Director, Liver Cancer Center, University of Pittsburgh Medical Center; Starzl Transplant Institute, Pittsburgh, Pennsylvania

DONALD J. GREEN, MD
Division of Acute Care Surgery, Department of Surgery, Arizona Health Sciences Center, University of Arizona, Tucson, Arizona

BRANDON T. GROVER, DO, FACS
Department of General and Vascular Surgery, Gundersen Health System, La Crosse, Wisconsin

JEFFREY M. HARDACRE, MD
Associate Professor, Department of Surgery, University Hospitals Case Medical Center, Cleveland, Ohio

TUN JIE, MD
Assistant Professor, Division of Hepatobiliary Surgery, Department of Surgery, Arizona Health Sciences Center, University of Arizona, Tucson, Arizona

KARA M. KEPLINGER, MD
General Surgery Resident, Department of Surgery, Wexner Medical Center, The Ohio State University, Columbus, Ohio

LAWRENCE M. KNAB, MD
Department of Surgery, Northwestern University Feinberg School of Medicine, Chicago, Illinois

SHANU N. KOTHARI, MD, FACS
Department of General and Vascular Surgery, Gundersen Health System, La Crosse, Wisconsin

NARONG KULVATUNYOU, MD
Assistant Professor, Division of Acute Care Surgery, Department of Surgery, Arizona Health Sciences Center, University of Arizona, Tucson, Arizona

DUSTIN D. LUCARELLI, MD
Department of General Surgery, Marshfield Clinic, Marshfield, Wisconsin

MINH B. LUU, MD
Assistant Professor, Department of General Surgery, Rush University Medical Center; Director of Undergraduate Surgical Education, Rush Medical College, Chicago, Illinois

DAVID M. MAHVI, MD
James R. Hines Professor of Surgery, Department of Surgery, Northwestern University Feinberg School of Medicine, Chicago, Illinois

JEFFREY M. MARKS, MD
Professor, Department of Surgery, University Hospitals Case Medical Center, Cleveland, Ohio

RONALD F. MARTIN, MD, FACS
Staff Surgeon, Department of Surgery, Marshfield Clinic, Marshfield; Clinical Associate Professor, University of Wisconsin School of Medicine and Public Health, Madison, Wisconsin; Colonel, Medical Corps, United States Army Reserve

KATHLEEN O'CONNELL, MD
Department of Surgery, Medical College of Wisconsin, Milwaukee, Wisconsin

EVAN S. ONG, MD
Associate Professor, Division of Hepatobiliary Surgery, Department of Surgery, Arizona Health Sciences Center, University of Arizona, Tucson, Arizona

SEAN B. ORENSTEIN, MD
University Hospitals Case Medical Center, Cleveland, Ohio

RICHARD R. SMITH, MD
Department of Surgery, Tripler Army Medical Center, Honolulu, Hawaii

LYGIA STEWART, MD
Professor of Clinical Surgery, Department of Surgery, San Francisco VA Medical Center, University of California San Francisco, San Francisco, California

JESSICA A. WERNBERG, MD, FACS
Adjunct Clinical Assistant Professor, Department of Surgery, University of Wisconsin, Madison; Department of General Surgery, Marshfield Clinic, Marshfield, Wisconsin

Contents

> Working knowledge of extrahepatic biliary anatomy is of paramount impor-
> tance to the general surgeon. The embryologic development of the extra-
> hepatic biliary tract is discussed in this article as is the highly variable
> anatomy of the biliary tract and its associated vasculature. The salient con-
> ditions related to the embryology and anatomy of the extrahepatic biliary
> tract, including biliary atresia, choledochal cysts, gallbladder agenesis,
> sphincter of Oddi dysfunction, and ducts of Luschka, are addressed.

> Biliary cystic disease has been known of for centuries. It has traditionally
> been classified as 5 major types of disease, each with different clinical pro-
> files and attributes. In this article, the basis for the existing classification
> schemes is reviewed and a simplified classification scheme and treatment
> regimen are suggested.

> Symptomatic cholelithiasis and functional disorders of the biliary tract
> present with similar signs and symptoms. The functional disorders of the
> biliary tract include functional gallbladder disorder, dyskinesia, and the
> sphincter of Oddi disorders. Although the diagnosis and treatment of
> symptomatic cholelithiasis are relatively straightforward, the diagnosis
> and treatment of functional disorders can be much more challenging.
> Many aspects of the diagnosis and treatment of functional disorders are
> in need of further study. This article discusses uncomplicated gallstone dis-
> ease and the functional disorders of the biliary tract to emphasize and up-
> date the essential components of diagnosis and management.

> Gallstone disease is the most common cause of acute pancreatitis in the
> Western world. In most cases, gallstone pancreatitis is a mild and self-
> limiting disease, and patients may proceed without complications to

cholecystectomy to prevent future recurrence. Severe disease occurs in about 20% of cases and is associated with significant mortality; meticulous management is critical. A thorough understanding of the disease process, diagnosis, severity stratification, and principles of management is essential to the appropriate care of patients presenting with this disease. This article reviews these topics with a focus on surgical management, including appropriate timing and choice of interventions.

Choledocholithiasis is a common manifestation of biliary disease. Intraoperative cholangiography can be performed in several ways. Common bile duct exploration can be safely performed but necessitates an advanced level of surgical experience to limit complications and improve success. An algorithm based on available resources and the physician skill set is vital for safe and effective management of choledocholithiasis. Endoscopic retrograde cholangiopancreatography requires the availability of an advanced endoscopist as well as significant equipment and resources. Current training of young surgeons is limited for open biliary procedures and common bile duct explorations. Educational guidelines are necessary to reduce this educational gap.

Because it offers several advantages over open cholecystectomy, laparoscopic cholecystectomy has largely replaced open cholecystectomy for the management of symptomatic gallstone disease. The only potential disadvantage is a higher incidence of major bile duct injury. Although prevention of these biliary injuries is ideal, when they do occur, early identification and appropriate treatment are critical to improving the outcomes of patients suffering a major bile duct injury. This report delineates the key factors in classification (and its relationship to mechanism and management), identification (intraoperative and postoperative), and management principles of these bile duct injuries.

Cholangiocarcinoma is an uncommon tumor with a poor prognosis. Presenting symptoms are often nonspecific, and jaundice appears late in the disease course. Surgical resection and liver transplant are the potentially curative treatments. Palliation can be performed by percutaneous, endoscopic, or surgical interventions.

Cholangiocarcinoma involving the distal common bile duct (distal cholangiocarcinoma [DCC]) is a periampullary neoplasm that is less common than, but often difficult to distinguish from, pancreatic adenocarcinoma

(PDA). Although the prognosis and cure rate of DCC is improved over that of PDA, it remains a highly lethal disease. While the pathophysiology of DCC is, in many instances, distinctly different form PDA, the diagnostic and therapeutic management of this disease is not dissimilar from pancreatic cancer. A multi-disciplinary approach toward DCC is important.

Gallbladder cancer remains a relatively rare malignancy with a highly variable presentation. Gallbladder cancer is the most common biliary tract malignancy with the worst overall prognosis. With the advent of the laparoscope, in comparison with historical controls, this disease is now more commonly diagnosed incidentally and at an earlier stage. However, when symptoms of jaundice and pain are present, the prognosis remains dismal. From a surgical perspective, gallbladder cancer can be suspected preoperatively, identified intraoperatively, or discovered incidentally on final surgical pathology.

Our understanding of bile metabolism and the molecular effects of bile acids has expanded in recent years. Bile acids, which are classically recognized for their involvement in dietary lipid absorption, are now known to be involved in many aspects of energy metabolism and disease processes in humans. Cholelithiasis, a consequence of altered bile metabolism, affects a significant number of American adults. An understanding of the disease process, risk factors, and complications of gallbladder disease is necessary for the development of novel targeted treatments and prophylactic therapies against the development of gallstones.

Extrinsic compression of the bile duct from gallstone disease is associated with bilio-biliary fistulization, requiring biliary-enteric reconstruction. Biliary-enteric fistulas are associated with intestinal obstruction at various levels. The primary goal of therapy is relief of intestinal obstruction; definitive repair is performed for selected patients. Hemobilia from gallstone-related pseudoaneurysms is preferentially controlled by selective arterial embolization. Rapidly increasing jaundice with relatively normal liver enzymes is a diagnostic hallmark of bilhemia. Acquired thoraco-biliary fistulas are primarily treated by percutaneous and endoscopic interventions.

The use of peroral endoscopy in the diagnosis of and therapy for biliary disorders has evolved immensely since the introduction of flexible fiberoptic endoscopes more than 50 years ago. Endoscopic retrograde cholangiopancreatography was introduced approximately a decade after flexible upper endoscopy and has evolved from a purely diagnostic procedure to almost exclusively a therapeutic procedure for managing biliary tract disorders. Endoscopic ultrasound, which continues to be a procedure of high diagnostic yield, is becoming a therapeutic modality for management of biliary diseases. This article discusses the diagnostic and therapeutic aspects of endoscopic retrograde cholangiopancreatography and endoscopic ultrasound for evaluation and treatment of biliary diseases.

Biliary disease is common in the obese population and increases after bariatric surgery. This article reviews management of the gallbladder at the time of bariatric surgery, as well as imaging modalities in the bariatric surgery population and prevention of lithogenesis in the rapid weight loss phase. In addition, diagnosis and treatment options for biliary diseases are discussed, including laparoscopic-assisted percutaneous transgastric endoscopic retrograde cholangiopancreatography in the patient having bariatric surgery.

The gold standard for the surgical treatment of symptomatic cholelithiasis is conventional laparoscopic cholecystectomy (LC). Although it has been associated with a slightly higher incidence of bile duct injury (BDI) in comparison with open cholecystectomy (OC), LC is considered a very safe operation. Prevention of BDI should be routinely performed in every LC. Recent trends include the performance of cholecystectomy through a single incision and NOTES (Natural Orifice Transluminal Endoscopic Surgery). However, lack of evidence of clinical advantages prevents their widespread adoption, and more data are needed to assess whether their use is warranted.

Acute cholecystitis is defined as inflammation of the gallbladder and is usually caused by obstruction of the cystic duct. Cholescintigraphy is the most sensitive imaging modality for cholecystitis. The gold standard treatment of acute cholecystitis is laparoscopic cholecystectomy. Operating early in the disease course decreases overall hospital stay and avoids increased complications, conversion to open procedures, and mortality. Cholecystitis during pregnancy is a challenging problem for surgeons. Operative intervention is generally safe for both mother and fetus, given the improved morbidity of the laparoscopic approach compared with open, although increased caution should be exercised in women with gallstone pancreatitis.

Postscript

For patients with small bowel and colonic perforations, a definitive diagnosis of the cause of perforation is not necessary before operation. Bowel obstruction and inflammatory bowel disease are the most common causes of nontraumatic intestinal perforations in industrialized countries, whereas infectious causes of intestinal perforations are more common in developing countries. Treatment of small bowel and colonic perforations generally includes intravenous antibiotics and fluid resuscitation, but the specific management of the bowel depends on the underlying cause of the perforation.

SURGICAL CLINICS
OF NORTH AMERICA

FORTHCOMING ISSUES

June 2014
Endocrine Surgery
Peter J. Mazzaglia, *Editor*

August 2014
Management of Burns
Robert L. Sheridan, *Editor*

October 2014
Surgical Infections
Robert G. Sawyer, and
Traci L. Hedrick, *Editors*

RECENT ISSUES

February 2014
Acute Care Surgery
George C. Velmahos, *Editor*

December 2013
Current Topics in Transplantation
A. Osama Gaber, *Editor*

October 2013
Abdominal Wall Reconstruction
Michael J. Rosen, *Editor*

August 2013
Vascular Surgery and Endovascular Therapy
Girma Tefera, *Editor*

ISSUE OF RELATED INTEREST

Surgical Oncology Clinics of North America April 2014 (Vol. 23, Issue 2)
Biliary Tract and Primary Liver Tumors
Timothy M. Pawlik, *Editor*

Foreword

Biliary Tract Surgery

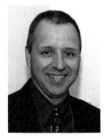

Ronald F. Martin, MD, FACS
Consulting Editor

I find myself once again writing a foreword to an issue of the *Surgical Clinics of North America* while deployed overseas for these ongoing conflicts. Being overseas in and of itself doesn't really matter that much, but the process of getting over here perhaps does. It may not be obvious to those who have never had to be "involuntarily mobilized" by federal authority or some other power beyond one's control, but the mere fact that one has to pack bags and disconnect from everyday life is usually quite trying. A litany of the tasks is not required but I would suggest that you consider this: if everything that you normally did, everything that represented your reason for getting up each day, suddenly needed to be done by other people—how would you feel about that?

Having had the opportunity to practice this, I can relay one sentiment on the matter— gratitude. I am deeply grateful for the people in my professional and private lives that step up and pick up the slack. I am also impressed by how supportive and willing to help these people are and have been. Many of them have done this time and again for me and some have just had the most recent opportunity.

It is easy, too easy, to become complacent and possibly even entitled when we are surrounded by all the necessities and luxuries to which many of us have become accustomed. Being removed from this somehow makes it simpler to focus on what matters.

The *Surgical Clinics of North America* has a cadence and a rhythm of its own. We develop and distribute six issues per year and each of these represents a minimum of one year of work, and often as much as two years, from concept to final printing. It is a wonderful process but one that requires a sustained and concerted effort to keep the schedule on pace. When I disappear for a while, I invariably put people in a position where they have to adjust and sometimes adjust a great deal. Mr John Vassallo, our guiding force at Elsevier, has always accommodated whatever we needed without complaint. Before his time working on this project, Ms Catherine Bewick did the same.

Surg Clin N Am 94 (2014) xiii–xiv
http://dx.doi.org/10.1016/j.suc.2014.02.001
0039-6109/14/$ – see front matter © 2014 Published by Elsevier Inc.

surgical.theclinics.com

Our surgical colleagues have bent over backwards to expedite plans for future issues and escalate timetables for delivering material to keep things going smoothly. My partners at Marshfield Clinic have unflinchingly taken on extra clinical responsibilities as well as nonclinical tasks. Perhaps, most importantly, my clinical partner, Dr Jessica Wernberg, has assembled the contributors and has shepherded this issue to completion with much less help from me than I originally promised her. And she has done an outstanding job of doing so.

Biliary surgery has increasingly become a specialty emerging from what was once among the most required skill sets of the generalist. Whether that is a good development or poor one—I shall let you decide. My observation has been that we are all redefining what are and are not the acceptable "comfort zones" for general surgeons. One can lament that or embrace it—I suggest the latter course. Independent of how one feels about biliary specialization, one needs a good grasp of the fundamentals and the not-so-fundamentals. This issue should be an excellent place to start on many of these topics.

One of the nice things about being deployed is that professional life condenses to its core: sustain the mission. The mission is being there for service members and others who need our help. There is little room for monetary concerns or ego or power struggles. It is not a perfect life but it does have its benefits.

Being removed from my everyday niceties always gives me a chance to remember what really matters. The petty squabbles recede and the acts of generosity and kindness seem to loom a bit larger. Many people thank me for my service when I travel in uniform, for which I am grateful, but rarely do people thank the people who prop up our lives and livelihoods when we are gone. It is not that they wouldn't thank them; it is just that those people are harder to identify in a crowd. I thank all of you who take care of us and manage our concerns while away.

I would like to see a day when no one needs to go abroad as a result of hostility but I am possibly too jaded to believe in such fantasies. Until then, I shall remain grateful for the support and help that others and I get when we do such things.

Please enjoy this issue for its very valuable clinical content but also consider the amount of pure effort and sharing that each of its contributors put into creating it. Take a moment to recognize those who make your life easier and better. It is all too easy to forget them.

Ronald F. Martin, MD, FACS
Department of Surgery
Marshfield Clinic
1000 North Oak Avenue
Marshfield, WI 54449, USA

E-mail address:
martin.ronald@marshfieldclinic.org

Preface

Biliary Tract Surgery

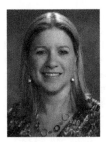

Jessica A. Wernberg, MD, FACS
Editor

This issue of *Surgical Clinics of North America* serves as an update on the multidisciplinary management of complex benign and malignant biliary tract disease, includes a simplified scheme for categorizing bile duct cysts, and functions as a basic review of the anatomy, physiology, and surgical techniques of the biliary tract.

Several contributing authors write about the need for individual and institutional expertise in biliary tract procedures, specifically commenting on the comfort level of the operating surgeon. As laparoscopic and endoscopic procedures become more sophisticated, there is perhaps a lesser, but still critical, role for open surgical exploration in this arena. Biliary surgeons are expected to be proficient in both open and laparoscopic techniques despite the declining number of procedures. Multidisciplinary management of complex biliary disease is paramount.

Only four liver cases are required for general surgery training and there are no defined requirements for complex biliary and pancreatic cases. General Surgery residents are often graduating without performing even a single common bile duct exploration. Developing an expertise in biliary tract surgery without fellowship training is unlikely. Even with fellowship training, early career mentorship from a senior surgeon is valuable.

I would like to take this opportunity to acknowledge Dr Marvin Kuehner, who died during the editing of this issue on Biliary Tract Surgery. He introduced me to hepatobiliary surgery and walked me through my early cases as a resident. His fearless nature and ingenuity never ceased to amaze me. I fondly remember one of his favorite mantras, "Anatomy strikes again!," which he regularly said as we proceeded through various advanced dissections. He trained in the era of independent surgical decision-making and predated routine endoscopic retrograde cholangiopancreatography, CT, and laparoscopy. He was devoted to his patients and continued to evolve as a skilled pancreaticobiliary surgeon. He and Dr Ron Martin served as invaluable mentors in complex foregut and hepatobiliary surgery when I returned to Marshfield Clinic as a new attending surgeon.

Surg Clin N Am 94 (2014) xv–xvi
http://dx.doi.org/10.1016/j.suc.2014.02.002
0039-6109/14/$ – see front matter © 2014 Published by Elsevier Inc.

surgical.theclinics.com

As the Assistant Program Director for General Surgery at our institution, I now mentor residents and new surgeons, but still rely on the expertise of colleagues and mentors. "See one, do one, teach one," or perhaps "see some, do some, teach some," will continue to mold future surgeons regardless of simulators and Web-based educational modules.

Participating in this project has clearly contributed to my lifelong learning. This edition of *Surgical Clinics of North America* could not have come together without the submissions from mentors, colleagues, and mentees and I truly appreciate their contributions to this issue.

Jessica A. Wernberg, MD, FACS
Department of General Surgery
Marshfield Clinic
1000 North Oak Avenue
Marshfield, WI 54449, USA

E-mail address:
wernberg.jessica@marshfieldclinic.org

Anatomy and Embryology of the Biliary Tract

Kara M. Keplinger, MD[a], Mark Bloomston, MD[b],*

KEYWORDS

- Gallbladder • Biliary tree • Portal triad • Anatomy • Embryology

KEY POINTS

- Variation in the anatomy of the extrahepatic biliary tree and its associated vasculature should be anticipated. When aberrant anatomy is encountered, other aberrancies should be expected.
- The embryologic development of the extrahepatic biliary tract is complex and incompletely understood; however, several important factors in cell signaling have been defined in recent years.
- Biliary atresia is an uncommon but serious cause of perinatal jaundice and requires operative intervention, usually a Kasai portoenterostomy. Liver transplant is often ultimately required.
- The symptoms of choledochal cysts may be nonspecific, but diagnosis is important in the face of increased risk of cholangiocarcinoma inherent to these patients.
- The replaced right hepatic artery is a common aberrancy of the hepatic vasculature and is found posterolateral in the portal triad. The replaced left hepatic artery can be found in the gastrohepatic ligament.
- Ducts of Luschka, perhaps better termed *subvesical ducts*, are an important cause of postcholecystectomy bile leak, a complication that may be avoided by cautious, shallow dissection of the gallbladder from the fossa.

INTRODUCTION

Working knowledge of extrahepatic biliary anatomy is of paramount importance to the general surgeon. The laparoscopic cholecystectomy is one of the most common surgical procedures in the United States. In surgical training, it is the procedure whereby learners often cut their teeth in the laparoscopic arena, first with the privilege of peeling the gallbladder from its fossa and later by dissecting out the cystic structures. The variation of the anatomy can be staggering. Depending on the disease process, the

Disclosures: None.
[a] Department of Surgery, Wexner Medical Center, The Ohio State University, 395 West 12th Avenue, Room 654, Columbus, OH 43210-1267, USA; [b] Surgical Oncology Fellowship, Division of Surgical Oncology, Department of Surgery, Wexner Medical Center, The Ohio State University, 320 West 10th Avenue, M256 Starling Loving Hall, Columbus, OH 43210-1267, USA
* Corresponding author.
E-mail address: Mark.Bloomston@osumc.edu

Surg Clin N Am 94 (2014) 203–217
http://dx.doi.org/10.1016/j.suc.2014.01.001
0039-6109/14/$ – see front matter © 2014 Elsevier Inc. All rights reserved.

setting of inflammation can significantly impair visualization and distort the usual locations of the regional structures. Congenital malformations are also a source of anatomic variation and can confuse or surprise the surgeon at the time of surgical exploration. Misunderstanding and underestimation of the anatomy can result in misdiagnosis and serious injury to the biliary tree in the operative setting. Although biliary injury is uncommon, its potential complications carry a high morbidity. In this article, the authors review the embryologic development of the extrahepatic biliary tract and gallbladder as well as its variable anatomy.

EMBRYOLOGY
General Biliary Embryology

Understanding of the biliary tract begins with the appreciation of its embryologic development. Beginning in the fourth week of gestation, the liver bud arises from the distal extent of the foregut. As the liver parenchyma develops, the cells between it and the foregut proliferate, forming the precursor to the bile duct.[1] Between the fourth and fifth weeks of gestation, the gallbladder primordium buds off the caudal extent of the bile duct giving rise to the gallbladder and cystic duct. This bud lies in close proximity to the ventral pancreatic bud. The shared stalk rotates posteriorly and medially to join the dorsal pancreatic bud (**Fig. 1**). The ventral pancreatic bud gives rise to the uncinate process; its duct, the duct of Wirsung, typically joins with the common bile duct (CBD). This confluence occurs at the ampulla of Vater, and they drain into the duodenum via the major papilla. Usually, the duct draining the dorsal pancreatic bud will fuse with the duct draining the ventral pancreatic bud. This duct, the duct of Santorini, may fail to fuse (known as *pancreas divisum*) and/or drain directly into the duodenum at the minor papilla.

The extrahepatic biliary tree develops in close concert with the hepatic artery. Further details of the development of the extrahepatic biliary tract remain nebulous. It was initially thought that the biliary tract lumen passed through a phase in which the lumen was obliterated by proliferating endothelial cells, and failure to recanalize resulted in biliary atresia in neonates, similar to the pathogenesis of duodenal atresia. This belief has been refuted by studies in human embryos showing that the lumen never obliterates during maturation.[2] The process of how the intrahepatic and extrahepatic biliary networks anastomose is not well understood, but they seem to be in continuity throughout development.

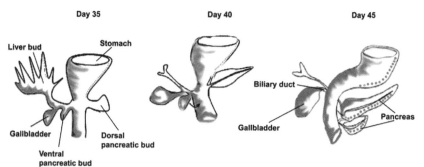

Fig. 1. Embryologic development of the biliary tree and pancreas. (*From* Sahu S, Joglekar MV, Yang SNY, et al. Cell sources for treating diabetes. In: Gholamrezanezhad A, editor. Stem Cells in Clinic and Research, 2011. InTech, http://dx.doi.org/10.5772/24174. Available at: http://www.intechopen.com/books/stem-cells-in-clinic-and-research/cell-sources-for-treating-diabetes.)

Cell Signaling in Biliary Development

The development of the liver and biliary tract is governed by many of the major pathways in cell signaling. These pathways include Notch, Wnt, sonic hedgehog, and transforming growth factor β.[3] Not surprisingly, these pathways have been implicated in the pathogenesis of biliary and pancreatic malignancies.[4–6] Although the development of intrahepatic bile ducts is fairly well understood, there seem to be distinctly different mechanisms regulating the development of the extrahepatic biliary tract. Current literature suggests that the development of the extrahepatic biliary tree is more closely related to the development of the duodenum and the pancreas.[7] Evidence of this includes the expression of Pdx1 in both biliary and pancreatic progenitor cells but not in the liver progenitor cells in the murine model.[8] Of particular importance are the transcription factors hepatic nuclear factor (HNF) 1β,[9] HNF6,[10] Sox17, and Hes1,[8] which when absent predispose to malformation of the extrahepatic biliary tree and gallbladder agenesis. Much of the difficulty in studying the embryologic development of the extrahepatic biliary tract stems from the essential nature of the cell signaling pathways regulating it. When these pathways are disturbed, it is often lethal to the embryo.

CONGENITAL DISORDERS OF THE BILIARY TRACT
Biliary Atresia

The pathogenesis of biliary atresia is a complicated process with multiple factors influencing development. The incidence of biliary atresia varies by region of the world and ranges from 1 in 5000 in Asian countries to 1 in 19,000 in European countries.[11] Around 20% of patients with biliary atresia also suffer from an additional congenital abnormality, including splenic abnormalities (most common), venous malformations, and syndromes driven by chromosomal abnormalities. The factors thought to influence the development of biliary atresia in the prenatal period include genetic dysregulation, immune dysfunction, and inflammation. Patients present with unresolving perinatal jaundice, cholestasis (pale stool and a direct hyperbilirubinemia), and progressive liver dysfunction. In this context, ultrasound showing no dilation of the bile ducts is suggestive of biliary atresia. Liver biopsy is usually necessary for diagnosis. Histologic examination of the bile ducts reveals "ductular reaction, bile plugs within bile ductules, portal tract edema, and portal fibrosis."[12] The natural history of biliary atresia is progression to cirrhosis and death by 2 years of age. The first-line treatment of biliary atresia is usually the Kasai portoenterostomy. The outcome is determined by the quality of biliary drainage. Regardless of drainage, cirrhosis will often progress over time, and liver transplant becomes necessary.

Choledochal Cysts

Choledochal cystic disease is another congenital condition whose pathophysiology remains incompletely understood. The incidence of choledochal cysts varies by region, occurring in about 1 per 1000 in Asia but only 1 per 100,000 to 150,000 in the Western world. Females are affected more often than males. The most commonly accepted theory for pathogenesis is pancreaticobiliary maljunction where the CBD and pancreatic duct share a long common channel. Pancreaticobiliary maljunction leads to the reflux of pancreatic enzymes up into the biliary tree. Subsequent inflammation and dilation occur. However, this theory does not completely account for other characteristics of the disease, including antenatal findings of dilation when pancreatic enzymes are not being produced in significant quantities.[13] The five types of choledochal cysts are depicted in **Fig. 2**. The most common presentation is fusiform dilation of the extrahepatic ducts, sometimes including the cystic duct (type I) representing 80% to 90% of cases.

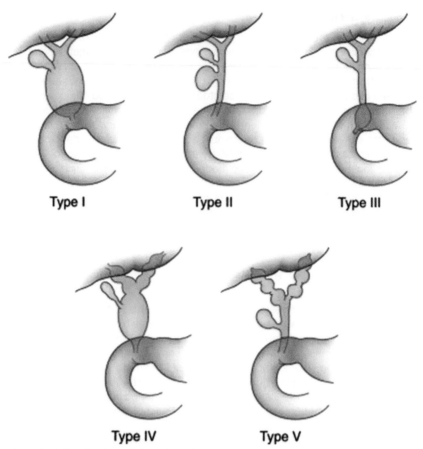

Fig. 2. Todani classification of choledochal cysts. (*From* Sabiston DC, Townsend CM. Sabiston textbook of surgery: the biological basis of modern surgical practice. 19th edition. Philadelphia: Elsevier Saunders; 2012; with permission.)

Presentation is variable. Patients usually present at childhood with symptoms that may classically include right upper quadrant pain, jaundice, and a palpable mass in the right upper quadrant. Patients may develop pancreatitis or cholangitis. Diagnosis is based on imaging, usually with either computed tomography (CT) or ultrasonography. Cholangiography is often necessary for surgical planning. Although the pathogenesis is not well defined, the complications that can result are. These complications include choledocholithiasis, cholecystitis, cholestasis, cirrhosis, and, most seriously, an increased risk of cholangiocarcinoma with age. The treatment of choledochal cystic disease is total cyst resection and biliary drainage, usually with a Roux-en-Y hepaticojejunostomy. Unfortunately, studies suggest that an increased risk for cancer persists despite resection, with up to 5% going on to develop cholangiocarcinoma.[14] Further details of choledochal cystic disease are discussed elsewhere in this issue.

Gallbladder Agenesis

As mentioned earlier, several signaling pathways and transcription factors have been shown to be of critical importance in the development of the gallbladder. It is estimated that congenital absence of the gallbladder occurs in 10 to 65 per 100,000 live births. This approximation may underestimate the true incidence because the malformation may go undetected.[15] Females are more likely to be diagnosed, but autopsy studies show an equal incidence between the sexes. Other congenital malformations or variants may be associated. Typically, there is little consequence of gallbladder agenesis; however, some patients develop symptoms of biliary colic.[16] Diagnosis is suggested by the absence of the gallbladder on right-upper-quadrant ultrasound. Further studies are usually required to confirm this and may include CT, magnetic resonance cholangiopancreatography, or the more invasive endoscopic retrograde cholangiopancreatography (ERCP) or endoscopic ultrasound. Cholescintigraphy in these patients may be misleading because nonvisualization of the cystic duct could lead the surgeon to diagnose cholecystitis, subjecting patients to an unnecessary procedure. Cases were often diagnosed intraoperatively after thorough exploration had failed to reveal the gallbladder. This situation occurs less commonly as a result of advances in imaging technology.[15] If at exploration the gallbladder is not easily visualized, intraoperative ultrasound can be used to avoid more aggressive exploration. Because sphincter of Oddi dysfunction (SOD) has been postulated to be one of the causes for biliary colic in these patients, endoscopic sphincterotomy may be helpful for symptomatic patients. This procedure is only pursued after medical management, such as with smooth muscle relaxants, has failed.

BILIARY ANATOMY
Classic Extrahepatic Biliary Anatomy

Perhaps the most consistent feature of biliary anatomy is its inconsistency. Aberrant anatomy should be expected and sought during any biliary surgery. Classically, the right and left hepatic ducts exit the liver and join to form the common hepatic duct, as seen in **Fig. 3**. The left hepatic duct courses from the base of the umbilical fissure along the inferior border of segment IV of the left lobe before joining the short right hepatic duct just below the infundibulum of the gallbladder. The longer length generally seen with the left hepatic duct allows for a more sufficient target for operative biliary decompression or bypass in cases of obstruction or for reconstruction in the face of malignancy. The close relationship between the confluence of the left and right hepatic ducts with the undersurface of the liver hilum emphasizes the need for extensive hepatic resection seen with hilar cholangiocarcinoma. Also, the short length of the right and left hepatic ducts provides a tumor in this location with ready access to intrahepatic secondary biliary radicals, often preventing curative resection.

The cystic duct may be of variable length and typically joins the common hepatic duct to form the CBD. The CBD courses down the hepatoduodenal ligament anterior to the portal vein and lateral to the hepatic artery. The CBD courses inferiorly, posterior to the first portion of the duodenum, then posterior to the pancreas in a groove, often covered by a thin layer of pancreas.[17] Finally, it enters into the second portion of the duodenum either alone or after joining the pancreatic duct.

The length of the CBD varies between 7 and 11 cm in length and has an internal diameter of up to 8 mm at a normal physiologic pressure.[18] Lining the lumen is a columnar epithelium that contains mucus-secreting cells. The main arteries supplying the CBD course along its lateral and medial walls and originate from the gastroduodenal and right hepatic arteries. This arterial anatomy is clinically relevant in iatrogenic injury of the CBD because compromise of this vascular network can lead to stenosis.

The hepatic artery is intimately associated with the biliary tree, situated medial to the CBD in the hepatoduodenal ligament. In the classic description, the celiac axis branches off of the aorta after it passes through the diaphragm. The celiac axis

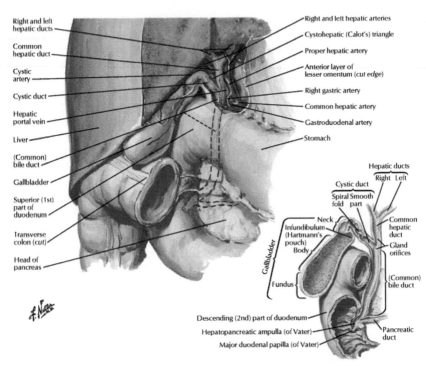

Fig. 3. Classic anatomy of the extrahepatic biliary ducts. (Netter illustration from www. netterimages.com. © Elsevier Inc. All rights reserved.)

trifurcates into the left gastric, splenic, and common hepatic arteries (**Fig. 4**). The common hepatic artery gives rise to the gastroduodenal and right gastric arteries before becoming the hepatic artery proper, which ascends in the hepatoduodenal ligament. The hepatic artery proper then bifurcates at a variable level into the left and right hepatic arteries before entering the liver. The left hepatic artery continues along the medial aspect of the hepatoduodenal ligament to enter the left liver through the

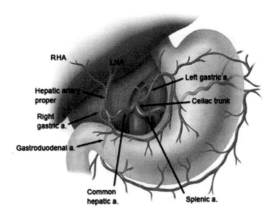

Fig. 4. Classic anatomy of the celiac axis. LHA, left hepatic artery; RHA, right hepatic artery. (*From* Geller DA, Goss JA, Tsung A. Liver. In: Brunicardi FC, Andersen DK, Billiar TR, et al, editors. Schwartz's principles of surgery. 9th edition. New York: McGraw-Hill Publishing; 2010; with permission.)

umbilical fissure. The right hepatic artery traverses from medial to lateral in the hepatoduodenal ligament, typically passing behind the common hepatic duct to enter the right liver. The cystic artery supplying the gallbladder usually branches off of the right hepatic artery. Thorough understanding of the relationships between these structures is imperative for general and hepatobiliary surgeons, particularly aberrant anatomy as described later.

The portal vein lies posterior to the CBD and the hepatic artery in the porta hepatis. It forms from the union of the superior mesenteric vein and the splenic vein, which receives venous blood from the inferior mesenteric vein. The left gastric (coronary) vein draining the lesser curve of the stomach empties into the portal vein near its origin. Similar to the hepatic artery proper, the portal vein branches bifurcate before entering the liver. The extrahepatic portal vein shows the least variation of the portal structures with the most common aberrancy being separate takeoffs of the anterior and posterior right portal branches from the main portal vein. Very little variation is seen in the left portal vein before entering the liver. The left, right, or both portal veins will provide blood supply to the caudate lobe.

Variations in Extrahepatic Biliary Anatomy

The right and left hepatic ducts run a short course outside of the liver parenchyma before forming the common hepatic duct. Rarely, the right and left ducts join within the liver. Alternatively, they may course separately and join lower in the hepatoduodenal ligament (**Fig. 5**).

Of particular importance is the first order branching of the right and left hepatic ducts within the liver. In a recent report based on radiographic imaging, there were atypical branching patterns of the right hepatic duct in 14% of patients, and there were atypical branching patterns of the left hepatic duct in 8%.[19] As shown in **Fig. 6**, the right anterior and posterior segmental branches can occur in many conformations, with the most worrisome being type A4 in which the right posterior segmental duct drains into the cystic duct. Ligating this duct may cause cholestasis in the

A   **B**   **C**

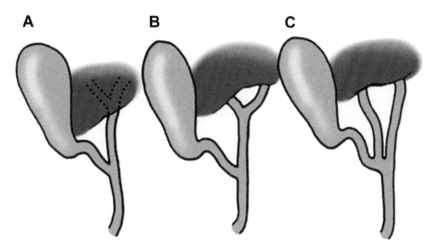

Fig. 5. Variation in confluence of right and left hepatic ducts. Intrahepatic (*A*), extrahepatic/typical (*B*), and low (*C*) confluence of the right and left hepatic ducts. (*From* Skandalakis JE, Branum GD, Colborn GL. Extrahepatic biliary tract and gallbladder. In: Skandalakis JE, Colburn GL, Weidman TA, editors. Skandalakis' Surgical Anatomy. Athens (Greece): Paschalidis Medical Publications, Ltd; 2004; with permission.)

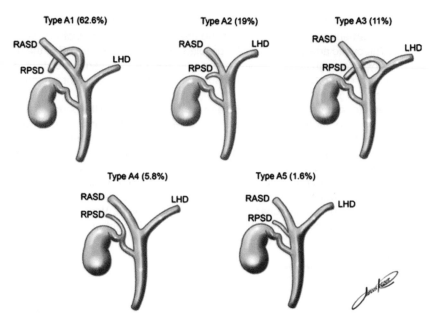

Fig. 6. Variations in sectoral drainage to right hepatic duct. LDH, left hepatic duct; RASD, right anterior hepatic duct; RPSD, right posterior hepatic duct. (*From* Chaib E, Kanas AF, Galvão FH, et al. Bile duct confluence: anatomic variations and its classification. Surg Radiol Anat 2013. [Epub ahead of print]; with permission.)

segment from which it drains. Given the wide variability in the conformation of these structures, intraoperative cholangiography can be immensely helpful in elucidating the anatomy and should be considered when unusual anatomy is encountered.

Variations in Hepatic Artery Anatomy

Only about 70% of patients have the classic hepatic arterial anatomy whereby the hepatic artery proper bifurcates to form the right and left hepatic arteries. Accessory right and left hepatic arteries may be found in addition to the usual right and left hepatic arteries (**Fig. 7**E–G) or the right or left hepatic arteries may be replaced, meaning they originate from another source entirely. Accessory arteries will usually supply a discreet segment of the liver; therefore, some argue that the nomenclature of the accessory hepatic artery is misleading. Rarely, the common hepatic artery derives completely from the superior mesenteric artery (SMA); this is known as the completely replaced common hepatic artery (see **Fig. 7**A).

The right hepatic artery usually courses posterior to the hepatic duct before entering the liver. In approximately one-fourth of patients, the right hepatic artery will lie anterior to the duct (see **Fig. 7**H). In 10%, the right hepatic artery will cross posterior to the portal vein (not pictured).[20] Nearly 20% of patients have a replaced right hepatic artery[21]; the most common origin of a replaced right hepatic artery is the SMA (see **Fig. 7**C). The replaced right hepatic artery can be found coursing upward posterior to the pancreas and portal vein. Approaching the level of the gallbladder, the right hepatic artery gives rise to the cystic artery, which can either course anteriorly or posteriorly to the hepatic duct. The replaced right hepatic artery then follows the usual course of the right hepatic artery into the liver hilum.[21] If a replaced right hepatic artery is ligated, the surgeon is obliged to perform a cholecystectomy because flow to the cystic artery is likely compromised. Ligation of the replaced right hepatic artery may

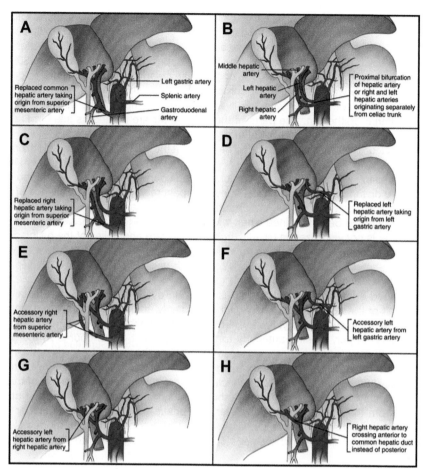

Fig. 7. Variations in hepatic arterial anatomy. (*From* Sabiston DC, Townsend CM. Sabiston textbook of surgery: the biological basis of modern surgical practice. 19th edition. Philadelphia: Elsevier Saunders; 2012; with permission.)

also be deleterious to a biliary enteric anastomosis because the loss of the blood supply to the bile duct predisposes the anastomosis to ischemia and leak.[22]

In approximately 15% of patients, a replaced left hepatic artery will be encountered (see **Fig. 7**D). In these patients, the left hepatic artery will most likely originate from the left gastric artery, course in the gastrohepatic ligament, and enter the liver at the hilum at the ligamentum teres. Although the replaced left hepatic artery is usually of little consequence in hepatic, biliary, and pancreatic surgery, it is relevant in gastric operations that require division of the gastrohepatic ligament. CT angiography can be of assistance in planning major surgeries in the region by delineating vascular aberrancies.

THE GALLBLADDER
Gallbladder Anatomy

The gallbladder is a muscular sac situated beneath the liver. Bile flowing from the liver drains to the CBD. The resting tone in the sphincter of Oddi prevents the flow of bile into the duodenum and allows the bile to fill the duct with subsequent retrograde filling of the cystic duct and gallbladder. There, the bile is concentrated by the gallbladder epithelium, which contains channels that actively transport sodium chloride. Water follows, thereby concentrating the bile. The typical capacity of the gallbladder is 30 mL but it can distend to hold up to 300 mL of fluid, particularly in the face of chronic distal obstruction. The wall of the gallbladder is composed of the visceral peritoneum (on areas not in direct contact with the liver), subserosa, muscularis, lamina propria, and columnar epithelium. The parts of the gallbladder are named as seen in **Fig. 8**. They are the fundus, body, infundibulum (Hartman pouch), and the neck.

The neck drains into the cystic duct. The lumen of the cystic duct is characterized by mucosal folds called the *spiral valves of Heister*. The cystic duct can run a very short course draining into the right hepatic duct or it can course alongside the common hepatic for a distance with insertion just above the pancreas. Congenital absence of the gallbladder is discussed earlier. Importantly, the gallbladder can be intrahepatic. This possibility should be entertained when working up gallbladder agenesis or when the gallbladder is not visualized in biliary surgery. Other rare anomalies of the gallbladder and cystic duct have been described, including duplication of the gallbladder as well as the left-sided gallbladder (draining into the left hepatic duct or common hepatic duct). These anomalies are exceedingly rare.

The blood supply to the gallbladder is from the cystic artery, which is usually a branch off of the right hepatic artery. Not surprisingly, there is significant variation in the course of the cystic artery. Rarely, it may branch from the left hepatic artery or hepatic artery proper, running anteriorly to the hepatic duct on its course to the gallbladder. It may arise from a replaced right hepatic artery from the SMA as mentioned earlier. **Fig. 9** shows the various conformations as well as their prevalence.

Venous drainage of the gallbladder includes veins that follow along the cystic and hepatic ducts to drain into the liver via the portal system as well as veins that drain directly from the gallbladder into the liver. Lymphatic vessels in the gallbladder are located in the subserosal layer and drain to the Calot node and lymph nodes along the porta hepatis. Lymphatic drainage can also course directly into the liver along

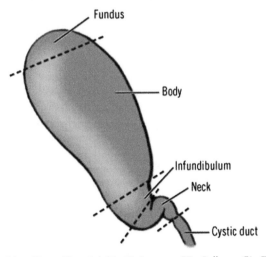

Fig. 8. The gallbladder. (*From* Skandalakis JE, Branum GD, Colborn GL. Extrahepatic biliary tract and gallbladder. In: Skandalakis JE, Colburn GL, Weidman TA, editors. Skandalakis' Surgical Anatomy. Athens (Greece): Paschalidis Medical Publications, Ltd; 2004; with permission.)

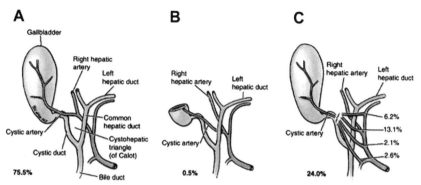

Fig. 9. Variations in cystic artery anatomy. (*A*) Most common configuration of the cystic artery, branching from right hepatic artery. (*B*) Less common, the cystic artery is seen branching from the right hepatic artery prior to crossing posterior to the common hepatic duct. (*C*) The cystic artery is seen branch from various arteries and courses anterior to the common hepatic duct. (*From* Agur AMR, Grant JCB. Grant's atlas of anatomy. 11th edition. Philadelphia: Lippincott Williams & Wilkins; 2005; with permission.)

segments V and IVB before reaching lymph nodes within the hepatoduodenal ligament. Hence, radical resection for gallbladder cancer routinely includes these segments of liver.

Contraction of the gallbladder is under the regulatory control of multiple signals. The major positive mediators of contraction are cholecystokinin (CCK) and parasympathetic innervation. CCK is a hormone secreted by the epithelium in the duodenum in response to intraluminal nutrients. CCK secretion results in postprandial gallbladder contraction to move bile into the duodenum for digestion. The hepatic branch of the vagus nerve supplies parasympathetic innervation, which also promotes contraction. Like the rest of the intestinal tract, the gallbladder is innervated by the enteric nervous system, promoting coordination with the migratory motor complex. There are also multiple modulators of gallbladder contraction. The gallbladder receives innervation by the sympathetic system via the celiac plexus. Sympathetic stimulation promotes relaxation of the gallbladder smooth muscle. Recent literature also supports that components of bile itself dampen gallbladder contractions through G-protein coupled receptors.[23] Stasis of bile in the gallbladder is thought to contribute to the formation of cholelithiasis.

Ducts of Luschka

One feared complication of the laparoscopic cholecystectomy is bile leak. Although the more common location for leak is the cystic duct stump, leak from a duct of Luschka is the second most common culprit. There is great controversy over the term *duct of Luschka*, and many researchers prefer the use of the term *subvesical bile duct*. In a recent systematic review of the literature, Schnelldorfer and colleagues[24] categorized subvesical bile ducts into 4 subtypes based on anatomic characteristics:

- Accessory segmental subvesical bile duct: an intrahepatic duct running along gallbladder fossa draining a segment of the liver that is drained by another intrahepatic duct
- Segmental subvesical bile duct: an intrahepatic duct running along gallbladder fossa draining a discreet segment of the liver

- Aberrant subvesical bile ducts: a network of ducts that end blindly in the connective tissue surrounding the gallbladder but that are in continuity with hepatic ducts, suggesting embryologic origin
- Hepaticocholecystic bile duct: a duct that drains from the liver directly into the gallbladder

Prevalence of these subtypes is not known; however, accessory segmental and segmental subvesical bile ducts are likely common, whereas aberrant subvesical bile ducts and hepaticocholecystic bile ducts are rare.[24] Injury occurs during the removal of the gallbladder from the fossa when the plane of dissection is too deep into the liver bed. Theoretically, the leak can be identified by direct visualization of the gallbladder fossa with identification of bilious drainage. More often, however, these leaks are identified in the postoperative period. Imaging may be helpful in defining the type of duct that has been injured; however, the main principle of treatment is drainage of the bile. In patients whose bile leak fails to improve, endoscopic sphincterotomy and stenting may be necessary to decrease luminal biliary pressures.[25]

AMPULLARY ANATOMY AND PHYSIOLOGY

Much like the rest of the biliary tract, the ampulla of Vater has variable anatomy. Classically, the CBD is described as coursing along the pancreatic groove, curving, then traversing the wall of the duodenum obliquely. The CBD joins with the pancreatic duct to form a short common channel that drains into the duodenum at the major papilla (**Figs. 10B and 11**). This anatomy is present in about 60% of patients. Most other patients will have ducts that remain separate through the wall of the duodenum but share an opening at the papilla, the so-called double barrel (see **Fig. 10A**). Rarely, the ducts empty into the duodenum separately.[26] The sphincter of Oddi surrounds the ducts in the wall of the duodenum.

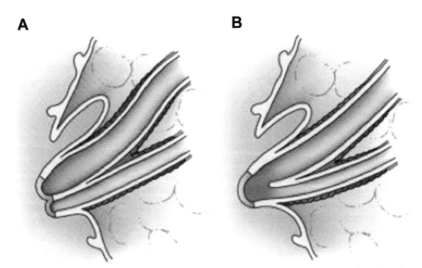

A **B**

Fig. 10. Variable anatomy of biliary drainage into the duodenum. (*A*) Double barrel opening of CBD and pancreatic duct. (*B*) Common channel shared by CBD and pancreatic duct. (*From* Sabiston DC, Townsend CM. Sabiston textbook of surgery: the biological basis of modern surgical practice. 19th edition. Philadelphia: Elsevier Saunders; 2012; with permission.)

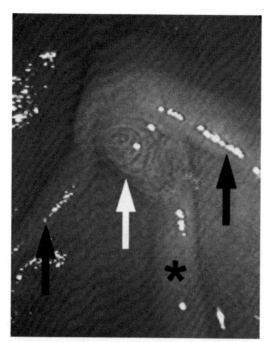

Fig. 11. Major papilla (*white arrow*), transverse mucosal folds (*black arrows*), longitudinal mucosal fold (*asterisk*). (*From* Kim TU, Kim S, Lee JW, et al. Ampulla of Vater: comprehensive anatomy, MR imaging of pathologic conditions, and correlation with endoscopy. Eur J Radiol 2008;66(1):48–64.)

The sphincter of Oddi exhibits rhythmic contractions above a basal pressure greater than that in the duodenum. When stimulated by cholecystokinin, the sphincter relaxes and allows the flow of bile into the digestive tract. In addition to CCK, the sphincter is regulated by the autonomic nervous system and the enteric nervous system. As the migratory motor complex causes contraction in the duodenum, the tone of the sphincter likewise increases.[27] When the CBD and pancreatic duct share a long common channel, the sphincter's contraction fails to occlude both ducts; the confluence allows regurgitation of pancreatic fluid into the biliary tree, a proposed mechanism for the formation of choledochal cystic disease as mentioned earlier. Regurgitation is also thought to lead to pancreatitis in some patients.

SOD

In patients with abdominal pain characterized by biliary colic in the absence of gallbladder pathology (eg, cholelithiasis and biliary dyskinesia) or in patients with recurrent idiopathic pancreatitis, the diagnosis of SOD should be entertained. Patients presenting with biliary pain may exhibit abnormal liver function testing (defined as greater than twice normal on 2 occasions) and/or may have a dilated CBD. The 2 main causes are stenosis and physiologic dysfunction of the sphincter.[28] SOD can be classified as one of 3 types according to the Milwaukee classification:

Type I: biliary colic, elevated liver enzymes, bile duct dilation, and delayed drainage of contrast from duct on ERCP

Type II: biliary colic and 1 or 2 of elevated liver enzymes, bile duct dilation, or de-layed drainage of contrast on ERCP

Type III: biliary colic only

Manometry can be useful and is often necessary to make the diagnosis. A basal pressure of greater than 40 mm Hg meets the criteria for SOD.[28] Manometry carries a significant risk of pancreatitis. Especially for those with type II or type III SOD, diagnosis can be challenging; many treatment options have limited data to support their use. Medical treatment, such as with calcium channel blockers or nitrates, may or may not be helpful; most options carry limiting side-effect profiles. According to a 2001 Cochrane Review, sphincterotomy is most likely to be helpful if manometry reveals elevated biliary basal pressures.[29]

SUMMARY

The anatomy of the biliary tract exhibits a wide degree of variation. The embryologic development of the biliary tract is highly complicated. It is better understood today than even just 5 years ago, but significant gaps in knowledge still exist. Therefore, the cause of congenital abnormalities, including biliary atresia and choledochal cystic disease, remains poorly understood and will continue to require surgical intervention.

Knowledge of anatomic variation is important in the operative setting. When the usual appearance of structures is not encountered, it can be tempting to fit abnormal findings within the paradigm of what is normal. This practice can lead to errors and injury. Intraoperative cholangiography can be helpful in interpreting the anatomy and should be used liberally. Similarly, the variation in hepatic vasculature can represent a challenge, and inadvertent ligation or injury can lead to poor outcomes. Recognition of variable anatomy is crucial in avoiding complication and achieving optimal outcomes for patients. When one anatomic variant is encountered, the surgeon must be on the lookout for others.

REFERENCES

1. Sadler TW, Langman J. Langman's medical embryology. 10th edition. Philadelphia: Lippincott Williams & Wilkins; 2006. p. 371, xiii.
2. Tan CE, Moscoso GJ. The developing human biliary system at the porta hepatis level between 29 days and 8 weeks of gestation: a way to understanding biliary atresia. Part 1. Pathol Int 1994;44(8):587–99.
3. Strazzabosco M, Fabris L. Development of the bile ducts: essentials for the clinical hepatologist. J Hepatol 2012;56(5):1159–70.
4. Yoon HA, Noh MH, Kim BG, et al. Clinicopathological significance of altered Notch signaling in extrahepatic cholangiocarcinoma and gallbladder carcinoma. World J Gastroenterol 2011;17(35):4023–30.
5. White BD, Chien AJ, Dawson DW. Dysregulation of Wnt/beta-catenin signaling in gastrointestinal cancers. Gastroenterology 2012;142(2):219–32.
6. Shen FZ, Zhang BY, Feng YJ, et al. Current research in perineural invasion of cholangiocarcinoma. J Exp Clin Cancer Res 2010;29:24.
7. Zong Y, Stanger BZ. Molecular mechanisms of bile duct development. Int J Biochem Cell Biol 2011;43(2):257–64.
8. Spence JR, Lange AW, Lin SC, et al. Sox17 regulates organ lineage segregation of ventral foregut progenitor cells. Dev Cell 2009;17(1):62–74.

9. Coffinier C, Gresh L, Fiette L, et al. Bile system morphogenesis defects and liver dysfunction upon targeted deletion of HNF1beta. Development 2002;129(8):1829–38.

10. Clotman F, Lannoy VJ, Reber M, et al. The onecut transcription factor HNF6 is required for normal development of the biliary tract. Development 2002;129(8):1819–28.

11. Hartley JL, Davenport M, Kelly DA. Biliary atresia. Lancet 2009;374(9702):1704–13.

12. Ovchinsky N, Moreira RK, Lefkowitch JH, et al. Liver biopsy in modern clinical practice: a pediatric point-of-view. Adv Anat Pathol 2012;19(4):250–62.

13. Jablonska B. Biliary cysts: etiology, diagnosis and management. World J Gastroenterol 2012;18(35):4801–10.

14. Ohashi T, Wakai T, Kubota M, et al. Risk of subsequent biliary malignancy in patients undergoing cyst excision for congenital choledochal cysts. J Gastroenterol Hepatol 2013;28(2):243–7.

15. Kasi PM, Ramirez R, Rogal SS, et al. Gallbladder agenesis. Case Rep Gastroenterol 2011;5(3):654–62.

16. Hershman MJ, Southern SJ, Rosin RD. Gallbladder agenesis diagnosed at laparoscopy. J R Soc Med 1992;85(11):702–3.

17. Kune GA. Surgical anatomy of common bile duct. Arch Surg 1964;89:995–1004.

18. Schwartz SI, Brunicardi FC. Schwartz's principles of surgery. 9th edition. New York: McGraw-Hill, Medical Pub. Division; 2010. p. 1866, xxi.

19. Chaib E, Kanas AF, Galvaō FH, et al. Bile duct confluence: anatomic variations and its classification. Surg Radiol Anat 2013. [Epub ahead of print].

20. Agur AM, Grant JC. Grant's atlas of anatomy. 11th edition. Philadelphia: Lippincott Williams & Wilkins; 2005. p. 848, xv.

21. Skandalakis J, Colborn G, Weidman T, et al. Extrahepatic biliary tract and gallbladder. In: Colborn G, Skandalakis JE, Weidman TA, et al, editors. Skandalakis' surgical anatomy. Athens (Greece): Paschalidis Medical Publications Ltd; 2004.

22. Shukla PJ, Barreto SG, Kulkarni A, et al. Vascular anomalies encountered during pancreatoduodenectomy: do they influence outcomes? Ann Surg Oncol 2010;17(1):186–93.

23. Lavoie B, Balemba OB, Godfrey C, et al. Hydrophobic bile salts inhibit gallbladder smooth muscle function via stimulation of GPBAR1 receptors and activation of KATP channels. J Physiol 2010;588(Pt 17):3295–305.

24. Schnelldorfer T, Sarr MG, Adams DB. What is the duct of Luschka?–A systematic review. J Gastrointest Surg 2012;16(3):656–62.

25. Spanos CP, Syrakos T. Bile leaks from the duct of Luschka (subvesical duct): a review. Langenbecks Arch Surg 2006;391(5):441–7.

26. Kim TU, Kim S, Lee JW, et al. Ampulla of Vater: comprehensive anatomy, MR imaging of pathologic conditions, and correlation with endoscopy. Eur J Radiol 2008;66(1):48–64.

27. Tanaka M. Function and dysfunction of the sphincter of Oddi. Dig Surg 2010;27(2):94–9.

28. Hall TC, Dennison AR, Garcea G. The diagnosis and management of sphincter of Oddi dysfunction: a systematic review. Langenbecks Arch Surg 2012;397(6):889–98.

29. Craig AG, Toouli J. Sphincterotomy for biliary sphincter of Oddi dysfunction. Cochrane Database Syst Rev 2001;(3):CD001509.

Biliary Cysts
A Review and Simplified Classification Scheme

Ronald F. Martin, MD[a,b],*

KEYWORDS

- Biliary cysts • Review • Classification scheme • Simplified

KEY POINTS

- Various biliary cystic conditions that have been considered together really represent markedly different disorders in terms of embryologic and anatomic considerations, and they also carry different risks of both neoplastic and nonneoplastic complications.
- Modern imaging techniques, as well as advances in operative technique and our ability to manage patients in the perioperative period, have likely altered and simplified the necessary classification schemes and treatment algorithms.

INTRODUCTION

If one has no real knowledge of biliary cysts, then one should study them. After a short time, it becomes clear that much is known about cystic abnormalities of the biliary system. If one continues to study theses oddities, perhaps for a long time, then it becomes even clearer that we do not know much at all about biliary cysts. There are competing views of how they come to be. There are competing views of how to classify them. There are even competing views of whether or not they are cysts.[1]

Despite the lack of agreement on many things, we can agree on a few things, and that is a start. We do know that there is a collection of entities in which a part or several parts of the biliary tree are abnormal in size or shape. We do know that some of these conditions can be associated with other problems, at least in some people. We do know that some people with some of these conditions are at increased risk for cancer. We know that collectively, these entities are more common in women than in men and that many, if not all, of these have a congenital component to their development.[1,2]

The fact that we cannot agree on how to classify these entities or agree on their significance or even agree whether or not they are cysts should not demoralize us. On the contrary, it should inspire us and make us curious. It matters not whether we call these entities biliary cysts or congenital choledochal malformations. It does not matter if we

[a] Marshfield Clinic and Saint Joseph's Hospital, 1000 North Oak Avenue, Marshfield, WI 54449, USA; [b] University of Wisconsin School of Medicine and Public Health, 640 Highland Avenue, Madison, WI, USA
* Marshfield Clinic and Saint Joseph's Hospital, 1000 North Oak Avenue, Marshfield, WI 54449.
E-mail address: martin.ronald@marshfieldclinic.org

Surg Clin N Am 94 (2014) 219–232
http://dx.doi.org/10.1016/j.suc.2014.01.011
0039-6109/14/$ – see front matter © 2014 Elsevier Inc. All rights reserved.

include every historical example into 1 classification scheme or another. All that matters is that we carefully assess what we do know and, perhaps more importantly, do not know about these clinical problems.

The purpose of this article is to review the information that is available and analyze through the prism of what else we have learned. At the conclusion of this article, I suggest an alternative scheme to the most widely accepted classifications. The purpose of this alternative scheme is to better match the anatomic findings with the required treatment based on what we have learned to date.

CLASSIFICATION SCHEMES

Under most circumstances, when one is writing an article such as this, one would begin with a description of the anatomy and physiology of the organs in question. It is a time-honored tradition and usually makes sense. In the case of biliary cysts or congenital choledochal malformations it is probably not so useful, perhaps even counterproductive. By definition, all of the cystic abnormalities either are or derive from anatomic variations. Furthermore, some of the defects may be the direct result of a physiologic abnormality, either de novo or as a result of anatomic variation. So, in the case of biliary cystic conditions, it makes more sense to review the standard schemes first (even if they are probably unhelpful) to understand how we got to where we are in our understanding of these entities. Once we have a grasp of the classification schemes, we can break down the entities into agreed subtypes to be followed by a, it is hoped, more useful grouping based on clinical significance.

Biliary cysts have been recognized for some time. Before the development of computed tomography (CT), fiber-optic flexible endoscopy, transcorporeal ultrasonography (US), endoscopic US, and magnetic resonance imaging (MRI), these abnormalities were identified at the time of operation, sometimes with a preoperative suspicion of their presence, other times not. The main evaluative tools were the surgeon's wits and intraoperative cholangiography. All of these diagnostic tools are readily available in many centers, as well as some variations on the themes. It is rare to stumble into a situation in which a biliary cyst is present if one is careful in one's preoperative evaluation.

The most common classification scheme currently used is the 1977 Todani modification of the 1959 Alonso-Lej classification. Alonso-Lej's original classification provided for 4 types of biliary cysts,[3] and Todani added the fifth category (**Figs. 1 and 2**).[4] In this classification, type I cysts are the extrahepatic cystic dilatations of the common duct (**Fig. 3**). They can be fusiform or spherical and can extend from the confluence of the biliary radicals to the pancreaticobiliary junction. Type II cysts are the biliary diverticula. (I am not convinced these even exist, or if they do exist that they are cysts at all. More on that to follow.) Type III lesions are the choledochoceles (**Fig. 4**).[5] The choledochoceles are frequently and erroneously referred to as type III choledochoceles. That is just wrong. One can either refer to them as a type III choledochal (or biliary) cyst or a choledochocele. There is a different, further subclassification of choledochoceles that is explored later, but it is not part of Alonso-Lej's or Todani's schemes. Type III biliary cysts are completely located within the duodenal wall and may have separate or combined entrances of the distal bile duct and ventral portion of the pancreatic duct (PD). Type IV choledochal cysts are present as multiple cysts, and at least 1 of them involves the extrahepatic bile duct. If more than 1 cystic area exists, the classification is used and further divided into type IVa and type IVb. Type IVa biliary cyst refers to cysts of the extrahepatic bile duct seen in conjunction with at least 1 intrahepatic biliary cyst. Type IVb biliary cyst refers to multiple

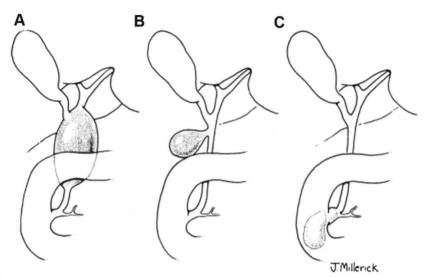

Fig. 1. Types I (*A*), II (*B*), and III (*C*) biliary cysts. (*From* Deziel DJ, Rossi RL, Munson JL, et al. Cystic disease of the bile ducts: surgical management and reoperation. Probl Gen Surg 1985;22(4):468; with permission.)

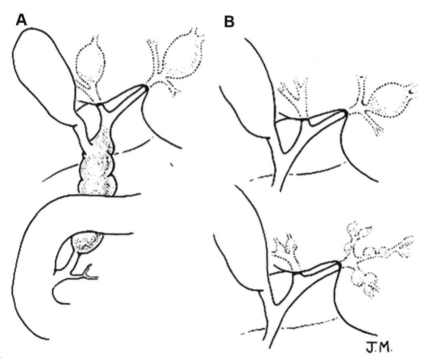

Fig. 2. Type IV (*A*) and V (*B*) biliary cysts. (*From* Deziel DJ, Rossi RL, Munson JL, et al. Cystic disease of the bile ducts: surgical management and reoperation. Problem Gen Surg 1985;22(4):469; with permission.)

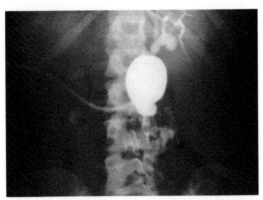

Fig. 3. Cholangiogram of type I biliary cyst. (*From* Mesleh M, Deziel DJ. Bile duct cysts. Surg Clin North Am 2008;88(6):1373; with permission.)

extrahepatic biliary cysts with no evidence of intrahepatic biliary cyst. This category would have concluded Alonso-Lej's classification scheme. Todani's modification added in type V biliary cysts. Type V biliary cyst(s) can include 1 or more intrahepatic biliary cysts but are not associated with extrahepatic biliary cysts. They may be distributed in a portion of the liver or be distributed throughout the liver. Type V biliary cyst is also known as Caroli disease (**Fig. 5**).

CAUSE

There are a few theories about the cause of choledochal cysts. Agreement on them is far from unanimous. The fact that the anatomic and physiologic aberrations exist

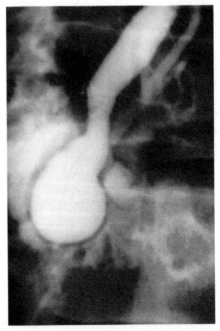

Fig. 4. Cholangiogram of type III biliary cyst. (*From* Mesleh M, Deziel DJ. Bile duct cysts. Surg Clin North Am 2008;88(6):1374; with permission.)

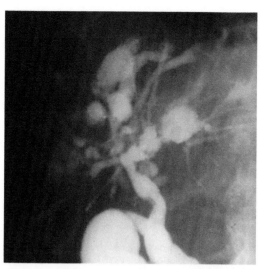

Fig. 5. Cholangiogram of type V biliary cysts. (*From* Mesleh M, Deziel DJ. Bile duct cysts. Surg Clin North Am 2008;88(6):1374; with permission.)

more so in some of the subtypes than in others leads to the increased confusion on the topic.

The main theme in most of the theories is one of an altered pressure-compliance situation. Essentially, something happens that makes the biliary structure more distensible, therefore more compliant, and this may or may not be associated with abnormally high biliary pressures within that structure. Increased compliance, as manifested by weakening of the muscular portion of the bile duct wall, could also lead to dilation in the setting of normal biliary pressure. The most often cited theory is one that Babbit[6] proposed in 1969 (**Fig. 6**). He reported a series of patients with anomalous junction of the pancreaticobiliary ducts, sometimes also referred to as anomalous pancreaticobiliary junction (APBJ), who were found to have associated type I choledochal cysts. In Babbit's model, the distal common bile duct (CBD) inserts into the PD in a more or less T-shaped arrangement, which places the pancreaticobiliary junction proximal to the main sphincter mechanisms of the ampulla of Vater and the main PD sphincter (perhaps all or in part) (**Fig. 7**).[5] The resultant anatomic variation produces a situation in which pancreatic juice can freely reflux into the bile duct, because pancreatic secretory pressure exceeds hepatic biliary secretory pressure. The theory further goes on to suppose that this reflux of pancreatic juice causes mechanical distention of the bile duct as well as inflammatory changes accompanied by degradation of the mucosa and even muscular wall that make the bile duct more distensible. Others have suggested that protein plugs that form in pancreatic juice may be a contributing factor to obstruction of outflow.[7,8] Evidence that supports these theories is increased pancreatic enzyme concentration in the cyst contents, measured pressure gradients between the PD and biliary cyst, and loss of mucosa and inflammation.[9,10] The prevalence of APBJ is reported to be 60% to 90% in patients with biliary cysts. The main weaknesses of these theories are, of course, that many patients who have biliary cysts do not have the proposed anatomic derangement. Also, the chemical studies may show association but not necessarily causation. Also, there are virtually no data on the denominator of people with APBJ who may not have an associated biliary cyst.

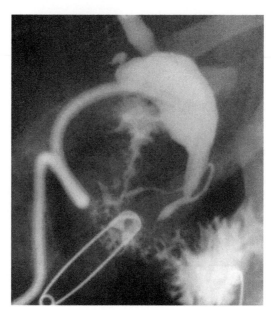

Fig. 6. Cholangiogram showing APBJ. (*From* Deziel DJ, Rossi RL, Munson JL, et al. Cystic disease of the bile ducts: surgical management and reoperation. Probl Gen Surg 1985;22(4):467–80; with permission.)

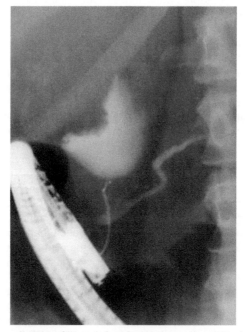

Fig. 7. Cholangiogram showing filling defect from cancer. (*From* Mesleh M, Deziel DJ. Bile duct cysts. Surg Clin North Am 2008;88(6):1379; with permission.)

Other theories of cause that do not rely completely on anomalous anatomy rely on more fundamental hydraulic principles of flow and resistance, yielding increased pressure and dilation. Animal studies have shown dilation in response to experimental ductal occlusion.[8,11,12] Others have suggested that webs or sphincter of Oddi dysfunction may be causative.[13] Embryologic variations have also been proposed. It has been postulated that the malformation of intrahepatic bile ducts in Caroli disease has been associated with faulty remodeling of the embryonic ductal plate,[14] and a maldistribution of epithelial cells within the bile duct may result in cyst formation. Motility disorders, or possible motility disorders, have also been put forth as explanatory. Tyler and colleagues[15] found that some patients with biliary cysts have fewer ganglion cells than would be expected. These investigators proposed that there might have been viral damage to the ganglion cells based on reoviral RNA levels found in patients with biliary cysts.[15] In a series of patients with type III biliary cysts, we postulated that there may be a motility disorder or motilitylike disorder associated with anomalous arrangement of the main ampullary sphincter to the distal common duct sphincter and the main PD sphincter but were unable to definitively show that.[16]

None of the etiologic theories is far fetched nor is it completely convincing. Also, none of the theories seems to tie the various types of biliary cysts (as described earlier) together. In the author's opinion, these observations make a better case for looking at the types of biliary cysts in a different way than has traditionally been described.

RISK OF MALIGNANCY

Irwin and Morrison[17] first reported the occurrence of malignancy and stones within a biliary cyst in 1944. Flanigan in 1977[18] reported a series of patients with biliary carcinomas, in whom slightly more than half had malignancy within the cyst itself (**Fig. 8**), and the others were distributed throughout the biliary system.[18] This finding led many to believe that there is a field defect associated with the presence of biliary cysts. I recommend that this assertion be taken with a large pinch of salt, because most of the cancers seen within cysts or associated with concurrent or antecedent cysts are seen in the setting of the type I or type IV cysts (ie, those with involvement of the extrahepatic duct and more likely to be associated with APBJ). Cancers are also seen in some patients with Caroli disease. The reported incidence of cancer in patients with Caroli disease is 7%.[19] Unlike the situation in type I and IV cysts with ABPJ and pancreatic reflux, patients with Caroli disease are believed to have

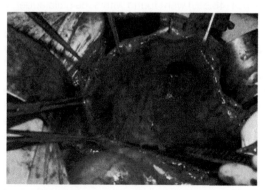

Fig. 8. Open type I cyst. (*From* Mesleh M, Deziel DJ. Bile duct cysts. Surg Clin North Am 2008;88(6):1380; with permission.)

increased risk of cancer from biliary stasis, chronic inflammation, and prolonged expo-sure of the bile duct epithelium to high concentrations of unconjugated, secondary bile acids.[20]

The remaining cysts are the type II and type III biliary cysts. Type II biliary cysts, or biliary diverticula, are extremely rare, bordering on nonexistent. There really is no good information on them in general and even less in regard to their association with malig-nancy. Type III choledochal cysts, or choledochoceles, are probably the most misun-derstood of the lot of biliary cysts, which leads to confusion in any assessment of malignancy risk. The risk of cancer associated with type III cysts seems to be low. In a review by Levy and Rohrmann in 2003,[2] only 4 known cases of malignancy asso-ciated with choledochoceles were reported. A more recent review by Ziegler and Zyromski in 2011[21] found fewer than 10 such reported. In their series of 146 patients of all types of biliary cysts, these investigators reported 6 patients with associated neoplasm, but none in the group of type III cysts.

TYPE I CYSTS

Type I biliary cysts, or extrahepatic biliary cysts, are uncommon but not unheard of in the general population. They are the most common of the biliary cysts. Their incidence is estimated at 1:100,000 to 1:150,000 in Western countries and higher in Japan, at 1:1,000.[22] The knowledge of their presence dates back to Vater in 1723.[23] Douglas in 1852[24] suggested the congenital nature of the cyst. The clinical presentation of pa-tients with type I biliary cysts may include abdominal pain, jaundice, an abdominal mass, or some combination of these. In children, pain may be the only presenting symptom. Given modern imaging techniques (and perhaps declining physical exami-nation skills of physicians and increasing levels of obesity), palpable abnormalities preceding image identification are fairly uncommon.

As mentioned earlier, altered anatomy in conjunction with reflux of pancreatic juice or perhaps other obstructions to biliary outflow is believed to lead to the development of cystic dilatation. The type I cysts are the most common of all the biliary cysts. They are 3 times more common in females than in males[25] and may present at any age. Although mainly presenting with jaundice or pain, they may present in association with gallstones in any part of the biliary tract, cholangitis, biliary cirrhosis, portal hyper-tension, or malignancy.[26] The risk of associated malignancy seems to increase with age, with reported incidence ranging from 2.5% to 28%.[27–29] Todani and colleagues[29] found in their series that about half (49.8%) of the cancers that they saw were in the cyst itself and about half (46.5%) were found within the gallbladder, with the remaining 3.7% equally distributed within the liver or pancreas.

The diagnosis of biliary cyst can be made clinically, or at least suspected, but is usu-ally confirmed by some imaging technique. Transcorporeal US is probably the most common initial imaging modality used, but with the almost ubiquitous use of CT, that may no longer be true. Almost any imaging modality raises the flag of suspicion, and many can be used to identify what is important. Body imaging such as CT, MRI, and US are all potentially useful and may define the extent of ductal involvement and presence or absence, of remote disease. If further delineation of the ductal system is required to plan treatment, endoscopic retrograde cholangiopancreatography (ERCP), magnetic resonance cholangiopancreatography, or percutaneous transhe-patic cholangiography can all be used. I have not found radionuclide studies to be of major help in planning treatment or diagnosis.

The treatment of type I cysts is removal of the cyst and restoration of biliary conti-nuity. Exceptions to this principle include patients with suspected malignancy outside the cyst or patients who are considered unacceptable operative candidates for other reasons. Reconstruction almost always requires hepaticojejunostomy, although rarely, a reconstruction above the biliary confluence is required. This operation can be tedious and does require excellent attention to detail and operative planes. However, the operation can be performed safely, with little to no mortality and low complication rates.[30–34] The fundamental rules of biliary surgery are no different than for other operations: at the conclusion of the case, all liver segments need to have unobstructed flow of bile into the lumen of the gastrointestinal tract. This requirement implies that all steps are taken to ensure that variant anatomy is not overlooked, and all debris is removed from the remaining ducts during the conduct of the operation. The distal limit of resection also needs careful attention. Most commonly, one can inspect through the open or divided cyst and see the narrowing of the intrapancreatic portion of the bile duct. Mesleh and Deziel[5,31] emphasize oversewing the distal duct to prevent possible pancreatic fistula and also advocate the placing of drains, both suggestions with which I wholeheartedly concur. In situations in which one is concerned about maintaining the integrity of the pancreaticobiliary junction, it may be advisable to place a nasopancreatic tube before the operation. It can offer several benefits, such as being able to see or feel the tube in addition to being able to inject the tube with either radiographic contrast or optically detectable fluid during the operation if necessary. Lily[35] has suggested limited resection of the cyst to spare the portion adherent to the portal vein. Personally, I have never encountered a situation in which this would have been helpful or even easier. Careful dissection has invariably produced a safe plan between the bile duct and the portal vein that has allowed for complete excision of the cyst.

Attempts at cyst drainage procedures should be of historical interest only. The only good reason I can think of to address them in this article is that the reader may encounter a patient who has had one already. Anastomoses of the cyst to the stomach, duodenum, or jejunum without excision have all been performed, and all fail to address the main concerns of biliary cysts. The problem of pancreatic juice reflux is left unaltered completely. These procedures tend to be complicated by stricture, stone formation, and recurrent cholangitis. When one encounters a patient who has undergone a previous limited drainage procedure, the approach is the same as if it were a de novo presentation. The major differences are in technical issues regarding evaluation and treatment based on how the anatomy has already been altered.

TYPE II CYSTS

Type II cysts, or biliary diverticula, are rare. They are so rare that, in my opinion, it would be best to discontinue including them in the discussion of biliary cysts. The differential diagnosis includes duplication of the gallbladder. Intersphincteric diverticula may represent a herniation of bile duct mucosa and, therefore, be false diverticula akin to sigmoid diverticula, whereas the more proximal diverticula are believed to be congenital true diverticula. The only published cholangiograms showing what one could construe as a biliary diverticulum that I have ever found are contained in a report from the Armed Forces Institute of Pathology.[2]

The treatment of these lesions needs to be based on fundamental principles as opposed to any real data. We have no idea if they represent a malignant risk or, if left alone, anything of adverse consequence would occur. Therefore, the main reason to intervene would be if someone were to present with symptoms or signs of clinical problems attributable to the diverticula. In that case, excision with either maintenance of biliary drainage or restoration of biliary continuity would be in order. In my opinion, if we all collectively decided to exclude this entity from discussion, the net impact would be negligible.

TYPE III CYSTS

Type III cysts, or choledochoceles, are located within the duodenal wall. The term choledochocele was coined by Wheeler in 1940.[36] It is believed to be the second least common of the biliary cysts, although I think that we should reserve judgment on that. The differential diagnosis includes duodenal duplications and other cystic abnormalities of adjacent anatomic structures. Further confusing the topic is that some investigators include cystic abnormalities with duodenal mucosa[37] as well as biliary mucosa.[38,39] The cysts range in size from small to large enough to palpate on examination. The very large ones can obstruct the duodenum, whereas others may present with jaundice or persistent or recurrent acute pancreatitis.

Scholz and colleagues[37] described a scheme for choledochoceles that differentiates based on separate insertions of the CBD and PD or a common channel of CBD and PD inserting into the cyst: types A and B, respectively. Sarris and Tsang[40] proposed a more complicated scheme of choledochoceles, which combines common and noncommon channels as well as intramural versus intraluminal characteristics for classification. In our series, we found that all of the choledochoceles that we encountered had biliary mucosa and a separate entrance of the CBD and PD.[16] We also discovered a radiographic finding of parallel folds within the cysts, which we referred to as Biber lines. We postulated that there was a defect in the crossing fibers of the sling mechanisms between the sphincter of Oddi and the main CBD and main PD sphincters that allows for bulging between the sphincters, allowing for a bulging cyst to develop. We were not able to prove this theory, because we did not have mannometric data or deep wall biopsies to show altered ganglion presence or dropout of the muscular sling.

It seems logical that the duodenal mucosa–lined cysts (duplications) and biliary mucosa–lined cysts (probably what we think of as a choledochocele) should behave differently. As stated earlier, the relationship, if any, to neoplasia or proper cancer is entirely unclear, and it is at most rare. Lesions that are large enough to cause obstruction of the duodenum may need to be managed by operative means, usually with transduodenal excision, which may or may not require reimplantation of the CBD and PD. Smaller lesions may be managed via unroofing only, via operative means or via endoscopic means, as was performed in our series.[16]

I have previously suggested that we may not know the true incidence of choledochoceles. The reason I suggest this is, since the advent of readily available flexible fiber-optic endoscopy and ERCP, it is entirely likely that many bulging papillas that have been managed with endoscopic retrograde sphincterotomy or needle-knife papillotomy may have been early or small choledochoceles. Even if so, the distinction would be largely academic and of no true clinical significance.

TYPE IV CYSTS

Type IV biliary cysts are classified separately, because multiple cysts are present, at least one of which must be extrahepatic. If the multiple cysts are extrahepatic and intrahepatic, they are considered type IVa cysts, and if the multiple cysts are all extrahepatic, they are considered type IVb cysts. This is probably an unnecessary classification, because it adds little to help us. In the category of the type IVb cysts, everything that can be said about type I cysts also applies without exception. In the category of the type IVa cysts, what is said about type I cysts applies as well to the extrahepatic component, and what is stated about type V biliary cysts (Caroli disease) applies to the intrahepatic portion.

I refer the reader to the sections on type I and type V cysts, because repeating the information here is counterproductive. This is 1 more reason why I add my support to the abandonment of this classification scheme later in this article.

TYPE V CYSTS

Caroli disease is also known as communicating ectasia of the intrahepatic bile ducts. It is a rare autosomal-recessive disorder described by Caroli and others in 1958.[41] As mentioned earlier, it is a result of embryologic ductal plate malformations that occur during remodeling. The resultant defect can cause fibrosing and scarring of bile ducts large or small. When the scarring is limited to the smaller duct, the effect may be negligible, but when the scarring involves the larger ducts, the large cystic collections that define Caroli disease can form.

Renal cysts are seen with disorders with the ductal plate, and renal developmental abnormalities can be caused by the same genetic determinants.[20] Autosomal-dominant and autosomal-recessive polycystic kidney, as well as medullary sponge and medullary cystic kidney, can be seen in association with Caroli disease.[2]

The treatment of Caroli disease is based on removing the portion of the liver containing the cysts and any residual impediment to biliary drainage of remaining segments. The treatment needs to be tailored to the patient being considered.[14,42] Factors that need to be taken into account are the extent and distribution of the cysts and associated strictures, any associated malignancy, as well as the underlying function of what will be the residual liver. Of course, the general medial condition of the patient may be determinant in the patient's ability to withstand a significant operation. Transplantation is the fallback position when there is either pan-lobar involvement or predicted inadequate functional residual liver after partial liver resection. If the distribution of disease is such that it can be eliminated with segmental resection or multiple segmental resections, yielding adequate residual liver mass, then this should be preferable to transplantation. There are insufficient data to suggest that any given operative approach to these resections is better than another, whether performed by conventional operative means or videoscopic or robotic means.

A SIMPLIFIED APPROACH

I submit to you, dear reader, that from this discussion, we have enough information to generate a simpler approach to biliary cystic disease than is currently used. In no way do I wish to denigrate the work of all those who have toiled before us. After all, it was their work that allowed us to study these disorders and learn what we have. Now, it is time to make use of that effort. I am not the first nor will I likely be the last to suggest an alternative classification scheme, but I provide one for us to consider.

The basis of the change is simple. Based on what we know to date, the type I to V classification scheme is overly complicated and occasionally confusing. If we begin by eliminating the biliary diverticula altogether, because they are exceedingly rare to the point of near nonexistence, that leaves us with 4 residual classes of cysts. (For anyone who fears or laments the loss of the type II cysts, we can give them a new place in surgical discourse away from here, much the way that Pluto lost its planetary status; Pluto, after all, is still there; it is just not called a planet anymore.) The type IV class of cysts is at best redundant. The type IVb are really just odd type I cysts with all the same clinical consequences and same treatment options. The type IVa cysts

Table 1
Simplified classification scheme for biliary cysts

Type	Treatment
Intrahepatic cysts	Segmental resection where possible and the patient is an adequate operative candidate; consider transplantation if inadequate liver reserve is expected
Extrahepatic bile duct cysts	Resection of extrahepatic bile ducts (including complete resection of cyst(s)) with restoration biliary continuity
Intraduodenal cysts	If small cyst unroofing by endoscopic or operative means if possible; if larger or unroofing not possible, resect cyst via transduodenal approach, possibly requiring reimplantation of CBD or PD

are just rare combinations of type I and type V cysts, which may be related abnormalities or coincidental abnormalities. Whatever advice is used for type I or type V cysts can be used to guide one when treating patients with these cysts. That leaves us with intrahepatic cysts and extrahepatic cysts. Honestly, that is it. The last point we need to address is whether or not to include the choledochoceles or type III cysts. Ziegler and Zyromski[21] have made a compelling argument for the exclusion of choledochoceles from the list of biliary cysts. Perhaps because of my previous work, or just not knowing where else to orphan these entities (because they are more prevalent than type II cysts), I support keeping them in for now.

If one keeps to this system, one is left with a scheme that includes intrahepatic cysts, extrahepatic cysts, and intraduodenal cysts. The treatment paradigm that would follow is shown in **Table 1**. For intrahepatic lesions, resect as little liver as possible to eliminate the cysts and accompanying strictures; however, as little as possible may require complete liver resection and transplantation. For extrahepatic lesions, resect the bile duct(s) that are involved and restore biliary drainage. For patients with both intrahepatic and extrahepatic cysts, follow each of these algorithms. For patients with intraduodenal lesions, unroof those smaller lesions by either endoscopic or operative means if possible. For larger lesions, resection via transduodenal approach with possible reimplantation of CBD or PD may be required.

SUMMARY

There is much known, and there is much unknown, about biliary cystic disease. Several classification schemes have been developed and modified over the last 70 years or so. What seems to be true is that the various biliary cystic conditions that have been considered together represent markedly different disorders in terms of embryologic and anatomic considerations, and they also carry different risks of both neoplastic and nonneoplastic complications. Modern imaging techniques, as well as advances in operative technique and our ability to manage patients in the perioperative period, have likely altered and simplified the necessary classification schemes and treatment algorithms.

As I stated at the beginning of this article, if you know nothing about biliary cysts, study a little, and you will know a lot. If you study a lot, you will soon realize how little we really do know, probably a metaphor for life. I have tried to demystify this situation as best as possible. Time will tell if I have oversimplified this or have completely missed the point. I look forward to the day that one of you revises this article and tells us how far off the mark I was.

REFERENCES

1. Makin E, Davenport M. Understanding choledochal malformation. Arch Dis Child 2012;97:69–72.
2. Levy AD, Rohrmann CA Jr. Biliary cystic disease. Curr Probl Diagn Radiol 2003; 32:233–63.
3. Alonzo-Lej F, Revor WB, Pessagno DJ. Congenital choledochal cyst, with a report of 2, and an analysis of 94 cases. Int Abstr Surg 1959;108:969–72.
4. Todani T, Watanabe Y, Narusue M, et al. Congenital bile duct cysts: classification, operative procedures, and review of thirty-seven cases including cancer arising from choledochal cyst. Am J Surg 1977;134:263–9.
5. Mesleh M, Deziel DJ. Bile duct cysts. Surg Clin North Am 2008;88:1369–84.
6. Babbitt DP. Congenital choledochal cysts: new etiological concept based on anomalous relationships of the common bile duct and the pancreatic bulb. Ann Radiol (Paris) 1969;12:231–40.
7. Kaneko K, Ando H, Seo T, et al. Proteomic analysis of protein plugs: causative agent of symptoms in patients with choledochal cyst. Dig Dis Sci 2007;52: 1979–86.
8. Miyano T, Suruga K, Chen SC. A clinicopathologic study of choledochal cyst. World J Surg 1980;4:231–8.
9. Babbit DP, Starshak RJ, Clemett AR. Choledochal cyst: a concept of etiology. Am J Roentgenol Radium Ther Nucl Med 1973;119:57–62.
10. Tanaka M, Ikeda S, Kawakami K, et al. The presence of a positive pressure gradient from pancreatic duct to choledochal cyst demonstrated by duodeno-scopic microtransducer manometry: clue to pancreaticobiliary reflux. Endoscopy 1982;14:45–7.
11. Ohkawa H, Sawaguchi S, Yamazaki Y, et al. Experimental analysis of the ill effect of anomalous pancreaticobiliary ductal union. J Pediatr Surg 1982;17: 7–13.
12. Deziel DJ, Rossi RL, Munson JL, et al. Cystic disease of the bile ducts: surgical management and reoperation. Probl Gen Surg 1985;2:467–79.
13. Metcalfe MS, Wemyss-Holden SA, Maddern GJ. Management dilemmas with choledochal cysts. Arch Surg 2003;138:333–9.
14. Ulrich F, Pratschke J, Pascher A, et al. Long-term outcome of liver resection and transplantation for Caroli disease and syndrome. Ann Surg 2008;247:357–64.
15. Tyler KL, Sokol RJ, Oberhaus SM, et al. Detection of reovirus RNA in hepatobiliary tissues from patients with extrahepatic biliary atresia and choledochal cysts. Hepatology 1998;27:1475–82.
16. Martin RF, Biber BP, Bosco JJ, et al. Symptomatic choledochoceles in adults. Endoscopic retrograde cholangiopancreatography recognition and management. Arch Surg 1992;127:536–8.
17. Irwin ST, Morison JE. Congenital cyst of the common bile duct containing stones and undergoing cancerous change. Br J Surg 1944;32:319–21.
18. Flanigan DP. Biliary carcinoma associated with biliary cysts. Cancer 1977;40: 880–3.
19. Bloustein PA. Association of carcinoma with congenital cystic conditions of the liver and bile ducts. Am J Gastroenterol 1977;67:40–6.
20. D'Agata ID, Jonas MM, Perez-Atayde AR, et al. Combined cystic disease of the liver and kidney. Semin Liver Dis 1994;14:215–28.
21. Ziegler KM, Zyromski NJ. Choledochoceles: are they choledochal cysts? Adv Surg 2011;45:211–24.

22. De Vries JS, De Vries S, Aronson DC, et al. Choledochal cysts: age of presentation, symptoms, and late complications related to Todani's classification. J Pediatr Surg 2002;37:1568–73.
23. Vater A. Dissertation in auguralis medica, poes diss. Qua Scirris viscerum dissert, C. S. Ezlerus. Edinburg (TX): University Library; 1723.
24. Douglas AH. Case of dilatation of the common bile duct. Monthly J Med Sci (Lond) 1852;14:97.
25. Yamaguchi M. Congenital choledochal cyst. Analysis of 1,433 patients in the Japanese literature. Am J Surg 1980;140:653–7.
26. Savader SJ, Benenati JF, Venbrux AC, et al. Choledochal cysts: classification and cholangiographic appearance. AJR Am J Roentgenol 1991;156:327–31.
27. Rossi RL, Silverman ML, Braasch JW, et al. Carcinomas arising in cystic conditions of the bile ducts. A clinical and pathologic study. Ann Surg 1987;205: 377–84.
28. Nagorney DM, McIlrath DC, Adson MA. Choledochal cysts in adults: clinical management. Surgery 1984;96:656–63.
29. Todani T, Toki A. Cancer arising in choledochal cyst and management. Nippon Geka Gakkai Zasshi 1996;97:594–8.
30. Chaudhary A, Dhar P, Sachdev A, et al. Choledochal cysts–differences in children and adults. Br J Surg 1996;83:186–8.
31. Deziel DJ, Rossi RL, Munson JL, et al. Management of bile duct cysts in adults. Arch Surg 1986;121:410–5.
32. Stain SC, Guthrie CR, Yellin AE, et al. Choledochal cyst in the adult. Ann Surg 1995;222:128–33.
33. Liu CL, Fan ST, Lo CM, et al. Choledochal cysts in adults. Arch Surg 2002;137: 465–8.
34. Chaudhary A, Dhar P, Sachdev A. Reoperative surgery for choledochal cysts. Br J Surg 1997;84:781–4.
35. Lilly JR. The surgical treatment of choledochal cyst. Surg Gynecol Obstet 1979; 149:36–42.
36. Wheeler W. An unusual case of obstruction of the common bile duct (choledochocele?). Br J Surg 1940;27:446–8.
37. Scholz FJ, Carrera GF, Larsen CR. The choledochocele: correlation of radiological, clinical and pathological findings. Radiology 1976;118:25–8.
38. Kagiyama S, Okazaki K, Yamamoto Y. Anatomic variants of choledochocele and manometric measurements of pressure in the cele and the orifice zone. Am J Gastroenterol 1987;82:641–9.
39. Venu RP, Geenen JE, Hogan WJ, et al. Role of endoscopic retrograde cholangiopancreatography in the diagnosis and treatment of choledochocele. Gastroenterology 1984;87:1144–9.
40. Sarris GE, Tsang D. Choledochocele: case report, literature review, and a proposed classification. Surgery 1989;105:408–14.
41. Caroli J, Soupault R, Kossakowski J, et al. Congenital polycystic dilation of the intrahepatic bile ducts; attempt at classification. Sem Hop 1958;34:488–95 [in French].
42. Lendoire J, Barros Schelotto P, Alvarez Rodriguez J, et al. Bile duct cyst type V (Caroli's disease): surgical strategy and results. HPB (Oxford) 2007;9:281–4.

Symptomatic Cholelithiasis and Functional Disorders of the Biliary Tract

Danielle E. Cafasso, DO, MPH*, Richard R. Smith, MD

KEYWORDS

- Gallstones • Cholelithiasis • Biliary colic • Gallbladder dyskinesia
- Sphincter of Oddi dysfunction

KEY POINTS

- Symptomatic cholelithiasis is uncomplicated gallstone disease that can be diagnosed through abdominal ultrasound and is treated surgically with cholecystectomy.
- Functional disorders of the biliary tract include functional gallbladder disorder, functional biliary, pancreatic, and combined sphincter of Oddi disorders.
- Functional gallbladder disorder, also known as gallbladder dyskinesia, is associated with decreased gallbladder ejection fraction and is also managed surgically with cholecystectomy.
- The sphincter of Oddi disorders have subclassifications based on anatomy, laboratory analysis, and imaging findings.
- The sphincter of Oddi disorders are typically evaluated with manometry and, in general, managed with endoscopic sphincterotomy when basal sphincter pressures are elevated.

SYMPTOMATIC CHOLELITHIASIS

Gallstone disease is one of the most common and costly conditions in the United States. An estimated 20 million Americans, 6.3 million men and 14.2 million women, have gallbladder disease.[1] The cost of gallstone disease has been estimated at $6.5 billion per year worldwide.[2] The epidemiology and risk factors for gallstones have become well published over the last several decades. Ultrasonography has become the gold standard in diagnosis. Laparoscopic cholecystectomy is the standard treatment.

No Disclosures.
The views expressed herein are those of the authors and do not reflect the official policy or position of the Department of the Army, the Department of Defense, or the US Government.
Department of Surgery, Tripler Army Medical Center, 1 Jarrett White Road, Honolulu, HI 96859, USA
* Corresponding author.
E-mail address: danielle.e.cafasso.mil@mail.mil

Epidemiology

The formation of gallstones and gallbladder disease is likely multifactorial and involves an interaction between genetic and environmental factors. Identified risk factors include ethnicity; age; gender; lifestyle; medications; and genetics. The third National Health and Nutrition Examination Survey surveyed a representative sample of greater than 14,000 people in the United States and conducted gallbladder ultrasonography to determine the ethnic distribution of gallstone disease. African American men and women had the lowest prevalence at 5.3% and 13.9%, respectively, whereas Mexican American men and women had a prevalence of 8.9% and 26.7%, respectively, with most other ethnicities falling somewhere in between.[1] Of note, Native Americans have the highest prevalence in North America, with 73% of female Pima Indians over 25 years of age having gallstones.[3] A multicenter, population-based Italian study known as the Multicenter, Population-based Italian study on Epidemiology of Chole-lithiasis project identified female gender and increasing age and body mass index as the most significant risk factors for gallstone disease.[4] In addition to obesity, rapid weight loss is also associated with gallstone formation and this patient population is more likely to be symptomatic as well.[5] The higher rates of gallstone disease in women are likely a result of pregnancy and sex steroids.[1,3,6] Moreover, the risk of developing cholesterol gallstones increases with the number of pregnancies. One study reported an increase in the prevalence of gallstones from 1.3% in nulliparous women to 12.2% in multiparous women.[7] A strong familial predisposition also exists for gallstone formation. First-degree relatives of gallstone patients were found to have gallstones over 4 times more often than in a matched control population.[8] Interestingly, mutations in the adenosine triphosphate-binding cassette, subfamily B, member 4 (ABCB4) gene are related to symptomatic cholelithiasis at a younger age (<40 years).[9] Finally, comorbidities such as diabetes mellitus, cirrhosis, hypertriglyceridemia, Crohn, disease, and conditions that lead to bile stasis are associated with gallstone formation.[2]

Pathophysiology

Gallstones are divided into the 3 following types: cholesterol stones, black pigment stones, and brown pigment stones. Cholesterol stones (>50% cholesterol content) are the most common in the Western world and account for approximately 70% of all stones. Black pigment stones account for the remainder of stone carriers in the Western world and can be caused by hemolytic disorders or cirrhosis. Brown pigment stones are seen most commonly in East Asia and are associated with infection of the biliary tree. Currently the prevalence of cholesterol gallstones seems to be increasing worldwide as a result of socioeconomic changes and an increase in a more Western diet.[10] The formation of cholesterol gallstones has been illustrated since the 1960s with variations of Admirand's triangle, which is essentially an equilibrium diagram of bile salt, cholesterol, and lecithin (**Fig. 1**). Supersaturation with cholesterol, a decrease in the quantity of bile salt or lecithin, or a combination of these factors promotes gallstone formation.[11] Many of the previously mentioned risk factors alter the composition of bile, thus leading to the formation of gallstones.

Clinical Presentation

Most patients with gallstones are asymptomatic. The Simione study examined more than 1900 members of a small Italian town and found an incidence of cholelithiasis of 6.9%. Most were asymptomatic with only 22% reporting biliary pain over the previous 5-year period.[12] Only 16% of the asymptomatic patients then went on to develop symptoms over a 10-year follow-up.[13] In another study by Rome Group for the Epidemiology

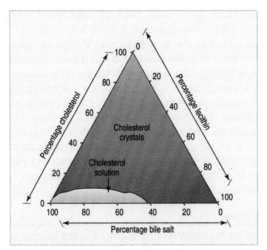

Fig. 1. Adaptation of Admirand's triangular coordinates relating cholesterol, bile salts, and lecithin concentration to cholesterol solubility. (*From* Johnson CD. ABC of the upper gastrointestinal tract. Upper abdominal pain: Gall bladder. BMJ 2001;323:1170; with permission.)

and Prevention of Cholelithiasis, initially asymptomatic patients with gallstones had a cumulative incidence of 26% for the development of biliary pain at 10 years.[14]

Uncomplicated gallstone disease typically presents with upper abdominal pain. A variety of other gastrointestinal complaints have been associated with uncomplicated gallstone disease, such as bloating, belching, nausea, and fatty food intolerance, but these other factors do not consistently discriminate between gallstone disease and other causes.[15] The symptoms are due to gallbladder contraction in the presence of gallstones, which then forces the stone against the outlet, cystic duct, leading to increased pressure in the gallbladder. This increase in pressure, or gallbladder distention, causes the pain, which subsides as the gallbladder relaxes, and the stone falls back from the cystic duct.[16]

Biliary colic is typically steady in quality rather than "colicky" as the name implies. The classic description is a constant, dull discomfort in the right upper quadrant that may radiate to the back. The pain is not relieved or exacerbated by movement, position, or bowel function. Typically, the pain will last greater than 30 minutes with the maximum time being 6 hours.[15] Many patients report postprandial pain; however, association with meals is not universal. In fact, in a significant proportion of patients the pain is nocturnal.[17,18] Recurrent attacks are common and can range from within hours to years.[19] Some patients may present with atypical symptoms such as chest pain, eructation, early satiety, dyspepsia, or nonspecific abdominal pain.

The physical examination and laboratory evaluation are typically benign. Upper abdominal tenderness is frequently noted on physical examination to include voluntary guarding but peritonitis is absent. Laboratory values in uncomplicated gallstone disease should be normal because any abnormalities, such as leukocytosis or elevated liver and pancreatic enzymes, suggest a complication of gallstone disease, including cholecystitis, cholangitis, or pancreatitis.[20]

Diagnostic Procedures

The diagnostic test for gallstone disease is ultrasonography. It is cost-effective, noninvasive, and accurate. Approximately 95% of gallbladder stones will be detected by ultrasound. Ultrasound can also detect findings associated with complicated gallbladder disease to assist in management. If there are no stones detected on ultrasound and a high suspicion exists, the ultrasound should be repeated.[21]

Ultrasonography findings in gallstones include single- or multiple-echo dense structures in the most dependent portion of the gallbladder. The stones produce a characteristic posterior shadowing due to reflection of the ultrasonic beam.[22] Gallbladder sludge, on the other hand, will not produce an acoustic shadow and is more viscous. It represents microlithiasis, which can also produce biliary colic or lead to complicated gallstone disease such as cholangitis or pancreatitis.[23,24] Endoscopic ultrasound (EUS) can be used to evaluate for occult cholelithiasis in patients with suspected gallstone disease but a negative transabdominal ultrasound. The sensitivity of 96% for occult cholelithiasis and choledocholithiasis exceeds both computed tomographic scan and transabdominal ultrasound.[25]

Treatment and Outcomes

The current standard for management of uncomplicated gallstone disease, or symptomatic cholelithiasis, is laparoscopic cholecystectomy. Medical management consists of oral dissolution therapy with oral bile acids and is reserved for symptomatic gallstone patients who are not a candidate for surgery and have small (equal to or less than 5 mm in size), uncalcified, cholesterol stones in a functioning gallbladder with a patent cystic duct. Oral litholysis uses oral hydrophilic bile acids for dissolution therapy for cholesterol gallstones. Ursodeoxycholic acid is currently used and leads to decreased biliary cholesterol secretion, increased solubility of cholesterol by forming liquid crystals, and reduced intestinal absorption. However this approach is successful only in a small subset of patients; recurrence is common (30%–50% at 5 years), and the cost-benefit ratio is unfavorable.[26] A variety of other medications and pathways have been studied in their effect on gallstone formation, including statins, aspirin, ezetimibe, and nuclear receptors that drive lipid homeostasis in the hepatobiliary and gastrointestinal systems.[27–30] Observational studies report that nutritional modification, such as increased dietary polyunsaturated or monounsaturated fatty acids, fiber, caffeine, vegetable protein, and a diet low in refined carbohydrates, may aid in reduction of symptoms.[31] Overall, most patients will undergo laparoscopic cholecystectomy as definitive and effective management for symptomatic cholelithiasis.[32]

Summary

Symptomatic cholelithiasis, or uncomplicated gallstone disease, is very common. Multiple risk factors exist and are associated with the balance of cholesterol, bile salts, and lecithin in the body. Biliary colic with otherwise normal examination findings and laboratory values and the findings of gallstones on ultrasound should alert the clinician to the likely diagnosis of symptomatic cholelithiasis. Although a small subset of patients may benefit from oral dissolution therapy, the gold standard for treatment is laparoscopic cholecystectomy. Additional avenues for medical management continue to be researched.

FUNCTIONAL DISORDERS OF THE BILIARY TRACT: BILIARY DYSKINESIA AND SPHINCTER OF ODDI DYSFUNCTION

Functional gastrointestinal disorders are defined by chronic or recurrent gastrointestinal symptoms that cannot be explained by structural or biochemical abnormalities. That is not to say that there are not physiologic abnormalities associated with functional disorders but that their presence may not coincide with symptoms or correction with relief of symptoms.[33] Given the lack of structural or biochemical abnormalities, these disorders must be identified by the pattern of symptoms they cause. These symptoms cluster into recognizable syndromes with symptoms centered on various gastrointestinal organs. These recognizable syndromes have been defined by the Rome criteria.[34] The 3 types of functional biliary disorders based on Rome III diagnostic criteria are functional gallbladder disorder (FGD) and functional biliary or pancreatic sphincter of Oddi disorder (SOD) (**Box 1**).[35] Diagnosis is made through clinical evaluation and imaging studies, which evaluate gallbladder contractility and ejection fraction for FGD and pressure differentials through manometry for SODs. The Rome III criteria were developed to minimize invasive procedures, such as endoscopic retrograde cholangiopancreatography (ERCP) in those patients who do not meet the diagnostic criteria, thereby limiting associated complications to those invasive procedures.[36] The current gold standard in treatment is laparoscopic cholecystectomy and endoscopic sphincterotomy (ES), respectively.[37]

FGD

Functional gallbladder disorder is the term currently accepted by the Rome classification for gallbladder dyskinesia. FGD is a motility disorder initially caused by either metabolic abnormalities or a primary motility alteration.[36] Synonyms for FGD include various names, such as gallbladder spasm, acalculous biliary disease, gallbladder dyskinesia, and cystic duct syndrome.[38,39] Objective data using the radionuclide gallbladder ejection fraction (GBEF) aid in diagnosis and most patients' symptoms are relieved with cholecystectomy.[37]

Box 1
Rome III criteria. Functional gallbladder and sphincter of Oddi disorders

Diagnostic criteria

  Episodes of right upper quadrant pain or epigastric pain and ALL of the following:

    Episodes lasting 30 min or longer

    Recurrent symptoms occurring at different intervals (not daily)

    The pain builds up to a steady level

    The pain is moderate to severe enough to interrupt the patient's daily activities or lead to an emergency department visit

    The pain is not relieved by bowel movements

    The pain is not relieved by postural change

    The pain is not relieved by antacids

    Exclusion of other structural disease than would explain the symptoms

Supportive criteria

  The pain may present with one or more of the following

    Associated nausea and vomiting

    Radiates to the back and/or right infra-subscapular region

    Awakens from sleep in the middle of the night

From Rome Foundation, Inc. Rome III diagnostic criteria for functional gastrointestinal disorders. Available at: http://www.romecriteria.org/criteria/. Accessed July 26, 2013.

Epidemiology

The true prevalence of FGD is unknown and varies per study. One large study reported the prevalence of biliary pain without stones to be about 2.4%.[12] Another Italian study evaluated biliary pain with normal transabdominal gallbladder ultrasound imaging in men and women and estimated the prevalence to be 8% and 21%, respectively.[40]

Pathophysiology

The true pathophysiology of FGD is unknown. The normal physiology of the gallbladder is regulated by neurohormonal mechanisms involving the vagus and splanchnic nerves and, most notably, the hormone cholecystokinin (CCK). The liver continuously secretes bile through the intrahepatic to the extrahepatic bile ducts. The sphincter of Oddi (SO) then aids in gallbladder filling and bile storage. The bile remains stored and concentrated in the gallbladder during the fasting state and then empties during the digestive phases. Vagus nerve (efferent fibers) stimulation and CCK release contracts the gallbladder, while splanchnic nerve stimulation relaxes the gallbladder. During the fasting state, nonpropulsive contractions also exist, likely to prevent bile stasis.[36] Abnormalities in any of these processes may be responsible for the symptoms observed.

Impaired gallbladder emptying, chronic inflammation, visceral hypersensitivity, and panenteric motility disorders have all been proposed as causes for FGD.[41] Impaired gallbladder emptying, or gallbladder hypokinesia/dyskinesia, may lead to supersaturation of bile with cholesterol monohydrate because of associated bile stasis.[42] Ineffective gallbladder contraction ultimately leads to a failure of gallbladder mixing and subsequent crystal formation, which then leads to chronic inflammation of the gallbladder wall. This theory was initially tested by Brugge and colleagues and reinforced by Velanovich, who studied patients with biliary-type pain, normal ultrasound imaging, and poor gallbladder emptying undergoing cholecystectomy. Intraoperative bile aspiration and postoperative pathologic abnormality were analyzed. Brugge illustrated that all those with preoperative crystals had chronic cholecystitis histologically. Velanovich reported 89% of patients without stones had crystals within their gallbladder walls and 94% of patients without stones had pathologic evidence of chronic cholecystitis. Both reports suggest acalculous gallbladder disease and dysmotility will eventually lead to gallstone formation and chronic inflammation.[43,44] However, some argue that the histologic changes are a cause, and not the effect, of poor gallbladder contractility.[42] Moreover, abnormal histology is not universal in patients with presumed FGD as studies report chronic inflammatory changes ranging from 44% to 100%.[45–47]

Clinical Presentation

The Rome III diagnostic criteria as listed in **Boxes 1** and **2**[35] define the clinical presentation of FGD. The criteria were developed by consensus and are not substantiated by any published evidence. The intent was to develop criteria to limit extensive investigations with invasive procedures and inappropriate endoscopic and surgical procedures.[36] They are generalizations that may not encompass every patient but should be used as a guideline when considering subjecting patients to potential harm.

Diagnostic Procedures

In the setting of biliary colic, other more common diagnoses, such as gastroesophageal reflux disease, irritable bowel syndrome, functional dyspepsia, and cholelithiasis, should be evaluated before considering FGD.[36] Abdominal ultrasonography is normal

---

Box 2
Rome III criteria. Functional gallbladder disorder

Diagnostic criteria

  Must include ALL of the following:

    Criteria for functional gallbladder and SOD

    Gallbladder is present

    Normal liver enzymes, conjugated bilirubin, and amylase/lipase

From Rome Foundation, Inc. Rome III diagnostic criteria for functional gastrointestinal disorders. Available at: http://www.romecriteria.org/criteria/. Accessed July 26, 2013.

---

in FGD. With that said, it is important to recognize the limitation of ultrasound in recognizing stones less than 3 to 5 mm in size and for stones or sludge within the common bile duct.[48] Upper gastrointestinal endoscopy is indicated once normal laboratory analysis and ultrasound imaging are obtained. Further evaluation with CCK and GBEF calculation is typically used as well.[49] Historically, the CCK provocation test was used but has fallen out of favor due to low sensitivity and specificity for FGD. Pain induced by CCK has been shown to be a function of the method of infusion not underlying disease.[50]

Endoscopic evaluation is used for FGD and other causes and for more specific testing to include bile sampling. Endoscopy can aid in the elimination of gastric or duodenal pathologic abnormality. Endoscopic bile sampling and EUS can aid in the detection of small gallbladder or bile duct stones. EUS allows for improved sensitivity for identifying small gallstones when compared with transabdominal ultrasound. Bile sampling can be done with standard endoscopy taking a sample from near the ampulla or directly from the bile duct by ERCP. The bile sample is used to evaluate for microlithiasis. To increase the sensitivity for microlithiasis, intravenous CCK is injected, and a sample of bile is obtained that has not been diluted by pancreatic and duodenal fluids. Cholesterol crystals identified in gallbladder bile is strongly associated with small gallbladder calculi and these patients typically benefit from cholecystectomy.[37] A prospective study by Dahan and colleagues[51] in which EUS and microscopic bile examination were compared reported a statistically significant higher sensitivity in the diagnosis of cholecystolithiasis by EUS, 97%, than by bile microscopy, 67%. Specificities were comparable. Furthermore, if both were negative, the likelihood of cholecystolithiasis was very low. Thorboll and colleagues[52] evaluated EUS as a solitary diagnostic method in patients with biliary colic and normal ultrasonography. EUS detected microlithiasis in 52.4% of patients with postoperative pathologic confirmation in 87% of patients. Another study by Mirbagheri and colleagues[53] confirmed the importance of EUS in the diagnosis of microlithiasis for patients with normal ultrasonography.

The functional assessment of gallbladder emptying by cholescintigraphy has become the test of choice for the evaluation of suspected FGD.[35,49] The hepatobiliary iminodiacetic acid (HIDA) cholecystokinin cholescintigraphy (CCK-CS) uses a radioactive biomarker, a gamma camera, and computer analysis to aid in estimating GBEF.[37] Technetium-99m-labeled iminodiacetic acid is administered, which has a high affinity for hepatic uptake and is readily excreted into the biliary tract and concentrated in the gallbladder. A fatty meal is ingested or CCK is administered to stimulate gallbladder emptying and serial observations of net change in gallbladder activity are reported as GBEF.[36]

A low GBEF is considered diagnostic of impaired gallbladder function. However, the accuracy of CCK-HIDA and GBEF is not without limitations. There is debate as to the dose, infusion rate, when to assess emptying, and what constitutes a low GBEF.[49] A low GBEF, or positive HIDA scan, is not specific for FGD. Many medical conditions to include diabetes, celiac disease, pregnancy, or irritable bowel syndrome, as well as many medications such as opioids, oral contraceptives, calcium channel blockers, benzodiazepines, and histamine-2-receptor antagonists, can cause low GBEF.[42] Regarding the controversy concerning the appropriate dose of CCK and infusion rate as well as timing of GBEF calculation, the pivotal study of GBEF by Yap and colleagues[54] used a CCK dose of 0.02 µg/kg/min infused over 45 minutes with a GBEF calculated at 60 minutes. They reported a normal GBEF of greater than 40% based on 40 asymptomatic patients. Multiple studies have evaluated infusion dose, rates, and times and GBEF since then. Essentially, shorter CCK infusion times are unreliable for predicting GBEF and longer infusion times of 30 to 60 minutes have less variation, which allows for the calculation of a normal GBEF to be $\geq 40\%$.[49] Ziessman and colleagues[55] then published a multicenter investigation to determine optimal infusion methods as well as establishment of normal GBEF values. The findings from this study prompted the delineation of a standard methodology for CCK-CS. In 2012 a multispecialty consensus panel published recommendations for CCK-CS to standardize a protocol and improve patient care. Current recommendations are to infuse 0.02 µg/kg of sincalide (CCK analogue) over 60 minutes. The panel also defined a normal GBEF of $\geq 38\%$. Finally, the panel also recommends a large, multicenter, randomized, prospective trial to establish the utility of CCK-CS in the diagnosis of FGD[56]; this is similar to the current Rome III recommendation of an abnormal ejection fraction of less than 40% after a continuous infusion of CCK greater than 30 minutes.[57]

Treatment and Outcomes

FGD or biliary dyskinesia has been commonly treated with cholecystectomy. Medical therapy is available, but has not been compared directly with cholecystectomy in a trial. Medications used include spasmolytics, choleretics, cholekinetics, and psychotropic drugs.[58] There is a single randomized trial examining surgery versus nonoperative treatment of FGD. Yap and colleagues[54] found a 91% symptomatic relief in the surgical group at a mean follow-up for 34 months and no patient with resolution of symptoms in the nonoperative group. Unfortunately, the trial accrued only 21 patients and a larger randomized trial has not been repeated. Two recent meta-analyses examined the effectiveness of surgical therapy for biliary dyskinesia. Ponsky and colleagues[59] evaluated 274 patients in 5 studies with biliary dyskinesia, as defined by biliary colic, without gallstones on ultrasound and GBEF less than 40%. Two hundred patients underwent cholecystectomy and 74 were treated nonoperatively. Symptomatic relief was reported in 98% of patients in the surgical group versus 32% in the nonoperative group. Mahid and colleagues[60] found similar results. The authors evaluated 10 studies with 462 patients and again compared cholecystectomy with nonoperative treatment of HIDA-positive biliary dyskinesia. Surgical treatment was 15-fold more likely than medical treatment to result in symptom improvement for patients without gallstones, with biliary colic, and a positive HIDA scan. Although available studies indicate generally good outcomes for cholecystectomy for FGD, the evidence is based on a single very small randomized trial and a series of chart reviews. Several authors have called for larger randomized controlled trials with some kind of active intervention for the nonoperative arm.[61,62] Further research is also supported by the estimate that approximately 30% of patients who undergo cholecystectomy for biliary dyskinesia will continue to have symptoms after surgery. Postprandial nausea and vomiting have been reported as a poor prognostic factor for surgery and a lower quality of life postoperatively, possibly due to a global gastrointestinal motility disorder.[63]

Summary

FGD is a diagnosis of exclusion whereby the patient experiences biliary colic in the absence of gallstones, with decreased GBEF. The functional assessment of the gallbladder by CCK-HIDA has become the most widely used imaging test, which has recently been standardized to improve patient evaluation and management. A single small randomized trial and several meta-analyses have shown symptomatic benefit with cholecystectomy for FGD; however, larger randomized trials would be beneficial to try and reproduce results, as some reports state approximately 30% of patients' symptoms will continue postoperatively.

FUNCTIONAL SOD

SOD is the term used for motility abnormalities of the SO associated with biliary and pancreatic pain, elevation of liver or pancreatic enzymes, common bile duct dilation, and recurrent episodes of pancreatitis.[36] SOD is one of the functional gastrointestinal disorders. Rome III diagnostic criteria defines both a biliary and a pancreatic SOD.[35] SOD is divided further into 3 categories (I, II, III) based on symptoms, radiologic findings, and serologic findings and these categories for biliary SOD are based on the Milwaukee criteria (**Table 1**).[64] SOD can occur with an intact gallbladder; however, most data are based on patients with continued symptoms following cholecystectomy and very few gastroenterologists will offer treatment, ES, before cholecystectomy.[65]

Epidemiology

SOD is estimated to affect 14% of patients with right upper quadrant pain after cholecystectomy and less than 1% of patients with an in situ gallbladder.[66,67] Biliary SOD

Table 1				
Milwaukee criteria related to the frequency of abnormal sphincter of Oddi manometry and pain relief by biliary sphincterotomy				
Patient Group Classification	Frequency of Abnormal Sphincter Manometry	Probability of Pain Relief by Sphincterotomy if Manometry		Manometry Before Sphincter Ablation
		Abnormal	Normal	
Biliary I (%) Biliary-type pain Abnormal AST or ALP > ×2 normal Delayed drainage of ERCP contrast from the biliary tree >45 min Dilated CBD >12 mm diameter	75–95	90–95	90–95	Unnecessary
Biliary II (%) Biliary-type pain Only 1 or 2 of the above criteria	55–65	85	35	Highly recommended
Biliary III (%) Only biliary-type pain	25–60	55–65	<10	Mandatory

Abbreviations: ALP, alkaline phosphatase; AST, aspartate aminotransferase; CBD, common bile duct.
From Cheon YK. How to interpret a functional or motility test—sphincter of Oddi manometry. J Neurogastroenterol Motil 2012;18:211–7.

is more common in women than men and is associated with a high incidence of disability, health care costs, and work absence.[68] As in FGD, other possible causes of the pain must be excluded, including costochondritis, nerve injury at trochar site, gastroparesis, irritable bowel syndrome, peptic ulcer disease, and other intra-abdominal causes.[66] Most patients present with the postcholecystectomy syndrome, persistent, right upper quadrant abdominal pain following gallbladder removal. Thus, the more common causes and complications related to the surgery, such as retained stones, bile leak, or bile duct injury, must also be ruled out.[69] Pancreatic SOD is associated with idiopathic recurrent acute pancreatitis (RAP). The estimated prevalence of pancreatic SOD is approximately 30% in patients with unexplained acute pancreatitis; however, that number ranges from 15% to 72% in studies.[70–74]

Pathophysiology

Anatomically, the SO is at the junction of the biliary and pancreatic ducts in the duodenum. Dysfunction can occur in either the biliary or the pancreatic portion or both. One study of more than 300 patients with pancreaticobiliary pain reported abnormal pancreatic sphincter pressure in 19%, abnormal biliary basal sphincter pressure in 11%, and combined biliary and pancreatic pressure elevations in 31%.[75] More than 100 years ago, Rugero Oddi first identified the sphincter and was also the first to write about possible dysfunction leading to symptoms.[37] Then, in 1937, Boyden described the anatomy of the SO in great detail.[76] The human SO has a well-defined musculature, is approximately 10 mm in length, and has intramural and extramural segments. Three relatively discrete zones of muscle are identified as minisphincters called the sphincter choledochus, the sphincter ampulla, and the sphincter pancreaticus (**Fig. 2**). The ampulla is a common channel formed by the junction of the pancreatic and common bile ducts and drains through the papilla of Vater into the duodenum.[77] The SO is independent from the duodenum with differing myoelectric and contractile patterns. The basal pressure of the SO ranges from 10 to 15 mm Hg with superimposed forceful contractions of up to 150 mm Hg.[78] The main functions of the SO include regulation of flow into the duodenum, reflux prevention from the duodenum to the bile and pancreatic duct, and gallbladder filling.[79] During fasting, most of the bile is diverted toward the gallbladder by resistance of the SO, whereas during the

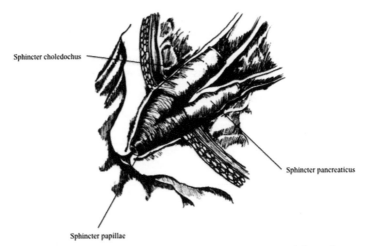

Sphincter choledochus

Sphincter pancreaticus

Sphincter papillae

Fig. 2. The sphincter of Oddi. (*Courtesy of* Robert B. Lim, MD Honolulu, HI.)

digestive phase, the gallbladder contracts and the SO relaxes, allowing release of bile into the duodenum for fat digestion and absorption. CCK leads to a coordinated contraction of the gallbladder and relaxation of the SO and duodenum, which ultimately leads to bile discharge into the duodenum. When the SO is severed, such as in sphincterotomy, there will be reflux of air and bile into the common bile duct.[78]

Clinical Presentation

The Rome III criteria also have established a set of guidelines for the diagnosis of functional biliary or pancreatic SOD. As shown in **Boxes 1, 3**, and **4**, both disorders must include the criteria for functional gallbladder and SO disorders, with normal amylase and lipase for biliary SOD or elevated amylase and lipase for pancreatic SOD. Biliary SOD patients typically present with biliary-type pain in the epigastrium or right upper quadrant with modifying factors as described previously. Biliary SOD is most commonly considered in the setting of postcholecystectomy pain. Pancreatic SOD patients have recurrent episodes of epigastric pain similar to biliary SOD patients, but radiation to the back can occur.[35] In addition, most patients with pancreatic SOD will present with recurrent episodes of pancreatitis.[80] In the absence of common causes of pancreatitis (stones, alcohol, triglycerides, pancreatic divisum), idiopathic recurrent pancreatitis or pancreatic SOD can be considered.[35] SOD is a notable disorder in the post-gastric bypass population and should be considered in these patients with biliary pain following cholecystectomy. A small series showed good relief of symptoms in post-gastric bypass patients with SOD who underwent transduodenal sphincterotomy.[81]

Diagnostic Procedures

Sphincter of Oddi manometry (SOM) is the gold standard for the diagnosis of SOD. Other imaging studies such as ultrasound, CCK-HIDA, or magnetic resonance cholangiopancreatography are used to evaluate for other causes. Other indirect tests have been used to avoid the invasive means of manometry; however, none of those studies produce the results that manometry can achieve through direct SO measurement.[36] Direct pressure measurements are obtained during ERCP in which a pressure catheter is inserted through the biopsy channel of the endoscope into the biliary or pancreatic duct. SOM has a significant risk of post-ERCP pancreatitis, which is higher than the risk with ERCP performed for other indications. Post-ERCP pancreatitis rates range from 10% to 40% in patients suspected of having SOD.[65,82] Patients with Milwaukee

---

Box 3

Rome III criteria. Functional biliary sphincter of Oddi disorder

Diagnostic criteria

   Must include BOTH of the following:

      Criteria for functional gallbladder and SOD

      Normal amylase/lipase

Supportive criteria

   Elevated serum transaminases, alkaline phosphatase, or conjugated bilirubin temporarily related to at least 2 pain episodes

From Rome Foundation, Inc. Rome III diagnostic criteria for functional gastrointestinal disorders. Available at: http://www.romecriteria.org/criteria/. Accessed July 26, 2013.

Box 4
Rome III criteria. Functional pancreatic sphincter of Oddi disorder

Diagnostic criteria

  Must include BOTH of the following:

    Criteria for functional gallbladder and SOD

    Elevated amylase/lipase

From Rome Foundation, Inc. Rome III diagnostic criteria for functional gastrointestinal disorders. Available at: http://www.romecriteria.org/criteria/. Accessed July 26, 2013.

---

classification SOD III are at the highest risk.[83] Recently placement of a pancreatic duct stent in patients suspected of having SOD has been shown to reduce the risk of post-ERCP pancreatitis.[84] SOM measurements include basal sphincter pressure, intraductal pressure, and phasic wave parameters.[75] Guelrud and colleagues[85] studied 50 asymptomatic healthy volunteer subjects to detail the characteristics of SO motor function and to help establish normal values. Findings are summarized in **Table 2**. Elevated basal sphincter pressures higher than 40 mm Hg are currently the gold standard to diagnose SOD.[66] However, other manometry abnormalities may include increased amplitude or frequency of phasic waves, paradoxic response to CCK, and increased quantity of retrograde waves.[36] Several factors, such as manometry technique and medications (nitrates, calcium channel blockers, anticholinergics, phosphodiesterase type 5 inhibitors, narcotics), can affect SO pressure and motility.[75]

SOM is not recommended for biliary type I SOD patients by many authors based on good results from ES independent of manometry findings.[66,72,86,87] Results of ES are not as universally good for biliary type II and particularly type III patients (see **Table 1**).[64] Complications for ES are also higher for patients with normal SOM, more frequently seen in biliary type II and most frequently in type III patients.[83] Based on this, SOM is recommended for biliary type II patients and is mandatory for all type III patients if sphincter ablation is considered.[66] In cases of suspected biliary SOD, SOM is typically only performed for the biliary sphincter.[88] However SOD may involve the biliary, the pancreatic, or both sphincters in patients with pancreaticobiliary pain and recurrent idiopathic pancreatitis.[89,90] Therefore manometry of both the biliary and the pancreatic sphincters is recommended by some authors in patients suspected of SOD undergoing SOM.[57,88] Particular consideration should be given in cases of type III SOD undergoing SOM because of the difficulty differentiating biliary

---

Table 2
Abnormal values for endoscopic SOM

Suggested Standard for Abnormal Values for Endoscopic SOM	
Basal sphincter pressure	>35 mm Hg
Phasic contractions	
Amplitude	>220 mm Hg
Duration	>8 s
Frequency	>10/min

Values were obtained by adding 3 SD to the mean.
From Guelrud M, Mendoza S, Rossiter G, et al. Sphincter of Oddi manometry in healthy volunteers. Dig Dis Sci 1990;35:38–46; with permission.

from pancreatic pain and generally poorer response to biliary ES (BES). Patients with failure to resolve symptoms after BES should also be considered for pancreatic SOM because up to 90% of these patients will have pancreatic SOD.[90] SOM is indicated in those with previously normal SOM studies but persistent symptoms consistent with SOD. A study of more than 5000 patients evaluated the frequency of SOD in persistently symptomatic patients with previously normal SOM studies, to determine if the short-term manometry recordings during ERCP reflect the 24-hour pathophysiology of the sphincter. Of 1037 patients with normal SOM studies, 30 underwent repeat ERCP with SOM for persistent symptoms and 60% of those patients were then diagnosed with SOD. Thus, repeat SOM may be warranted in patients with persistent debilitating symptoms and a high index of suspicion for SOD in which previous SOM is normal.[91]

Other potential diagnostic procedures are also available for further evaluation of SOD. Quantitative cholescintigraphy with a fatty meal or CCK administration can be used to evaluate for SOD. In postcholecystectomy patients, the flow of bile from the liver into the duodenum is primarily regulated by the SO and patients with SOD will show marked delay in transit into the duodenum.[92] However, precise criteria to define an abnormal study remain controversial. The hilum to duodenum transit time of greater than 10 minutes and the duodenal appearance time greater than 20 minutes are the most frequently used in studies.[93] In addition to the controversy over criteria, studies show varying results regarding correlation to SOM and no studies show correlation with outcome after ES. Where correlation occurs, it is most commonly with type I patients in whom it is frequently not necessary.[66,94,95] In patients with intact gallbladders, the criteria for diagnosis of SOD are based on delayed biliary visualization, intrahepatic biliary prominence, and biliary-bowel transit time.[96] The injection of secretin with subsequent measurement of the main pancreatic duct diameter has been studied in comparison with SOM. Ultrasound or magnetic resonance pancreatography has been used, but has not been shown to correlate with manometry or to predict outcomes.[97–99] Morphine-neostigmine provocation has also been suggested, but the low sensitivity and specificity have been disappointing.[100]

Treatment for Biliary SOD

The most well-known classification system for SOD was proposed by Hogan and Geenen[101] in 1988 and is known as the Milwaukee classification. Three groups of patients were identified and classified based on symptoms and laboratory or imaging abnormalities to include ERCP biliary drainage times. This classification has been revised by the Rome III project to use noninvasive methods, ultrasonographic measurement of the bile duct, over ERCP drainage times and can be seen in **Table 3**. Type I biliary SOD is also referred to as benign SO stenosis and type II and type III biliary SOD are also referred to as SO dyskinesia. SO dyskinesia is an intermittent symptomatic disease; thus, short-time SOM may not capture the pathologic abnormality.[102]

Sphincter ablation is the treatment for SOD. The traditional surgical approach is transduodenal biliary sphincteroplasty with a transampullary septoplasty (**Fig. 3**). The surgical approach has been replaced by endoscopic therapy in most instances and is based on decreased morbidity, mortality, and cost. Surgical therapy is reserved for endoscopic failures and in cases where endoscopic methods are not technically possible.[88]

It is generally accepted that type I biliary SOD patients have true papillary stenosis and should undergo ES without manometry; this is based on reported relief of symptoms after ES ranging from 90% to 95% regardless of manometry results, which are normal in 14% to 35% of cases.[86,103,104] Some argue that occult biliary microlithiasis

Table 3
Classic and revised classification for SOD

	Type	Classic	Revised
Biliary	I	Abnormal hepatic enzymes on 2 occasions + dilated CBD + delayed drainage >45 min	Abnormal hepatic enzymes + dilated CBD
	II	1 or 2 of abnormal hepatic enzymes ×2, dilated CBD, delayed drainage >45 min	Either abnormal hepatic enzymes or dilated CBD
	III	No laboratory or imaging abnormalities	
Pancreatic	I	Abnormal pancreatic enzymes on 2 occasions + dilated PD + delayed drainage >8 min	Abnormal pancreatic enzymes + dilated PD
	II	1 or 2 of abnormal pancreatic enzymes ×2, dilated PD, delayed drainage >8 min	Either abnormal pancreatic enzymes or dilated PD
	III	No laboratory or imaging abnormalities	

Biliary, all patients present with biliary type pain; Pancreatic, all patients present with recurrent pancreatitis or typical pancreatic pain.

Abbreviations: CBD, common bile duct; PD, pancreatic duct.

Adapted from Peterson BT. Sphincter of Oddi dysfunction, part 2: evidence-based review of the presentations, with "objective" pancreatic findings (types I and II) and of presumptive type III. Gastrointest Endosc 2004;59:670–87.

is actually the same clinical entity as type I SOD because they have similar clinical presentations and both show clinical improvement with endoscopic treatment.[105]

Type II SOD represents a functional sphincter disturbance. Patients should undergo SOM and those with elevated biliary sphincter pressures typically undergo ES for treatment.[66] The recommendation is based on 2 randomized controlled trials that showed improvement with ES for patients with elevated basal pressures. However several retrospective studies did not find symptom improvement was associated with abnormal SOM.[106] Geenen and colleagues[64] randomized 47 patients with type II SOD to ES or sham sphincterotomy. After randomization but before ES, SOM was performed. At 1-year follow-up ES resulted in clinical improvement in 10 of 11 patients who had elevated sphincter pressures versus improvement in only 3 of 12 patients in the sham group. Seven patients in the sham sphincterotomy group with elevated sphincter pressures crossed over and underwent ES. At 4-year follow-up, 17 of 18 patients with initially elevated sphincter pressures demonstrated symptom improvement after ES. Patients with normal SOM had no benefit from ES compared with sham sphincterotomy. Toouli and colleagues[107] randomized 81 patients with types I and II SOD to ES or sham sphincterotomy. SOM classified each into 3 categories: elevated basal pressures, dyskinesia (phasic contraction abnormalities), and normal. At 3 and 24 months, symptoms improved in 11 of 13 patients with elevated basal pressures treated by ES versus only 5 of 13 in the sham group. Results between ES and sham did not differ for the dyskinesia or normal groups. A recent review of available studies showed long-term symptom relief for type II SOD in up to 79% of patients.[66]

Several reports have evaluated ES for the subset of type III SOD and results are mixed. Botoman and colleagues[108] found symptom improvement at 3 years of 56% for SOD type III patients with elevated basal biliary sphincter pressures. Freeman and colleagues[82] found 62% symptom improvement at 2 years in SOD type III patients irrespective of SOM findings. Finally Wehrmann and colleagues[109] found only 8% of SOD type III patients with elevated basal biliary sphincter pressures had symptom

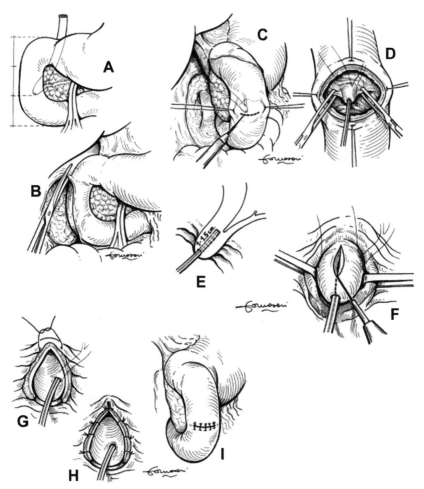

Fig. 3. The ampulla of Vater position in relation to the (*A*) second duodenal loop and (*B*) duodenal mobilization. Incision of the duodenum after the wall, opposite the ampulla of Vater, is exposed by (*C*) rotating the mobilized duodenum to the left; the papilla is exposed and (*D*) a grooved director is introduced into its proximal end. Following the guidance of the (*E*) grooved director, the (*F*) papilla is incised for 1 to 1.5 cm. After papillotomy, (*G*) sinus probe has been introduced into the proximal end of the Wirsung duct. Suture of the medial aspect of papillotomy (*H*) is completed. (*I*) Duodenal closure. (*From* Miccini M, Amore Bonapasta S, Gregori M, et al. Indications and results for transduodenal sphincteroplasty in the era of endoscopic sphincterotomy. Am J Surg 2010;200:247–51; with permission.)

improvement at 2.5 years after ES. Given the variations in outcomes among studies of ES in type III SOD, ES is only considered after all other potential causes have been evaluated and the patient has failed medical management. At this point SOM can be considered and ES, if basal biliary sphincter pressure is elevated. Medical therapy in type III SOD has been shown to be effective in decreasing symptoms in 71% of patients.[110] Furthermore, symptoms may resolve spontaneously in up to 69.8% of patients with type III disease.[66]

Medical therapy should be considered in all type III SOD and in mild type II SOD, before considering sphincterotomy. Because the SO is a smooth muscle sphincter, medical therapy has been aimed at smooth muscle relaxation. Calcium channel blockers and nitrates have been the subject of investigation. Sublingual nifedipine and nitrates have been shown to reduce basal sphincter pressures in healthy volunteers as well as in symptomatic patients.[111,112] Nifedipine is the most well-studied medical therapy and has been shown to be effective in symptomatic improvement of patients with documented SOD by manometry. Khuroo and colleagues[113] found in a prospective, randomized, placebo controlled crossover trial that 75% of patients with manometrically documented type II and III SOD had improvement in symptoms and Emergency Room visits with use of nifedipine and oral analgesics over the 12-week treatment period. Sand and colleagues[114] found similar findings over a 16-week trial in type II SOD patients. However, associated vasodilator effects such as headaches, flushing, and dizziness can limit long-term use and the studies with nifedipine have short follow-up. Vardenafil, a phosphodiesterase type 5 inhibitor, has been shown to significantly reduce mean basal sphincter pressure and mean phasic amplitude in patients undergoing SOM, but has not been evaluated for clinical response.[115] Lower levels of serum motilin and gastrin have been shown to be associated with hypomotility of the SO.[116] Trimebutine is a medication with antimuscarinic effects and is marketed for treatment of irritable bowel syndrome and other gastrointestinal disorders. A recent study treated 59 patients with SOD for 1 year with Trimebutine and clinically re-evaluated each patient after 30 months. At the end of follow-up, 62% of patients showed more than 50% improvement with medical management alone. The improvement rate was no different in patients who ultimately underwent ES after failure of medical management (64%).[117] Although promising, further trials with long-term data are needed to evaluate long-term effectiveness of medical SOD management. With that said, given the relative safety of medical therapy and the non-life-threatening nature of SOD, strong consideration should be given to initial treatment of all type III SOD and mildly symptomatic type II SOD patients before ES.[118]

Treatment for Pancreatic SOD

A classification system similar to the Milwaukee classification for biliary SOD has also been developed for pancreatic SOD (**Box 5**). The current recommendation for

---

Box 5
Modified classification of pancreatic type SOD

Type I

  Pancreatic-type pain

  Amylase/lipase >1.5–2 times normal

  Pancreatic duct diameter >6 mm in head or >5 mm in body

Type II

  Pancreatic-type pain and 1 of the following:

  Amylase/lipase >1.5–2 times normal

  Pancreatic duct diameter >6 mm in head or >5 mm in body

Type III

  Pancreatic-type pain only

From Prajapati DN, Hogan WJ. Sphincter of Oddi dysfunction and other functional biliary disorders: evaluation and treatment. Gastroenterol Clin North Am 2003;32:601–18.

pancreatic SOD with elevated basal pressures on SOM is ES. Many authors think complete division of the biliary and pancreatic sphincters is necessary, and the septum is required.[36,57,88,118] Toouli and colleagues[119] examined patients with idiopathic pancreatitis and found treatment aimed at the biliary sphincter failed in 10 of 16 patients, whereas therapy directed at the pancreatic sphincter was successful in 23 of 26 patients. Long-term follow-up was significant for no further episodes of pancreatitis in more than 90% of patients.[120] Park and colleagues[121] examined 313 patients with pancreaticobiliary pain and abnormal pressures in the biliary, pancreatic, or both sphincters. All patients underwent sphincterotomy of both sphincters (dual endoscopic sphincterotomy [DES]) at a single setting. Reintervention rates were then examined. There was no difference in reintervention rates between type II and type III SOD. The patient's reintervention rate was compared with historical controls that underwent only BES. Patients with an isolated abnormal pancreatic sphincter underwent reintervention at a significantly lower rate than historical controls. Patients with an isolated abnormal biliary sphincter or abnormality of both sphincters had similar reintervention rates. In the only randomized trial for RAP, Cote and colleagues[122] randomized 69 patients with idiopathic pancreatitis and elevated pancreatic sphincter pressures to DES versus BES. Another 20 patients with idiopathic pancreatitis and normal pancreatic sphincter pressures were randomized to BES or sham sphincterotomy. At a median of 78 months follow-up rates of RAP were significantly higher for the patients with abnormal SOM than patients with normal SOM. The rates for RAP in the DES were similar to the BES for patients with abnormal SOM and rates were similar between sham sphincterotomy and BES in the normal SOM group. The one caveat to this study is the percentage of patients in the BES group with abnormal biliary SOM was significantly higher than the DES group. The results of this randomized trial differ from most retrospective studies previously showing benefit to pancreatic sphincterotomy. Given these results and the risks associated with pancreatic sphincterotomy, it seems reasonable to begin with BES, particularly if biliary SOM is abnormal.

Summary

Functional disorders of the SO represent a group of disorders that are incompletely defined with variable responses to treatment. The SOD classification system is based on anatomy, symptoms, and objective findings and, although imperfect, continues to be the best way to group these disorders to aid in further investigation and management. Noninvasive diagnostic testing should be further investigated, but current results lack sensitivity or specificity to guide therapy. Type I SOD should be managed by ES without SOM. Type II SOD should have a trial of medical therapy before subjecting to risks of SOM. In patients where medical management fails, and with appropriate discussion of risk and benefits, SOM can be done and ES for abnormal results. Type III disease is pain alone without abnormal laboratory or imaging findings. Type III SOD should have extensive investigation for alternate diagnosis and be treated with medical therapy. Given the variability of response to ES in studies, the relatively high response to medical therapy, and the risks of SOM, SOM and ES for an abnormality should be used after exhausting all other avenues. Patients with pancreatic SOD and elevated SOM should undergo ES. Pancreatic SOD type III should be treated the same as biliary type III and likely are the same group.

REFERENCES

1. Everhart JE, Khare M, Hill M, et al. Prevalence and ethnic differences in gallbladder disease in the United States. Gastroenterology 1999;117(3):632–9.

2. Yoo EH, Lee SY. The prevalence and risk factors for gallstone disease. Clin Chem Lab Med 2009;47(7):795–807.
3. Sampliner RE, Bennett PH, Comess LJ, et al. Gallbladder disease in pima indians. Demonstration of high prevalence and early onset by cholecystography. N Engl J Med 1970;283(25):1358–64.
4. Festi D, Dormi A, Capodicasa S, et al. Incidence of gallstone disease in Italy: results from a multicenter, population-based Italian study (the MICOL project). World J Gastroenterol 2008;14(34):5282–9.
5. Amaral JF, Thompson WR. Gallbladder disease in the morbidly obese. Am J Surg 1985;149(4):551–7.
6. Maurer KR, Everhart JE, Ezzati TM, et al. Prevalence of gallstone disease in Hispanic populations in the United States. Gastroenterology 1989;96(2 Pt 1):487–92.
7. Valdivieso V, Covarrubias C, Siegel F, et al. Pregnancy and cholelithiasis: pathogenesis and natural course of gallstones diagnosed in early puerperium. Hepatology 1993;17(1):1–4.
8. Sarin SK, Negi VS, Dewan R, et al. High familial prevalence of gallstones in the first-degree relatives of gallstone patients. Hepatology 1995;22(1):138–41.
9. Denk GU, Bikker H, Lekanne Dit Deprez RH, et al. ABCB4 deficiency: a family saga of early onset cholelithiasis, sclerosing cholangitis and cirrhosis and a novel mutation in the ABCB4 gene. Hepatol Res 2010;40(9):937–41.
10. Venneman NG, van Erpecum KJ. Pathogenesis of gallstones. Gastroenterol Clin North Am 2010;39(2):171–83, vii.
11. Admirand WH, Small DM. The physicochemical basis of cholesterol gallstone formation in man. J Clin Invest 1968;47(5):1043–52.
12. Barbara L, Sama C, Morselli Labate AM, et al. A population study on the prevalence of gallstone disease: the Sirmione study. Hepatology 1987;7(5):913–7.
13. Bar-Meir S. Gallstones: prevalence, diagnosis and treatment. Isr Med Assoc J 2001;3:111–3.
14. Attilli AF, de Santis A, Capri R, et al. The natural history of gallstones: The GREPCO experience. Hepatology 1995;21(3):656–60.
15. Diehl AK, Sugarek NJ, Todd KH. Clinical evaluation for gallstone disease: Usefulness of symptoms and signs in diagnosis. Am J Med 1990;89(1):29–33.
16. Portincasa P, Moschetta A, Petruzzelli M, et al. Gallstone disease: Symptoms and diagnosis of gallbladder stones. Best Pract Res Clin Gastroenterol 2006; 20(6):1017–29.
17. Rigas B, Torosis J, McDougall CJ, et al. The circadian rhythm of biliary colic. J Clin Gastroenterol 1990;12(4):409–14.
18. Minoli G, Imperiale G, Spinzi GC, et al. Circadian periodicity and other clinical features of biliary pain. J Clin Gastroenterol 1991;13(5):546–8.
19. Festi D, Sottili S, Colecchia A, et al. Clinical manifestations of gallstone disease: Evidence from the Multicenter Italian Study on Cholelithiasis (MICOL). Hepatology 1999;30(4):839–46.
20. Nahrwold DL. Chronic cholecystitis and cholelithiasis. In: Sabiston DC Jr, editor. Textbook of Surgery: The Biological Basis of Modern Surgical Practice. Philadelphia: W.B. Saunders; 1991. p. 1057–63.
21. Johnson CD. ABC of the upper gastrointestinal tract. upper abdominal pain: Gall bladder. BMJ 2001;323(7322):1170–3.
22. Leopold GR, Amberg J, Gosink BB, et al. Gray scale ultrasonic cholecystography: a comparison with conventional radiographic techniques. Radiology 1976; 121(2):445–8.
23. Ko CW, Sekijima JH, Lee SP. Biliary sludge. Ann Intern Med 1999;130(4 Pt 1):301–11.

24. Lee SP, Nicholls JF, Park HZ. Biliary sludge as a cause of acute pancreatitis. N Engl J Med 1992;326(9):589–93.
25. Robinson O'neill DE, Saunders MD. Endoscopic ultrasonography in diseases of the gallbladder. Gastroenterol Clin North Am 2010;39(2):289–305.
26. Portincasa P, Ciaula AD, Bonfrate LE. Therapy of gallstone disease: what it was, what it is, what it will be. World J Gastrointest Pharmacol Ther 2012; 3(2):7–20.
27. Portincasa P, Di Ciaula A, Wang HH, et al. Medicinal treatments of cholesterol gallstones: old, current and new perspectives. Curr Med Chem 2009;16(12): 1531–42.
28. Di Ciaula A, Wang DQ, Wang HH, et al. Targets for current pharmacologic therapy in cholesterol gallstone disease. Gastroenterol Clin North Am 2010;39(2): 245–64, viii–ix.
29. Wang HH, Portincasa P, de Bari O, et al. Prevention of cholesterol gallstones by inhibiting hepatic biosynthesis and intestinal absorption of cholesterol. Eur J Clin Invest 2013;43(4):413–26.
30. Cariati A, Piromalli E. Limits and perspective of oral therapy with statins and aspirin for the prevention of symptomatic cholesterol gallstone disease. Expert Opin Pharmacother 2012;13(9):1223–7.
31. Gaby AR. Nutritional approaches to prevention and treatment of gallstones. Altern Med Rev 2009;14(3):258–67.
32. Gui GP, Cheruvu CV, West N, et al. Is cholecystectomy effective treatment for symptomatic gallstones? Clinical outcome after long-term follow-up. Ann R Coll Surg Engl 1998;80(1):25–32.
33. Corazziari E. Definitions and epidemiology of functional gastrointestinal disorders. Best Pract Res Clin Gastroenterol 2004;18(4):613–31.
34. Corazziari E. New Rome criteria for functional gastrointestinal disorders. Dig Liver Dis 2000;32(Suppl 3):S233–4.
35. Drossman DA. Rome III: the new criteria. Chin J Dig Dis 2006;7(4):181–5.
36. Behar J, Corazziari E, Guelrud M, et al. Functional gallbladder and sphincter of Oddi disorders. Gastroenterology 2006;130(5):1498–509.
37. Toouli J. Biliary motility disorders. Baillieres Clin Gastroenterol 1997;11(4): 725–40.
38. Rastogi A, Slivka A, Moser AJ, et al. Controversies concerning pathophysiology and management of acalculous biliary-type abdominal pain. Dig Dis Sci 2005; 50(8):1391–401.
39. Cozzolino HJ, Goldstein F, Greening RR, et al. The cystic duct syndrome. JAMA 1963;185:920–4.
40. The epidemiology of gallstone disease in Rome, Italy. Part I. Prevalence data in men. The Rome group for epidemiology and prevention of cholelithiasis (GREPCO). Hepatology 1988;8(4):904–6.
41. Penning C, Gielkens HA, Delemarre JB, et al. Gall bladder emptying in severe idiopathic constipation. Gut 1999;45(2):264–8.
42. Hansel SL, Dibaise JK. Functional gallbladder disorder: Gallbladder dyskinesia. Gastroenterol Clin North Am 2010;39(2):369–79.
43. Velanovich V. Biliary dyskinesia and biliary crystals: a prospective study. Am Surg 1997;63(1):69–74.
44. Brugge WR, Brand DL, Atkins HL, et al. Gallbladder dyskinesia in chronic acalculous cholecystitis. Dig Dis Sci 1986;31(5):461–7.
45. Shaffer E. Acalculous biliary pain: new concepts for an old entity. Dig Liver Dis 2003;35(Suppl 3):S20–5.

46. Barron LG, Rubio PA. Importance of accurate preoperative diagnosis and role of advanced laparoscopic cholecystectomy in relieving chronic acalculous cholecystitis. J Laparoendosc Surg 1995;5(6):357–61.

47. Patel NA, Lamb JJ, Hogle NJ, et al. Therapeutic efficacy of laparoscopic cholecystectomy in the treatment of biliary dyskinesia. Am J Surg 2004;187(2): 209–12.

48. Wilkinson LS, Levine TS, Smith D, et al. Biliary sludge: Can ultrasound reliably detect the presence of crystals in bile? Eur J Gastroenterol Hepatol 1996; 8(10):999–1001.

49. Francis G, Baillie J. Gallbladder dyskinesia: fact or fiction? Curr Gastroenterol Rep 2011;13(2):188–92.

50. Ziessman HA. Functional hepatobiliary disease: chronic acalculous gallbladder and chronic acalculous biliary disease. Semin Nucl Med 2006;36(2):119–32.

51. Dahan P, Andant C, Levy P, et al. Prospective evaluation of endoscopic ultrasonography and microscopic examination of duodenal bile in the diagnosis of cholecystolithiasis in 45 patients with normal conventional ultrasonography. Gut 1996;38(2):277–81.

52. Thorboll J, Vilmann P, Jacobsen B, et al. Endoscopic ultrasonography in detection of cholelithiasis in patients with biliary pain and negative transabdominal ultrasonography. Scand J Gastroenterol 2004;39(3):267–9.

53. Mirbagheri SA, Mohamadnejad M, Nasiri J, et al. Prospective evaluation of endoscopic ultrasonography in the diagnosis of biliary microlithiasis in patients with normal transabdominal ultrasonography. J Gastrointest Surg 2005;9(7): 961–4.

54. Yap L, Wycherley AG, Morphett AD, et al. Acalculous biliary pain: Cholecystectomy alleviates symptoms in patients with abnormal cholescintigraphy. Gastroenterology 1991;101(3):786–93.

55. Ziessman HA, Tulchinsky M, Lavely WC, et al. Sincalide-stimulated cholescintigraphy: a multicenter investigation to determine optimal infusion methodology and gallbladder ejection fraction normal values. J Nucl Med 2010;51(2):277–81.

56. DiBaise JK, Richmond BK, Ziessman HA, et al. Cholecystokinin-cholescintigraphy in adults: consensus recommendations of an interdisciplinary panel. Clin Nucl Med 2012;37(1):63–70.

57. Vassiliou MC, Laycock WS. Biliary dyskinesia. Surg Clin North Am 2008;88: 1253–72.

58. Simanenkov VI, Poroshina EG, Tikhonov SV. The use of tenoten preparation in complex therapy of hypomotoric biliary dyskinesia. Bull Exp Biol Med 2009; 148(2):349–50.

59. Ponsky TA, DeSagun R, Brody F. Surgical therapy for biliary dyskinesia: a meta-analysis and review of the literature. J Laparoendosc Adv Surg Tech A 2005; 15(5):439–42.

60. Mahid SS, Jafri NS, Brangers BC, et al. Meta-analysis of cholecystectomy in symptomatic patients with positive hepatobiliary iminodiacetic acid scan results without gallstones. Arch Surg 2009;144(2):180–7.

61. Bielefeldt K. The rising tide of cholecystectomy for biliary dyskinesia. Aliment Pharmacol Ther 2013;37(1):98–106.

62. Gurusamy KS, Junnarkar S, Farouk M, et al. Cholecystectomy for suspected gallbladder dyskinesia. Cochrane Database Syst Rev 2009;(1):CD007086. http://dx.doi.org/10.1002/14651858.CD007086.pub2.

63. Geiger TM, Awad ZT, Burgard M, et al. Prognostic indicators of quality of life after cholecystectomy for biliary dyskinesia. Am Surg 2008;74(5):400–4.

64. Geenen JE, Hogan WJ, Dodds WJ, et al. The efficacy of endoscopic sphincter-otomy after cholecystectomy in patients with sphincter-of-oddi dysfunction. N Engl J Med 1989;320(2):82–7.
65. Baillie J. Sphincter of Oddi dysfunction. Curr Gastroenterol Rep 2010;12(2): 130–4.
66. Hall TC, Dennison AR, Garcea G. The diagnosis and management of sphincter of Oddi dysfunction: a systematic review. Langenbecks Arch Surg 2012;397(6): 889–98.
67. Bar-Meir S, Halpern Z, Bardan E, et al. Frequency of papillary dysfunction among cholecystectomized patients. Hepatology 1984;4(2):328–30.
68. Drossman DA, Li Z, Andruzzi E, et al. U.S. householder survey of functional gastrointestinal disorders. prevalence, sociodemography, and health impact. Dig Dis Sci 1993;38(9):1569–80.
69. Hermann RE. The spectrum of biliary stone disease. Am J Surg 1989;158(3): 171–3.
70. Kaw M, Brodmerkel GJ Jr. ERCP, biliary crystal analysis, and sphincter of Oddi manometry in idiopathic recurrent pancreatitis. Gastrointest Endosc 2002;55(2): 157–62.
71. Coyle WJ, Pineau BC, Tarnasky PR, et al. Evaluation of unexplained acute and acute recurrent pancreatitis using endoscopic retrograde cholangiopancrea-tography, sphincter of Oddi manometry and endoscopic ultrasound. Endoscopy 2002;34(8):617–23.
72. Sherman S, Troiano FP, Hawes RH, et al. Frequency of abnormal sphincter of Oddi manometry compared with the clinical suspicion of sphincter of Oddi dysfunction. Am J Gastroenterol 1991;86(5):586–90.
73. Toouli J, Roberts-Thomson IC, Dent J, et al. Sphincter of Oddi motility disorders in patients with idiopathic recurrent pancreatitis. Br J Surg 1985;72(11):859–63.
74. Geenen JE, Nash JA. The role of sphincter of Oddi manometry and biliary micro-scopy in evaluating idiopathic recurrent pancreatitis. Endoscopy 1998;30(9): A237–41.
75. Cheon YK. How to interpret a functional or motility test—sphincter of Oddi manometry. J Neurogastroenterol Motil 2012;18(2):211–7.
76. Boyden EA. The sphincter of Oddi in man and certain representative mammals. Surgery 1937;1:25–37.
77. Boyden EA. The anatomy of the choledochoduodenal junction in man. Surg Gynecol Obstet 1957;104(6):641–52.
78. Behar J. Physiology and pathophysiology of the biliary tract: The gallbladder and sphincter of Oddi—A review. ISRN Physiol 2013;2013:15.
79. Toouli J. Sphincter of Oddi: function, dysfunction, and its management. J Gastroenterol Hepatol 2009;24(Suppl 3):S57–62.
80. Wehrmann T. Long-term results (≥10 years) of endoscopic therapy for sphincter of Oddi dysfunction in patients with acute recurrent pancreatitis. Endoscopy 2011;43(3):202–7.
81. Morgan KA, Glenn JB, Byrne TK, et al. Sphincter of Oddi dysfunction after roux-en-Y gastric bypass. Surg Obes Relat Dis 2009;5(5):571–5.
82. Freeman ML, Gill M, Overby C, et al. Predictors of outcomes after biliary and pancreatic sphincterotomy for sphincter of Oddi dysfunction. J Clin Gastroen-terol 2007;41(1):94–102.
83. Beltz S, Sarkar A, Loren DE, et al. Risk stratification for the development of post-ERCP pancreatitis by sphincter of Oddi dysfunction classification. South Med J 2013;106(5):298–302.

84. Saad AM, Fogel EL, McHenry L. Pancreatic duct stent placement prevents post-ERCP pancreatitis with suspected sphincter of Oddi dysfunction but normal manometry results. Gastrointest Endosc 2008;6(7):255–61.

85. Guelrud M, Mendoza S, Rossiter G, et al. Sphincter of Oddi manometry in healthy volunteers. Dig Dis Sci 1990;35(1):38–46.

86. Rolny P, Geenen JE, Hogan WJ. Post-cholecystectomy patients with "objective signs" of partial bile outflow obstruction: clinical characteristics, sphincter of Oddi manometry findings, and results of therapy. Gastrointest Endosc 1993; 39(6):778–81.

87. Thomas PD, Turner JG, Dobbs BR, et al. Use of (99m)tc-DISIDA biliary scanning with morphine provocation for the detection of elevated sphincter of Oddi basal pressure. Gut 2000;46(6):838–41.

88. Piccinni G, Angrisano A, Testini M, et al. Diagnosing and treating sphincter of Oddi dysfunction: a critical literature review and reevaluation. J Clin Gastroenterol 2004;38(4):350–9.

89. Raddawi HM, Geenen JE, Hogan WJ, et al. Pressure measurements from biliary and pancreatic segments of sphincter of Oddi: comparison between patients with functional abdominal pain, biliary, or pancreatic disease. Dig Dis Sci 1991;36(1):71–4.

90. Eversman D, Fogel EL, Rusche M, et al. Frequency of abnormal pancreatic and biliary sphincter manometry compared with clinical suspicion of sphincter of Oddi dysfunction. Gastrointest Endosc 1999;50:637–41.

91. Khashab MA, Watkins JL, McHenry L Jr, et al. Frequency of sphincter of oddi dysfunction in patients with previously normal sphincter of Oddi manometry studies. Endoscopy 2010;42(5):369–74.

92. Funch-Jensen P, Drewes AM, Madacsy L. Evaluation of the biliary tract in patients with functional biliary symptoms. World J Gastroenterol 2006;12(18): 2839–45.

93. Madacsy L, Middelfart HV, Matzen P, et al. Quantitative hepatobiliary scintigraphy and endoscopic sphincter of Oddi manometry in patients with suspected sphincter of Oddi dysfunction: assessment of flow-pressure relationship in the biliary tract. Eur J Gastroenterol Hepatol 2000;12(7):777–86.

94. Vijayakumar V, Briscoe EG, Pehlivanov ND. Postcholecystectomy sphincter of Oddi dyskinesia–a diagnostic dilemma–role of noninvasive nuclear and invasive manometric and endoscopic aspects. Surg Laparosc Endosc Percutan Tech 2007;17(1):10–3.

95. Craig AG, Peter D, Saccone GT, et al. Scintigraphy versus manometry in patients with suspected biliary sphincter of Oddi dysfunction. Gut 2003;52(3):352–7.

96. Santhosh S, Mittal BR, Arun S, et al. Quantitative cholescintigraphy with fatty meal in the diagnosis of sphincter of Oddi dysfunction and acalculous cholecystopathy. Indian J Gastroenterol 2012;31(4):186–90.

97. Di Francesco V, Brunori MP, Rigo L, et al. Comparison of ultrasound-secretin test and sphincter of Oddi manometry in patients with recurrent acute pancreatitis. Dig Dis Sci 1999;44(2):336–40.

98. Bolondi L, Gaiani S, Gullo L, et al. Secretin administration induces a dilatation of main pancreatic duct. Dig Dis Sci 1984;29(9):802–8.

99. Aisen AM, Sherman S, Jennings SG, et al. Comparison of secretin-stimulated magnetic resonance pancreatography and manometry results in patients with suspected sphincter of Oddi dysfunction. Acad Radiol 2008;15(5):601–9.

100. Chowdhury AH, Humes DJ, Pritchard SE, et al. The effects of morphine-neostigmine and secretin provocation on pancreaticobiliary morphology in

healthy subjects: A randomized, double-blind crossover study using serial MRCP. World J Surg 2011;35(9):2102–9.

101. Hogan WJ, Geenen JE. Biliary dyskinesia. Endoscopy 1988;20(Suppl 1): 179–83.
102. Tanaka M. Function and dysfunction of the sphincter of Oddi. Dig Surg 2010; 27(2):94–9.
103. Cicala M, Habib FI, Vavassori P, et al. Outcome of endoscopic sphincterotomy in post cholecystectomy patients with sphincter of Oddi dysfunction as predicted by manometry and quantitative choledochoscintigraphy. Gut 2002; 50(5):665–8.
104. Heetun ZS, Zeb F, Cullen G, et al. Biliary sphincter of Oddi dysfunction: response rates after ERCP and sphincterotomy in a 5-year ERCP series and proposal for new practical guidelines. Eur J Gastroenterol Hepatol 2011;23(4): 327–33.
105. Elmi F, Silverman WB. Biliary sphincter of Oddi dysfunction type I versus occult biliary microlithiasis in post-cholecystectomy patients: Are they both part of the same clinical entity? Dig Dis Sci 2010;55(3):842–6.
106. Kalaitzakia E, Ambrose T, Phillips-Hughes J, et al. Management of patients with biliary sphincter of Oddi disorder without manometry. BMC Gastroenterol 2010; 10:124–32.
107. Toouli J, Roberts-Thomson IC, Kellow J, et al. Manometry based randomised trial of endoscopic sphincterotomy for sphincter of Oddi dysfunction. Gut 2000;46(1):98–102.
108. Botoman VA, Kozarek RA, Novell LA. Long-term outcome after endoscopic sphincterotomy in patients with biliary colic and suspected sphincter of Oddi dysfunction. Gastrointest Endosc 1994;40:165–70.
109. Wehrmann T, Wiemer K, Lembcke B. Do patients with sphincter of Oddi dysfunction benefit from endoscopic sphincterotomy? A 5-year prospective trial. Eur J Gastroenterol Hepatol 1996;8:251–6.
110. Vitton V, Delpy R, Gasmi M, et al. Is endoscopic sphincterotomy avoidable in patients with sphincter of Oddi dysfunctyion? Eur J Gastroenterol Hepatol 2006;20: 15–21.
111. Kalloo AN, Pasricha PJ. Therapy of sphincter of Oddi dysfunction. Gastrointest Endosc Clin N Am 1996;6(1):117–25.
112. Guelrud M, Mendoza S, Rossiter G, et al. Effect of nifedipine on sphincter of Oddi motor activity: studies in healthy volunteers and patients with biliary dyskinesia. Gastroenterology 1988;95(4):1050–5.
113. Khuroo MS, Zargar SA, Yattoo GN. Efficacy of nifedipine therapy in patients with sphincter of Oddi dysfunction: a prospective, double-blind, randomized, placebo-controlled, cross over trial. Br J Clin Pharmacol 1992;33(5):477–85.
114. Sand J, Nordback I, Koskinen M, et al. Nifedipine for suspected type II sphincter of Oddi dyskinesia. Am J Gastroenterol 1993;88(4):530–5.
115. Cheon YK, Cho YD, Moon JH, et al. Effects of vardenafil, a phosphodiesterase type-5 inhibitor, on sphincter of Oddi motility in patients with suspected biliary sphincter of Oddi dysfunction. Gastrointest Endosc 2009;69(6):1111–6.
116. Zhang ZH, Wu SD, Wang B, et al. Sphincter of Oddi hypomotility and its relationship with duodenal-biliary reflux, plasma motilin and serum gastrin. World J Gastroenterol 2008;14(25):4077–81.
117. Vitton V, Ezzedine S, Gonzalez JM, et al. Medical treatment for sphincter of Oddi dysfunction: Can it replace endoscopic sphincterotomy? World J Gastroenterol 2012;18(14):1610–5.

118. Sherman S. What is the role of ERCP in the setting of abdominal pain of pancreatic or biliary origin (suspected sphincter of Oddi dysfunction)? Gastrointest Endosc 2002;56(6):S258–66.

119. Toouli J, Di Francesco V, Saccone G, et al. Division of the sphincter of Oddi for treatment of dysfunction associated with recurrent pancreatitis. Br J Surg 1996; 83(9):1205–10.

120. Toouli J. The sphincter of Oddi and acute pancreatitis–revisited. HPB (Oxford) 2003;5(3):142–5.

121. Park SH, Watkins JL, Fogel EL, et al. Long-term outcome of endoscopic dual pancreatobiliary sphincterotomy in patients with manometry-documented sphincter of Oddi dysfunction and normal pancreatogram. Gastrointest Endosc 2003;57:483–91.

122. Cote GA, Imperiale TF, Schmidt SE, et al. Similar efficacies of biliary, with or without pancreatic, sphincterotomy in treatment of idiopathic recurrent acute pancreatitis. Gastroenterology 2012;143(6):1502–9.e1.

Gallstone Pancreatitis: A Review

Daniel Cucher, MD[a], Narong Kulvatunyou, MD[b],
Donald J. Green, MD[b], Tun Jie, MD[c], Evan S. Ong, MD[c],*

KEYWORDS

- Gallstone pancreatitis • Biliary acute pancreatitis • Diagnosis • Management
- Early cholecystectomy

KEY POINTS

- Gallstone disease is the most common cause of acute pancreatitis in the Western world.
- The diagnosis of gallstone pancreatitis (GSP) is based on physical examination, with elevated serum pancreatic enzymes and imaging of biliary tract stones, in the absence of any other compelling etiology.
- The purpose of imaging in GSP is to detect the cause of the disease, identify complications, and gauge severity.
- Severity stratification is essential to ensure that appropriate supportive care and interventions are provided in moderate to severe cases while also not delaying care for patients with mild disease.
- The goal of cholecystectomy is to prevent recurrent GSP.
- Cholecystectomy within 48 hours of admission for mild GSP is safe and feasible.
- Patients with moderate to severe GSP and peripancreatic fluid collections should undergo delayed cholecystectomy to prevent serious infectious complications.
- Endoscopic retrograde cholangiopancreatography and laparoscopic explorations of the common bile duct are effective means of managing concomitant choledocholithiasis.

INTRODUCTION

Gallstone disease is the most common cause of acute pancreatitis in the Western world.[1–4] In most cases, gallstone pancreatitis (GSP) is a mild and self-limiting disease, and patients may proceed without complications to cholecystectomy to prevent future recurrence. Severe disease occurs in about 20% of cases and is associated

Disclosure: None.
[a] Department of Surgery, College of Medicine, University of Arizona, PO Box 245005, Tucson, AZ 85724, USA; [b] Division of Acute Care Surgery, Department of Surgery, Arizona Health Sciences Center, University of Arizona, 1501 North Campbell Avenue, PO Box 245063, Tucson, AZ 85724-5063, USA; [c] Division of Hepatobiliary Surgery, Department of Surgery, Arizona Health Sciences Center, University of Arizona, 1501 North Campbell Avenue, PO Box 245066, Tucson, AZ 85724, USA
* Corresponding author.
E-mail address: eong@surgery.arizona.edu

Surg Clin N Am 94 (2014) 257–280
http://dx.doi.org/10.1016/j.suc.2014.01.006
0039-6109/14/$ – see front matter © 2014 Elsevier Inc. All rights reserved.

with significant mortality, and meticulous management is critical. A thorough under-standing of the disease process, diagnosis, severity stratification, and principles of management is essential to the appropriate care of patients presenting with this com-mon disease. This article reviews these topics with a focus on surgical management, including the appropriate timing and choice of interventions.

EPIDEMIOLOGY

GSP is most common among women older than 60 years, and the number of cases reported annually is increasing worldwide, possibly as a result of the worsening obesity epidemic.[1,5] The incidence of acute pancreatitis is estimated at 40 per 100,000 people, and 40% to 50% of cases are biliary in etiology. The burden of acute pancreatitis from all causes in the United States exceeds $2.2 billion per year, with more than 300,000 inpatient admissions and 20,000 deaths annually.[6-8]

The prevalence of gallstone disease in the United States and Europe is 10% to 15%, and risk factors for GSP are similar to those for gallstone formation: age, gender, obesity, pregnancy, genetics and family history, fasting and rapid weight loss, and gallbladder stasis, among others.[9,10] Although symptomatic gallstones most commonly present as biliary colic and acute cholecystitis, the incidence of developing GSP is 3% to 8%, and symptomatic gallstones carry an annual risk for developing GSP of 0.04% to 1.5%.[11-14] Once gallstones are implicated in acute pancreatitis, the disease follows a mild course in 80% of patients, and mortality is 1% to 3%. How-ever, in 20% of patients the acute pancreatitis is severe, and mortality approaches 30%.[15]

PATHOPHYSIOLOGY

Gallstones have been detected in the feces of up to 90% of patients with GSP, sug-gesting that the causative stones usually pass into the duodenum spontaneously. The composition of these stones is primarily cholesterol, bile salts, and phospho-lipids.[16,17] When bile becomes supersaturated, overabundant cholesterol precipitates as crystals, which mix with bilirubinate and solidify to form biliary sludge, which may then aggregate to form gallstones.[18] Although gallstone migration into the common bile duct (CBD) may be a relatively common event, the stones cause GSP with far less regularity.[19]

Bernard and Prince first described the relationship of gallstones and acute pancre-atitis in 1852 and 1882, followed by Opie in 1901.[4,20-22] There is an impressive body of basic science research focused on the intricacies of this relationship and the exact mechanism by which gallstones cause acute pancreatitis. Risk factors include multi-ple small stones less than 0.5 mm in size, and a large cystic duct.[23-25] Multiple theories have been proposed to describe how gallstones set off the inflammatory response in acute pancreatitis, and a commonly accepted mechanism involves a transient obstruction of the bile or pancreatic duct by an impacted or passing stone. Alterna-tively, biliary sludge may cause cholestasis or irritate the sphincter of Oddi, causing edema and biliopancreatic outflow obstruction. This process initiates an intracellular activation of digestive enzymes within the pancreas, but the mechanism is not well un-derstood. Biliopancreatic reflux resulting from increased ductal pressure may contribute, but this theory has been challenged based on physiologic studies demon-strating a higher secretory pressure in the pancreatic duct than in the bile duct. In addi-tion, some researchers have observed that sterile bile under physiologic pressures is not harmful to the pancreas, although this has also been challenged.[26,27] Neverthe-less, increased intraductal pressure likely plays a role, because the extent of pancreatic injury is related to the duration of ampullary obstruction.[28,29] The pancreatic sphincter, exocrine secretions, mucosal barrier, and the delayed activation of trypsinogen in the duodenum are all protective elements of normal biliopancreatic physiology. In GSP, this homeostasis is altered and pancreatic injury is compounded by inflammatory cytokines, which may worsen pancreatic parenchymal damage and potentially incite the systemic inflammatory response syndrome (SIRS).

DIAGNOSIS
History and Physical Examination

Most patients presenting with GSP complain of typical symptoms of pancreatitis, and fewer may also provide a history of biliary colic. The most common complaint is sudden-onset epigastric or right upper quadrant abdominal pain that is unrelenting, and in 50% of cases radiates to the back.[10] Associated symptoms are nausea and vomiting. A strong history of alcohol abuse should raise a suspicion of alcoholic pancreatitis.[30] Physical examination usually demonstrates impressive abdominal tenderness, and patients with severe pancreatitis may also exhibit signs suggestive of an acute surgical abdomen. Immediate evaluation is necessary in patients with peritoneal findings, because the presentation of severe acute pancreatitis may mimic intestinal perforation. As with acute cholecystitis, the pain is exacerbated by eating or drinking. Peripancreatic inflammation may result in a generalized ileus, which causes hypoactive bowel sounds and anorexia. Patients with moderate to severe disease may also present with symptoms of SIRS, including pyrexia, tachycardia, and tachypnea.

Laboratory Evaluation

Laboratory analysis is indispensable in the initial diagnosis of acute pancreatitis. Upper abdominal pain with amylase or lipase 3-times the upper normal limit is diagnostic of acute pancreatitis in many cases, and the addition of cholelithiasis on imaging may sufficiently identify the cause as biliary. Lipase is highly sensitive (>90%) in acute pancreatitis and also has an advantage over amylase in specificity, because lipase is produced primarily by pancreatic acinar cells, whereas amylase is also found in saliva. The level of amylase typically increases within 2 to 12 hours after onset and normalizes within 3 to 5 days, whereas lipase peaks at 24 hours and may stay elevated for several days.[31] Of importance, the degree of elevation of amylase and lipase do not correlate with disease severity.[32] Despite this limitation, higher levels of amylase have been observed in gallstone pancreatitis in comparison with alcoholic pancreatitis.[33]

A complete blood count is likely to show leukocytosis. It has also been observed that hematocrit correlates modestly with disease severity.[15] A basic metabolic panel is useful in detecting metabolic derangements, and may also demonstrate mild hyperglycemia from decreased insulin secretion and increased glucagon.[7] Renal function is also important to consider in severe disease where organ failure is a potential sequela. In addition, patients with acute pancreatitis of any origin may present as hypovolemic, with acute kidney injury correctable by adequate volume resuscitation. Bicarbonate levels are also a marker of resuscitation and can correlate with disease severity (see Indices of Severity in the section Management).

Liver function tests are also essential in the initial evaluation. Because the underlying pathology in GSP may involve a biliary obstruction, albeit transitory in most cases, patients may present with elevated bilirubin and transaminases. Transaminases are usually only modestly elevated, unlike the high levels seen in viral hepatitis. However, in cases where a stone is impacted they may increase markedly, but normalize after resolution within days as opposed to weeks. Except in sustained choledocholithiasis, the bilirubin level is usually less than 15 mg/dL, because the obstruction is generally incomplete or intermittent.[34] In 10% of cases of GSP, liver function tests (LFTs) are normal.[35] Although poorly sensitive (48%), an alanine aminotransferase level more than 3 times the upper limit within 24 to 48 hours of onset is the best predictor of GSP, with a positive predictive value of 95%.[36] In addition, alkaline phosphatase and γ-glutamyl transpeptidase may be elevated, particularly if cholestasis persists.

Initial laboratory workup for acute pancreatitis should also include triglyceride and calcium levels for the consideration of hypertriglyceridemia and hypercalcemia as possible etiologic factors. In idiopathic pancreatitis, immunoglobulin G4 may help to identify autoimmune pancreatitis.

Imaging

The purpose of imaging in acute pancreatitis is 3-fold: to detect the cause of the disease (biliary stones, neoplasms, anatomic variances), to identify complications (fluid collections, pseudocysts, hemorrhage), and to gauge the severity of the disease (peripancreatic inflammation, pancreatic necrosis).

Ultrasonography

Every patient presenting with acute pancreatitis and no obvious alternative cause should undergo transabdominal ultrasonography to isolate gallstones as the possible cause. Ultrasonography is inexpensive, sensitive, and widely available. In the past decade the technology has evolved, allowing for portable ultrasound devices with vastly improved resolution. Ultrasonography spares patients the pain of an invasive test and the ionizing radiation of computed tomography (CT). Of note, ultrasonography studies are obtained by trained technicians and are operator dependent.

In general, the presence of cholelithiasis or sludge on ultrasonography (**Fig. 1**), in the absence of other likely causes, is sufficient evidence to diagnose GSP when combined with a typical presentation and elevated pancreatic enzymes. Ultrasonography is 95% sensitive for cholelithiasis, but in GSP, overlying bowel gas attributable to ileus may decrease sensitivity to 60% to 80%.[32,37] In the detection of choledocholithiasis, ultrasonography is reported to be 25% to 60% sensitive.[38–40] Ultrasonography is useful in detecting dilated intrahepatic and extrahepatic bile ducts, which may indicate obstruction, but is less sensitive in the context of GSP because the obstruction is

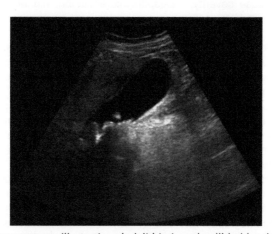

Fig. 1. Typical ultrasonogram illustrating cholelithiasis and gallbladder sludge.

acute. Ultrasonography may also fail to detect stones smaller than 4 mm, and small stones are a known risk factor for GSP.[41] Despite its limitations, ultrasonography remains the standard imaging study in the diagnosis of GSP, and in imaging terms is sufficient for most patients with mild disease.

Computed tomography

The utility of CT in GSP is to detect the anatomic changes that correlate with complications and mortality.[42] CT is often not an essential study in mild GSP, but provides more useful information in moderate to severe cases. CT is 85% to 97% sensitive and 88% to 96% specific for common duct stones when contrast is used (**Fig. 2**).[43–45] The use of CT for stratification of severity and to direct management requires appropriate timing and technique. Pancreatic necrosis is best visualized on CT at 2 to 3 days after the onset of symptoms.[46] If an initial CT was obtained during diagnosis, it may need to be repeated at 3 days if the patient's pain is severe and persistent, and laboratory values fail to trend toward normal. To optimize radiographic evaluation of the pancreas, a pancreatic protocol should be specified, comprising 2- to 3-mm cuts through the pancreas, intravenous contrast, and both pancreatic and venous phases of imaging. Oral contrast should be avoided, as it causes artifact in the duodenum that limits the study. The Balthazar CT severity index was developed to help stratify patients with acute pancreatitis (see Indices of Severity in the section Management).

Magnetic resonance imaging

To understand the role of magnetic resonance imaging (MRI), it is important to differentiate between abdominal MRI and magnetic resonance cholangiopancreatography (MRCP). Whereas abdominal MRI refers to series of images of the abdomen, MRCP describes a specific protocol designed to enhance fluid within the biliary system. It is a noninvasive imaging technique that serves diagnostic aims similar to those of endoscopic retrograde cholangiopancreatography (ERCP) with comparable accuracy. MRCP produces images that clearly define the biliary and pancreatic duct anatomy to delineate anatomic abnormalities, such as pancreas divisum, a disruption of the pancreatic duct, or filling defects that may represent tumors or gallstones. MRCP is reported to be 85% to 90% sensitive in detecting CBD stones, with 93%

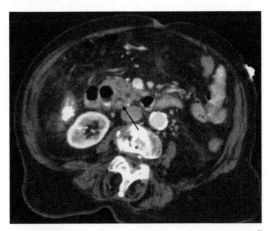

Fig. 2. Computed tomography scan demonstrating peripancreatic inflammatory changes and an obstructing stone (*arrow*) in a dilated distal common bile duct (CBD).

to 95% specificity.[47,48] An advantage of MRCP is the ability to detect stones as small as 2 mm, although this modality still has limited sensitivity for most stones smaller than 5 mm. MRCP is likely to confirm choledocholithiasis, and is commonly used by clinicians to help select patients for ERCP.

Although more expensive and less available than CT, MRI is excellent at visualizing choledocholithiasis, and is particularly useful in evaluating the complications of GSP. MRI is capable of distinguishing pancreatic fluid collections from liquefied necrosis, and is also helpful in diagnosing pancreatic hemorrhage (**Fig. 3**).[10,49] The effective use of MRI relies heavily on updated technology and experts in radiology who are facile at interpreting the data.

Endoscopic ultrasonography

Endoscopic ultrasonography (EUS) is a diagnostic modality with substantial utility in diagnosing hepatobiliary abnormalities. It is performed by advancing a specialized endoscopic ultrasound probe into the upper gastrointestinal tract. The close proximity to biliopancreatic structures allows for visualization superior to that of transabdominal ultrasonography. Diagnostically, EUS is 93% to 98% sensitive and 97% to 100% specific for choledocholithiasis.[47,50] It has a negative predictive value of 93% to 100%, and may spare patients without common duct stones unnecessary ERCP.[51–53] EUS has also been used to exclude choledocholithiasis in pregnant patients with GSP, and in patients who have contraindications to MRCP such as implanted metallic devices. The safety profile of EUS is superior to diagnostic ERCP, and its use in the pretherapeutic ERCP setting has been strongly advocated.[51]

MANAGEMENT

A central principle in determining the best course of management is predicting the severity of the disease. GSP is a disease with a broad spectrum of severity, ranging from mild pancreatic inflammation that resolves within 24 hours to fulminant infected pancreatic necrosis. Self-limited pancreatitis has a mortality of 1% to 3%, and describes 80% of cases. In 15% to 25% of patients with all forms of acute pancreatitis the disease may progress to pancreatic necrosis, and some of these patients will progress further to infected pancreatic necrosis with a mortality of 30%.[15] It is therefore essential to determine the severity of the disease early in the hospital course to ensure that appropriate supportive care and interventions are provided while also

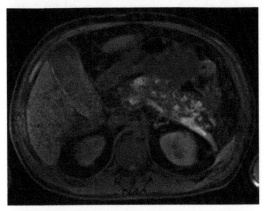

Fig. 3. Precontrast T1-weighted magnetic resonance image demonstrating severe hemorrhagic pancreatitis as extensive pancreatic enhancement.

not delaying care for patients with mild disease. Several models have been developed to assist in risk stratification and predict mortality in patients presenting with acute pancreatitis.

Indices of Severity

The Ranson score is still among the most widely used severity indices in the United States, and is calculated based on 11 parameters at the time of admission and at 48 hours. A modification of this index specifically for biliary pancreatitis uses 10 parameters, and reflects a different threshold (**Table 1**). A Ranson score of 3 or greater classifies a patient with severe disease. The positive predictive value has been reported to range from 37% to 70%, and one study demonstrated that the predictive power of the Ranson criteria is similar to good clinical judgment.[56–59]

The APACHE-II score was developed to predict mortality in patients in the intensive care unit (ICU), and has been widely applied to patients with acute pancreatitis (**Box 1**). APACHE-II at 48 hours is reported to have a higher positive predictive value than the Ranson score.[56] In addition, the APACHE-II score may be calculated at any time during admission, and an increase or decrease in this score has been found to correlate with clinical improvement or deterioration.[60,61] An APACHE-II score of 8 or greater indicates severe disease.

The bedside index for severity in acute pancreatitis (BISAP) is based on 5 parameters, 1 of which is the presence of SIRS. A score of 3 or greater is associated with higher mortality, and is reported to have accuracy similar to that of the Ranson and APACHE-II scores.[57]

The revised Atlanta Classification of acute pancreatitis (2012) is a means of categorizing the severity of acute pancreatitis based on clinical and radiographic data. It describes an early phase, which defines the early local and systemic responses to pancreatic injury, and a late phase of acute pancreatitis, which is limited to moderate and severe pancreatitis. The classification is divided into mild, moderate, and severe pancreatitis based on the presence of local and systemic complications, and the

Table 1
Ranson criteria

Parameter	All Causes of Pancreatitis	Gallstone Pancreatitis
On Admission		
Age	>55	>70
White blood cell count	>16,000	>18,000
Serum glucose (mg/dL)	>200	>220
Serum AST (IU/L)	>250	>250
Serum LDH (IU/L)	>350	>400
Within 48 h		
Base deficit (mmol/L)	>4	>5
Hematocrit decrease	>10%	>10%
BUN increase (mmol/L)	>5	>2
Pao$_2$ (mm Hg)	<60	—
Sequestration of fluids (L)	>6	>4
Serum calcium (mg/dL)	<8	<8

Abbreviations: AST, aspartate aminotransferase; BUN, blood urea nitrogen; LDH, lactate dehydrogenase; Pao$_2$, partial pressure of arterial oxygen.
Data from Refs.[14,54,55]

Box 1
APACHE-II parameters
Age
History of organ insufficiency
History of immunocompromise
Rectal temperature
Mean arterial temperature
Heart rate
Respiratory rate
Oxygenation
Serum sodium
Serum potassium
Serum creatinine
Hematocrit
Arterial pH
White blood count

presence and persistence of organ failure. The revised Atlanta Classification was proposed to facilitate communication between clinicians and to serve as an index of severity based on an understanding of the disease process.[62] This classification takes into account the difference in mortality between transient and persistent organ failure, which is an important distinction because organ failure of less than 48 hours is associated with low mortality, whereas organ failure of more than 48 hours has a predicted mortality of 36%.[63]

Balthazar and colleagues[64] introduced the CT severity index (CTSI) that grades severity of acute pancreatitis based on morphologic features including gland enlargement, peripancreatic inflammation, fluid collections, retroperitoneal gas, and degree of pancreatic necrosis, with prognostic implications (**Table 2**). Whereas clinical scores, such as Ranson, APACHE-II, and Glasgow, may have more utility in predicting

Table 2			
Balthazar CT severity index and prognosis			
Grade and CT Findings	**Score**	**Mortality (%)**	**Degree of Necrosis (%)**
A: Normal pancreas	0	3	None
B: Focal or diffuse pancreatic enlargement	1		None
C: Pancreatic/peripancreatic inflammation	2	6	<33
D: Single pancreatic/peripancreatic fluid collection	3		33–50
E: Multiple fluid collections/ retroperitoneal gas	4	17	>50

Data from Balthazar EJ, Ranson JH, Naidich DP, et al. Acute pancreatitis: prognostic value of CT. Radiology 1985;156:767–72; and Balthazar EJ, Robinson DL, Megibow AJ, et al. Acute pancreatitis: value of CT in establishing prognosis. Radiology 1990;174(2):331–6.

the course of disease early, the CTSI may be more helpful in managing patients with established disease and determining the appropriate future, as opposed to immediate, care.[65]

Other predictors of severity of interest include biochemical markers. C-reactive protein has been shown to correlate with severe disease, and has been advocated as a useful single biochemical marker.[66] Other potential serum levels such as those of interleukin-6 and macrophage migration inhibitory factor have been evaluated, and further investigation may help incorporate these parameters into novel indices to predict clinical severity.

There are no perfect or universally accepted scoring methods to predict the severity of GSP, particularly early in the disease when the clinician must decide between ICU monitoring or whether to proceed with cholecystectomy. Among all patients with predicted mild pancreatitis, as many as 15% progress to severe disease.[57,66] It is therefore incumbent on clinicians who choose to use these indices to do so selectively in combination with clinical acumen to determine the best course of management. Regardless of the method, it serves the clinician and patient well to stratify GSP as mild, moderate, or severe.

Initial Management

The general guidelines in managing acute pancreatitis apply equally to GSP. The basis of supportive care is to provide pain control, correct metabolic derangements, aggressively resuscitate with intravenous fluids, and prevent hypoxemia. Patients with an ileus may require a nasogastric tube for decompression. Those with severe disease are best served by a multidisciplinary team approach in the ICU, including gastroenterologists with ERCP capabilities, surgeons comfortable with hepatobiliary surgery, physicians with experience in critical care, and interventional radiologists. Patients with mild disease may require only adequate hydration and pain control before early cholecystectomy.

Nutrition

Patients admitted with acute pancreatitis are typically kept nil by mouth initially. However, those with mild disease benefit from a shorter length of stay in hospital with immediate oral feeding.[67] GSP patients are no exception, unless early feeding interferes with early cholecystectomy. Patients with severe disease have been shown to benefit from enteral feeding within 48 hours, without exacerbation of illness. Total parenteral nutrition is less safe, less effective, and more expensive, and should be reserved for patients who cannot tolerate enteral feeding. Jejunal feeding is preferred, but gastric feeding has also been shown to be safe.[68]

Antibiotics

Appropriate broad-spectrum antibiotics are indicated pending a workup for sepsis and in infected pancreatic necrosis. In sterile pancreatic necrosis, the use of prophylactic antibiotics is controversial. There are several large studies that disagree as to whether prophylactic antibiotics impart a benefit in pancreatic sepsis and mortality, and recent literature does not recommend antibiotic use in sterile necrosis.[69–71] It has been shown that prolonged use of broad-spectrum antibiotics increases the risk of developing a fungal infection, so judicious use is imperative.[15]

Interventions

Unlike alcoholic acute pancreatitis, whereby the management is primarily to provide supportive care, the management of GSP includes several modalities that are specific to the disease's underlying cause. These measures include cholecystectomy, exploration of the CBD, ERCP with sphincterotomy, and specific interventional radiology procedures. The goals of these procedures range from mitigating disease severity to preventing the recurrence of GSP.

Cholecystectomy

The goal of cholecystectomy is to prevent recurrence of GSP by removing the source of secondary gallstones. Although 1% to 2% of patients may recur even after cholecystectomy, the rate of recurrence in untreated patients with GSP is up to two-thirds of patients within 3 months of index presentation.[72–75] Recurrent GSP may be graver than the initial presentation, as between 4% and 50% of cases are reported as severe, and mortality and morbidity is reported in up to 10% and 40%, respectively.[13,76,77]

Stratifying patients as mild, moderate, or severe has a profound impact on surgical management. Historically, the recommendation was to delay cholecystectomy for 6 to 8 weeks after an attack of acute pancreatitis to allow the inflammation to subside.[78] High readmission rates for patients waiting for cholecystectomy lead to new guidelines. Although several early studies showed lower morbidity and mortality in delayed operations, the data from some of these studies is interpreted irrespective of patient stratification.[11,78] Early cholecystectomy in GSP has now been advocated in mild disease for several decades, but what defines early timing, and the challenge of stratifying patients, have led to a great deal of discussion.

Published recommendations and references to early cholecystectomy in mild pancreatitis range from within 48 hours to within 2 to 4 weeks of presentation.[11,58,72,79,80] Most surgical literature, however, advocates cholecystectomy during the same hospital admission. Whereas many surgeons wait for resolution of abdominal pain and normalization of pancreatic enzymes, Aboulian and colleagues[81] found that laparoscopic cholecystectomy performed within 48 hours of admission for mild pancreatitis, regardless of pain or laboratory values, results in a shorter length of stay in hospital without compromising patient safety or unjustifiably challenging the surgeon's technical ability.[82] Several other studies support performing laparoscopic cholecystectomy within 48 hours of admission in mild cases, and many others advocate early cholecystectomy within the same hospital admission.[83,84] It is common practice for surgeons to wait for laboratory values to normalize. However, there are data demonstrating a shorter length of stay in hospital without increased morbidity when surgery is undertaken as laboratory values begin to trend toward normal.[85] Waiting for complete normalization of pancreatic enzymes may cause a delay in care and an increased length of stay.

There are compelling reasons to recommend cholecystectomy following idiopathic acute pancreatitis, as many patients may have undocumented biliary sludge or microlithiasis. This view is supported by evidence that biliary sludge and microlithiasis are also responsible for the pathologic process cited in GSP.[86,87] Thus, for the purposes of this review, all acute pancreatitis caused by gallstones, microlithiasis, and biliary sludge is termed GSP.

Despite the compelling data to support early cholecystectomy, compliance is poor and many patients are discharged for interval cholecystectomy. In the Western world, the rate of index cholecystectomy for appropriate surgical candidates is between 10% and 60%.[88–94] Factors associated with patients who do not undergo early cholecystectomy in the United States include old age, black race, admission to a nonsurgical service, comorbid conditions, and lack of a surgical consultation.[94] Access to appropriate medical care in certain populations may play a role.[95] Surveys of surgeons who do not perform early cholecystectomy cite reasons such as busy operating rooms, budgetary concerns, lack of resources, and concern for a more difficult dissection.[90,96] Contrary to these concerns, the feasibility of cholecystectomy during index admission, and at most within 2 weeks, has been studied and found to be cost neutral and practical.[97] In addition, the surgeons involved in one cohort study reported the dissection more difficult during delayed, as opposed to early, laparoscopic cholecystectomy.[98] Of note is a study with atypical findings from a busy public hospital. Clarke and colleagues[99] reported that performing index cholecystectomies put an undue strain on hospital resources, and the length of stay was in fact higher in inpatients waiting for index cholecystectomy than in patients directed toward discharge and elective surgical admission. The morbidity was the same in both groups, but 6.5% of patients in the interval laparoscopic cholecystectomy group had unplanned readmissions for mild recurrent pancreatitis.

Severe GSP is associated with significantly higher morbidity and mortality, and the disease process is such that the surgical management follows a more conservative course. Much of the morbidity and mortality reported in early studies that cautioned against early cholecystectomy is attributable to patients with severe forms of GSP. In one such study, Ranson[14] excluded patients with mild pancreatic edema and only considered patients who underwent surgery with pancreatic inflammation in addition to fat necrosis or pancreatic hemorrhage, and reported high mortality. Other studies have reported similar findings whereby high rates of morbidity and mortality in patients undergoing early cholecystectomy were attributable to those patients with moderate and severe disease.[100]

Once a patient is stratified as having moderate or severe GSP, the initial management is supportive care and management of complications. Follow-up care includes interval cholecystectomy, delayed at least 3 weeks after resolution, if clinical circumstances permit. Early cholecystectomy is contraindicated in moderate and severe GSP, and is associated with increased infectious complications and sepsis.[101]

Peripancreatic fluid collections are well recognized on CT and, when correlated to GSP severity, should dramatically influence management.[64,102] Nealon and colleagues[103] reported that among patients with moderate to severe GSP who underwent early cholecystectomy, regardless of CT-proven peripancreatic fluid collections, 63% required reoperation and 44% had postoperative complications. Most of the reoperations were for definitive management of pseudocysts, and the infectious complications were presumably a result of pseudocysts that were sterile but became infected at the time of early cholecystectomy. These investigators thus advocate delaying cholecystectomy until it is possible to operatively manage the gallbladder and pseudocysts simultaneously. By virtue of exclusion, almost all investigators advocating early cholecystectomy specify patients with mild disease, and caution against operating too early on those with moderate or severe GSP.

Pseudocysts occur in acute pancreatitis as a result of disruption of the pancreatic duct and extravasated pancreatic excretory fluid. A fluid collection may or may not communicate with the pancreatic duct, and a fibrous wall ultimately forms around the collection (**Fig. 4**). Pseudocysts may be adequately diagnosed with contrast CT or MRI. A general rule is to wait 6 weeks before intervening to allow the pseudocyst wall to mature.[103,104] Exceptions to this are cases of infected or symptomatic pseudocysts, when earlier intervention may be indicated. However, there are no universally accepted guidelines for post-GSP pseudocyst management, and a complete discussion of pseudocyst management is beyond the scope of this article. In general, the management is conservative because many of these pseudocysts will resolve spontaneously, especially if there is no patency between the pseudocyst and the pancreatic duct. Because GSP patients with peripancreatic fluid collections or

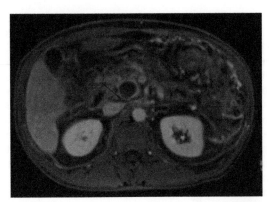

Fig. 4. Well-circumscribed pseudocyst in the pancreatic head (*arrow*) causing mechanical obstruction of the CBD.

pseudocysts are often discharged for interval cholecystectomy, appropriate follow-up is critical.

Interventional management of pseudocysts with mature walls most commonly includes gastric or proximal enteric drainage by open or endoscopic techniques. Several studies have demonstrated comparable pseudocyst resolution rates in both techniques, and the endoscopic method is favored in simple pseudocysts accessible from the gastric or duodenal lumens.[105–110] Surgical internal drainage may be indicated in complex pseudocysts and in those not readily accessible endoscopically. The use of EUS may enhance visualization and make otherwise inaccessible pseudocysts manageable with endoscopic drainage.[105,111] Percutaneous drainage has a role in infected pseudocysts and in symptomatic cases where endoscopic and surgical options are limited. However, this technique risks creating a controlled pancreaticocutaneous fistula, which may persist for an extended period.[108,112]

Cholecystostomy
In high-risk patients it may be necessary to resort to other means of decompressing the biliary system. Elderly, comorbid, and/or severely ill patients may be deemed unsuitable candidates for either surgery or ERCP, yet still require emergent management of obstructing common duct stones causing biliary sepsis or aggravating acute pancreatitis. In these patients, interventional radiologists may perform percutaneous cholecystostomy, often through the use of ultrasonography and fluoroscopy. This procedure uses the Seldinger technique, and is a minimally invasive method of decompressing the biliary system. However, patients who require this degree of interventional minimalism tend to have a poor prognosis, and 30-day mortality has been reported to be as high as 15.4% in patients undergoing percutaneous cholecystostomy for acute cholecystitis.[113]

Intraoperative cholangiography
The role of intraoperative cholangiography (IOC) in GSP is controversial, and its use varies widely among surgeons.[114] Some surgeons perform IOC routinely, whereas others do so only when there is a high suspicion for a common duct stone (**Fig. 5**). Although IOC is reported to be 94% specific and 98% sensitive for biliary stones, one study has demonstrated that air bubbles in the ducts can mimic stones in appearance, and routine use may be associated with a substantial false-positive rate.[115] Many surgeons will perform an IOC if there is indirect evidence of choledocholithiasis, such as an obstructive pattern on LFTs or a relatively large common duct on

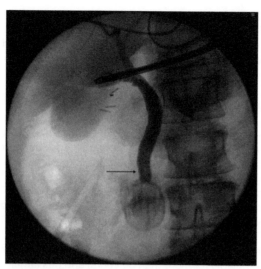

Fig. 5. Intraoperative cholangiogram demonstrating an irregular lucency in the CBD (*arrow*), representing a stone.

ultrasonography. The diagnosis of GSP should be considered poor indirect evidence of a duct stone, as most stones causing acute pancreatitis pass into the duodenum spontaneously. Nevertheless, the diagnosis of GSP is associated with an increased use of IOC.[114] Johnson and Walsh[116] found that patients with GSP who undergo IOC during cholecystectomy were more likely to have postoperative ERCP or CBD exploration during surgery, but without influencing the outcome of the pancreatitis. These findings are supported in the literature, as a recent systematic review of IOC use did not identify sufficient evidence to demonstrate a benefit.[117] This issue is controversial and requires further investigation.

Laparoscopic exploration of common bile duct

Gallstones passing into the common duct are the offending agents in GSP, and although most pass spontaneously into the duodenum without incident, 7% to 28% of the time stones may remain in the common duct.[21,118–121] Given sufficient evidence for choledocholithiasis coexistent with mild pancreatitis, it is safe and effective to remove the stone at the time of cholecystectomy by laparoscopic CBD exploration (LCBDE).[122] Impacted stones causing cholangitis or aggravating severe GSP are generally removed emergently by ERCP, discussed in the next section.

LCBDE has been used for more than 2 decades, and the technology available to safely and effectively perform the procedure has evolved substantially, helping to make it as effective as ERCP in some hands.[123–125] However, owing to the risks involved in manipulating the CBD and the exceptional level of skill required, most surgeons do not perform this procedure. LCBDE is most commonly performed by surgeons with additional hepatobiliary or laparoscopic training.

Transcystic and transcholedochal approaches are possible laparoscopically. The transcystic method is the favored approach among most surgeons performing LCBDE, and is most suitable for small stones in a small common duct. Choledochotomy is reported to be better for larger, multiple stones in a dilated common duct. Although technically more challenging, LCDBE by choledochotomy may be a more definitive approach.[116,123,126] Refer to the article by Hardacre and colleagues, elsewhere in this issue for a detailed description of bile duct exploration.

The success of stone clearance by LCBDE has been reported in several studies to be equivalent to ERCP, with decreased morbidity, lower cost, and shorter length of stay.[127–131] When LCBDE is not an option and patients are either diagnosed with or suspected of having common duct stones, ERCP is favored, in most cases, over open CBD exploration.

Endoscopic retrograde cholangiopancreatography

ERCP refers to the contrast imaging of the biliary and pancreatic ducts (cholangiopancreatography) using a side-viewing endoscope and fluoroscopy. When the ampulla of Vater is accessed in this manner and the CBD cannulated with a guide wire, an endoscopist may then perform endoscopic sphincterotomy or balloon dilatation of the biliary sphincter followed by extraction of stones using a balloon or basket for stones that do not pass spontaneously (**Fig. 6**). For particularly large stones, there are devices available to perform intraluminal lithotripsy to assist in extraction. For diagnostic purposes, the sensitivity of ERCP for choledocholithiasis is 90% to 97%, with 95% to 100% specificity.[132] This diagnostic performance is similar to that of MRCP, which is noninvasive. The success rate of ERCP in extracting stones is around 95%.

ERCP has been available for more than 30 years, and has largely replaced surgical CBD exploration in cases of isolated choledocholithiasis. The role of ERCP in GSP has been discussed extensively, and it is widely accepted that in mild cases of GSP without evidence of biliary obstruction or cholestasis there is no utility for ERCP for diagnostic or therapeutic purposes.[133–135] Most patients presenting with transiently elevated pancreatic enzymes without a sustained elevation of bilirubin may proceed to early cholecystectomy without either preoperative or postoperative ERCP. Although earlier reports advocated ERCP within 24 hours for all-comers with GSP, this strategy has been formidably challenged.[136] There is now widely accepted evidence that ERCP in patients with GSP, but without cholestasis or cholangitis, confers no benefit in terms of complications or mortality.[137,138]

In patients with severe GSP and evidence of choledocholithiasis, including increasing LFTs, persistently elevated bilirubin, persistent pain, or visualization on

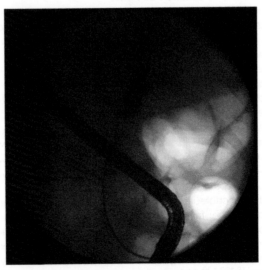

Fig. 6. Fluoroscopic image of endoscopic retrograde cholangiopancreatography during balloon extraction of a large stone.

MRCP, performing ERCP within 72 hours decreases the rate of sepsis, mortality, and complications, including pancreatic necrosis.[134,139–142] In all patients with GSP, additional evidence of common duct stones warranting intervention includes bile-free gastric aspirate and an increasing level of serial bilirubin. Performing ERCP within 48 hours in these patients may decrease morbidity.[143] Acute cholangitis may complicate GSP in up to 10% of cases, and early ERCP is indicated to decompress the biliary system in these patients.[58]

ERCP serves a role in mild GSP in patients who are unfit or unwilling to undergo surgery. Although it is well established that patients with GSP have a high rate of recurrence without cholecystectomy, ERCP with sphincterotomy is protective against recurrence of acute pancreatitis. However, because the gallbladder is left in situ, the rates of acute cholecystitis and biliary colic remain elevated.[2,72,144,145] ERCP is thus indicated in patients with GSP who cannot undergo cholecystectomy, or will experience a prolonged delay before cholecystectomy.

Complications of ERCP include pancreatitis, hemorrhage, perforation, cholangitis, and stenosis of the sphincter of Oddi.[127,146] Although an increased risk of cholangiocarcinoma after ERCP has been discussed in the literature, there is currently insufficient evidence to confirm this concern.

Special patient populations

As the incidence of GSP increases in the adult population, a similar increase in gallstone disease is being observed in the pediatric population. The recommendation for index-admission cholecystectomy prevails in children with mild GSP, as in adults.[147,148]

Pregnancy is a risk factor for gallstone formation, and as many as one-third of pregnant patients presenting with biliary complaints require surgical intervention.[149–151] Gallstone disease underlies 65% to 70% of cases of acute pancreatitis occurring during pregnancy.[152] Previous recommendations warned against performing laparoscopy on pregnant patients during the first trimester, and cited limitations of intra-abdominal visualization caused by the third-trimester uterus. Thus pregnant patients presenting during the first and third trimester underwent delayed cholecystectomy. However, guidelines within the last decade endorsed by the Society of American Gastrointestinal and Endoscopic Surgeons cite substantial evidence in support of safely performing laparoscopic procedures during any trimester of pregnancy. The recommendations additionally state that the indications for laparoscopic cholecystectomy for biliary disease should also be honored in pregnancy.[153] Delaying cholecystectomy in pregnant patients carries a formidable risk of recurrent GSP, for both the patient and the fetus, which likely outweighs the poorly quantified risk of spontaneous abortion. EUS or MRCP without gadolinium contrast may be safely used in pregnancy to select pregnant patients for further intervention, including ERCP or LCBDE, if choledocholithiasis is suspected or confirmed.

It is estimated that 30% of patients older than 70 years have gallstones, and the incidence of choledocholithiasis in the elderly population is up to 20%.[154,155] Because older patients are more likely to have gallstones and bile ducts of increased diameter, this population also has a higher incidence of GSP.[156] Several studies demonstrate the safety of performing laparoscopic cholecystectomy in elderly patients, yet less than 57% of older patients undergo index cholecystectomy, and it is estimated that compliance can be improved to greater than 70% while still maintaining appropriate patient selection.[94,157,158] Recurrent GSP should be prevented in the young and elderly populations with index cholecystectomy in mild GSP, when clinically feasible.

SUMMARY

GSP is a disease with a wide spectrum of severity. Diagnosis and management have evolved over the past several decades with the advent of new and improved technology. Advancements in imaging techniques have limited the need for invasive diagnostic procedures in many cases, and diverse therapeutic options are becoming more widely available. The paradigm continues to shift toward earlier operation in mild cases, with more judicious interventions in severe disease. Risk stratification is essential to provide the best possible care for all patients, and good clinical judgment is paramount in selecting the most pertinent invasive and diagnostic procedures at the most appropriate time.

REFERENCES

1. Whitcomb DC. Acute pancreatitis. N Engl J Med 2006;354(20):2142–50.
2. Ito K, Ito H, Whang EE. Timing of cholecystectomy for biliary pancreatitis: do the data support current guidelines? J Gastrointest Surg 2008;12(12):2164–70.
3. Frossart JL, Steer ML, Pastor CM. Acute pancreatitis. Lancet 2008;372(9607):143–52.
4. Baillie J. Treatment of acute biliary pancreatitis. N Engl J Med 1997;336(4):286–7.
5. Yadav D, Lowenfels AB. Trends in the epidemiology of the first attack of acute pancreatitis: a systematic review. Pancreas 2006;33(4):323–30.
6. Steinberg W, Tenner S. Acute pancreatitis. N Engl J Med 1994;330(17):1198–210.
7. Cappell MS. Acute pancreatitis: etiology, clinical presentation, diagnosis, and therapy. Med Clin North Am 2008;92(4):889–923.
8. Fagenholz PJ, Fernandez-del CC, Harris NS, et al. Direct medical costs of acute pancreatitis hospitalizations in the United States. Pancreas 2007;35:302–7.
9. Sandler RS, Ecerhart JE, Donowitz M, et al. The burden of selective digestive diseases in the United States. Gastroenterol 2002;122:1500–11.
10. Attasaranya S, Fogel EL, Lehman GA. Choledocholithiasis, ascending cholangitis, and gallstone pancreatitis. Med Clin North Am 2008;92(4):925–60.
11. Uhl W, Müller CA, Krähenbühl L, et al. Acute gallstone pancreatitis: timing of laparoscopic cholecystectomy in mild and severe disease. Surg Endosc 1999;13(11):1070–6.
12. Armstrong CP, Taylor TV, Torrance HB. Effects of bile, infection, and pressure on pancreatic duct integrity. Br J Surg 1985;72:792–5.
13. Moreau JA, Zinsmeister AR, Melton LJ 3rd, et al. Gallstone pancreatitis and the effect of cholecystectomy: a population based cohort study. Mayo Clin Proc 1988;63:466–73.
14. Ranson JH. The timing of biliary surgery in acute pancreatitis. Ann Surg 1979;189:654–63.
15. Banks PA, Freeman ML. Practice guidelines in acute pancreatitis. Am J Gastroenterol 2006;101(10):2379–400.
16. Diehl AK. Epidemiology and natural history of gallstone disease. Gastroenterol Clin North Am 1991;20:11–9.
17. Friedman GD. Natural history of asymptomatic and symptomatic gallstones. Am J Surg 1993;165:399–404.
18. Portincases P, Moschetta A, Palasciano G. Cholesterol gallstone disease. Lancet 2006;368:230–9.

19. Ko CE, Lee SP. Epidemiology and natural history of common bile duct stones and prediction of diseases. Gastrointest Endosc 2002;56(Suppl 6):S165–9.

20. Prince M. Pancreatic apoplexy with a report of two cases. Boston Med Surg J 1882;107:28–32.

21. Raraty MG, Finch M, Neoptolemos JP. Acute cholangitis and pancreatitis secondary to common duct stones: management update. World J Surg 1998; 22(11):1155–61.

22. Opie EL. The aetiology of acute haemorrhagic pancreatitis. Bull Johns Hopkins Hosp 1901;12:182.

23. Venneman NG, Buskens E, Besselink MG, et al. Small gallstones are associated with increased risk of acute pancreatitis: potential benefits of prophylactic cholecystectomy? Am J Gastroenterol 2005;100:2540–50.

24. Sugiyama M, Atomi Y. Risk factors for acute biliary pancreatitis. Gastrointest Endosc 2004;60:210–2.

25. Diehl AK, Holleman DR Jr, Chapman JB, et al. Gallstone size and risk of pancreatitis. Arch Intern Med 1997;157:1674–8.

26. Lerch M, Aghdassi A. The role of bile acids in gallstone-induced pancreatitis. Gastroenterol 2010;138(2):426–9.

27. Muili KA, Wang D, Orabi AI, et al. Bile acids induce pancreatic acinar cell injury and pancreatitis by activating calcineurin. J Biol Chem 2012;288(1):570–80.

28. Acosta JM, Pellegrini CA, Skinner DB. Etiology and pathogenesis of acute biliary pancreatitis. Surgery 1980;88:118–25.

29. Hirano T, Manabe T. A possible mechanism for gallstone pancreatitis: repeated short-term pancreaticobiliary duct obstruction with exocrine stimulation in rats. Proc Soc Exp Biol Med 1993;202:246–52.

30. Yadav D, Papachristou GI, Whitcomb DC. Alcohol-associated pancreatitis. Gastroenterol Clin North Am 2007;36(2):219–38.

31. Zieve L. Clinical value of determinations of various pancreatic enzymes in serum. Gastroenterol 1964;46:62–7.

32. Wang SS, Lin XZ, Tsai YT, et al. Clinical significance of ultrasonography, computed tomography, and biochemical tests in the rapid diagnosis of gallstone-related pancreatitis: a prospective study. Pancreas 1988;3:153–8.

33. Fogel EL, Sherman S. Acute biliary pancreatitis: when should the endoscopist intervene? Gastroenterol 2003;125:229–35.

34. Nathwani RA, Kumar SR, Reynolds TB, et al. Marked elevation in serum transaminases: an atypical presentation of choledocholithiasis. Am J Gastroenterol 2005;100:295–8.

35. Dholakia K, Pitchumoni CS, Agarwal N. How often are liver function tests normal in acute biliary pancreatitis? J Clin Gastroenterol 2004;38:81–3.

36. Tenner S, Dubner H, Steinberg W. Predicting gallstone pancreatitis with laboratory parameters: a meta-analysis. Am J Gastroenterol 1994;89:1863–6.

37. Neoptolemos JP, Hall AW, Finlay DF, et al. The urgent diagnosis of gallstones in acute pancreatitis: a prospective study of three methods. Br J Surg 1984;71:230–3.

38. Sugiyama M, Atomi Y. Endoscopic ultrasonography for diagnosing choledocholithiasis: a prospective comparative study with ultrasonography and computed tomography. Gastrointest Endosc 1997;45:143–6.

39. Amouyal P, Amouyal G, Levy P, et al. Diagnosis of choledocholithiasis by endoscopic ultrasonography. Gastroenterol 1994;106:1062–7.

40. O'Connor HJ, Hamilton I, Ellis WR, et al. Ultrasound detection of choledocholithiasis: prospective comparison with ERCP in the postcholecystectomy patient. Gastrointest Radiol 1986;11(2):161–4.

41. Thorboll J, Vilmann P, Jacobsen B, et al. Endoscopic ultrasonography in detection of cholelithiasis in patients with biliary pain and negative transabdominal ultrasonography. Scand J Gastroenterol 2004;39:267–9.
42. Balthazar EJ, Ranson JH, Naidich DP, et al. Acute pancreatitis: prognostic value of CT. Radiology 1985;156:767–72.
43. Polkowski M, Palucki J, Regula J, et al. Helical computed tomographic cholangiography versus endosonography for suspected bile duct stones: a prospective blinded study in non-jaundiced patients. Gut 1999;45:744–9.
44. Cabada Giadas T, Sarria Octavio de Toledo L, Martinez-Berganza Asensio MT, et al. Helical CT cholangiography in the evaluation of the biliary tract: application to the diagnosis of choledocholithiasis. Abdom Imaging 2002;27:61–70.
45. Kim HJ, Park DI, Park JH, et al. Multidetector computed tomography cholangiography with multiplanar reformation for the assessment of patients with biliary obstruction. J Gastroenterol Hepatol 2007;22:400–5.
46. Balthazar EJ. Acute pancreatitis: assessment of severity with clinical and CT evaluation. Radiology 2002;223:603–13.
47. Verma D, Kapadia A, Eisen GM, et al. EUS vs MRCP for detection of choledocholithiasis. Gastrointest Endosc 2006;64:248–54.
48. McMahon CJ. The relative roles of magnetic resonance cholangiopancreatography (MRCP) and endoscopic ultrasound in diagnosis of common bile duct calculi: a critically appraised topic. Abdom Imaging 2008;33(1):6–9.
49. Hirota M, Kimura Y, Ishiko T, et al. Visualization of the heterogeneous internal structure of so-called "pancreatic necrosis" by magnetic resonance imaging in acute necrotizing pancreatitis. Pancreas 2002;25:63–7.
50. Buscarini E, Tansini P, Vallisa D, et al. EUS for suspected choledocholithiasis: do benefits outweigh costs? A prospective, controlled study. Gastrointest Endosc 2003;57:510–8.
51. De Lisi S, Leandro G, Buscarini E. Endoscopic ultrasonography versus endoscopic retrograde cholangiopancreatography in acute biliary pancreatitis. Eur J Gastroenterol Hepatol 2011;23(5):367–74.
52. Amouyal P, Palazzo L, Amouyal G, et al. Endosonography: promising method for diagnosis of extrahepatic cholestasis. Lancet 1989;2:1195–8.
53. Norton SA, Alderson D. Prospective comparison of endoscopic ultrasonography and endoscopic retrograde cholangiopancreatography in the detection of bile duct stones. Br J Surg 1997;84:1366–9.
54. Ranson JH, Rifkind KM, Roses DF. Prognostic signs and the role of operative management in acute pancreatitis. Surg Gynecol Obstet 1974;139:69–81.
55. Ranson JH. Etiologic and prognostic factors in human acute pancreatitis: a review. Am J Gastroenterol 1982;77:633–8.
56. Yeung YP, Kit Lam BY, Chun Yip AW. APACHE system is better than Ranson system in the prediction of severity of acute pancreatitis. Hepatobiliary Pancreat Dis Int 2006;5(2):294–9.
57. Papachristou GI, Muddana V, Yadav D, et al. Comparison of BISAP, Ranson's, APACHE-II, and CTSI scores in predicting organ failure, complications, and mortality in acute pancreatitis. Am J Gastroenterol 2009;105(2):435–41.
58. Forsmark CE, Baillie J. AGA Institute technical review on acute pancreatitis. Gastroenterol 2007;132(5):2022–44.
59. De Bernardinis M, Violi V, Roncoroni L, et al. Discriminant power and information content of Ranson's prognostic signs in acute pancreatitis: a meta-analytic study. Crit Care Med 1999;27(10):2272–83.

60. Wilson C, Heath DI, Imrie CW. Prediction of outcome in acute pancreatitis: a comparative study of APACHE-II, clinical assessment and multiple factor scoring systems. Br J Surg 1990;77:1260–4.
61. Khan AA, Parekh D, Cho Y, et al. Improved prediction of outcome in patients with severe acute pancreatitis by the APACHE II score at 48 hours after hospital admission compared with APACHE II score at admission. Arch Surg 2002;137: 1136–40.
62. Banks PA, Bollen TL, Dervenis C, et al. Classification of acute pancreatitis— 2012: revision of the Atlanta classification and definitions by international consensus. Gut 2013;62(1):102–11.
63. Johnson CD, Abu-Hilal M. Persistent organ failure during the first week as a marker of fatal outcome in acute pancreatitis. Gut 2004;53:1340–4.
64. Balthazar EJ, Robinson DL, Megibow AJ, et al. Acute pancreatitis: value of CT in establishing prognosis. Radiology 1990;174(2):331–6.
65. Alhajeri A, Erwin S. Acute pancreatitis: value and impact of CT severity index. Abdom Imaging 2007;33(1):18–20.
66. Dambrauskas Z, Gulbinas A, Pundzius J, et al. Value of the different prognostic systems and biological markers for predicting severity and progression of acute pancreatitis. Scand J Gastroenterol 2010;45(7–8):959–70.
67. Eckerwall GE, Tingstedt BB, Bergenzaun PE, et al. Immediate oral feeding in patients with mild acute pancreatitis is safe and may accelerate recovery—a randomized clinical study. Clin Nutr 2007;26(6):758–63.
68. Eatock FC, Chong P, Menezes N, et al. A randomized study of early nasogastric versus nasojejunal feeding in severe acute pancreatitis. Am J Gastroenterol 2005;100:432–9.
69. Bassi C, Larvin M, Villatoro E. Antibiotic therapy for prophylaxis against infection of pancreatic necrosis in acute pancreatitis. Cochrane Database Syst Rev 2003;(4):CD002941.
70. Isenmann R, Runzi M, Kron M, et al. Prophylactic antibiotic treatment in patients with predicted severe acute pancreatitis: a placebo-controlled, double-blind trial. Gastroenterol 2004;126:997–1004.
71. Dellinger EP, Tellado JM, Soto NE, et al. Early antibiotic treatment for severe acute necrotizing pancreatitis: a randomized, double-blind, placebo-controlled study. Ann Surg 2007;245:674–83.
72. Van Baal MC, Besselink MG, Bakker OJ, et al. Timing of cholecystectomy after mild biliary pancreatitis: a systematic review. Ann Surg 2012;255(5):860–6.
73. Cameron DR, Goodman AJ. Delayed cholecystectomy for gallstone pancrea- titis: re-admissions and outcomes. Ann R Coll Surg Engl 2004;86:358–62.
74. Nebiker CA, Frey DM, Hamel CT, et al. Early versus delayed cholecystectomy in patients with biliary acute pancreatitis. Surg 2009;145:260–4.
75. Delhaye M, Matos C, Deviere J. Endoscopic technique for the management of pancreatitis and its complications. Best Pract Res Clin Gastroenterol 2004;18: 155–81.
76. Lankisch PG, Bruns A, Doobe C, et al. The second attack of acute pancreatitis is not harmless. Pancreas 2008;36:207–8.
77. Hernandez V, Pascual I, Almela P, et al. Recurrence of acute gallstone pancre- atitis and relationship with cholecystectomy or endoscopic sphincterotomy. Am J Gastroenterol 2004;99:2417–23.
78. Pellegrini CA. Surgery for gallstone pancreatitis. Am J Surg 1993;165(4):515–8.
79. Working Party of the British Society of Gastroenterology, Association of Sur- geons of Great Britain and Ireland, Pancreatic Society of Great Britain and

Ireland, et al. UK guidelines for the management of acute pancreatitis. Gut 2005;54(Suppl 3):iii1–9.

80. El-Dhuwaib Y, Deakin M, David G, et al. Definitive management of gallstone pancreatitis in England. Ann R Coll Surg Engl 2012;94(6):402–6.

81. Aboulian A, Chan T, Yaghoubian A, et al. Early cholecystectomy safely decreases hospital stay in patients with mild gallstone pancreatitis. Ann Surg 2010;251(4):615–9.

82. Larson SD, Nealon WH, Evers BM. Management of gallstone pancreatitis. Adv Surg 2006;40:265–84.

83. De Virgilio C. Early laparoscopic cholecystectomy for mild gallstone pancreatitis: time for a paradigm shift. Arch Surg 2012;147(11):1031–5.

84. Rosing DK, de Virgilio C, Yaghoubian A, et al. Early cholecystectomy for mild to moderate gallstone pancreatitis shortens hospital stay. J Am Coll Surg 2007; 205(6):762–6.

85. Taylor E, Wong C. The optimal timing of laparoscopic cholecystectomy in mild gallstone pancreatitis. Am Surg 2004;70(11):971–5.

86. Lee SP, Nicholls JF, Park HZ. Biliary sludge as a cause of acute pancreatitis. N Engl J Med 1992;326:589–93.

87. Ros E, Navarro S, Bru C, et al. Occult microlithiasis in 'idiopathic' acute pancreatitis: prevention of relapses by cholecystectomy or ursodeoxycholic acid therapy. Gastroenterol 1991;101(6):1701–9.

88. Nguyen GC, Tuskey A, Jagannath SB. Racial disparities in cholecystectomy rates during hospitalizations for acute gallstone pancreatitis: a national survey. Am J Gastroenterol 2008;103:2301–7.

89. Sandzen B, Rosenmuller M, Haapamaki MM, et al. First attack of acute pancreatitis in Sweden 1988-2003: incidence, aetiological classification, procedures and mortality—a register study. BMC Gastroenterol 2009;9:18.

90. Campbell EJ, Montgomery DA, Mackay CJ. A national survey of current surgical treatment of acute gallstone disease. Surg Laparosc Endosc Percutan Tech 2008;18:242–7.

91. Senapati PS, Bhattarcharya D, Harinath G, et al. A survey of the timing and approach to the surgical management of cholelithiasis in patients with acute biliary pancreatitis and acute cholecystitis in the UK. Ann R Coll Surg Engl 2003;85:306–12.

92. Chiang DT, Thompson G. Management of acute gallstone pancreatitis: so the story continues. ANZ J Surg 2008;78(1–2):52–4.

93. Sanjay P, Yeeting S, Whigham C, et al. Management guidelines for gallstone pancreatitis. Are the targets achievable? JOP 2009;10(1):43–7.

94. Trust MD, Sheffield KM, Boyd CA, et al. Gallstone pancreatitis in older patients: are we operating enough? Surg 2011;150(3):515–25.

95. Everhart JE. Gallstones and ethnicity in the Americas. J Assoc Acad Minor Phys 2001;12(3):137–43.

96. Lankisch PG, Weber-Dany B, Lerch MM. Clinical perspectives in pancreatology: compliance with acute pancreatitis guidelines in Germany. Pancreatology 2005; 5:591–3.

97. Monkhouse SJ, Court EL, Dash I, et al. Two-week target for laparoscopic cholecystectomy following gallstone pancreatitis is achievable and cost neutral. Br J Surg 2009;96(7):751–5.

98. Sinha R. Early laparoscopic cholecystectomy in acute biliary pancreatitis: the optimal choice? HPB (Oxford) 2008;10(5):332–5.

99. Clarke T, Sohn H, Kelso R, et al. Planned early discharge-elective surgical readmission pathway for patients with gallstone pancreatitis. Arch Surg 2008; 143(9):901.

100. Kelly TR, Wagner DS. Gallstone pancreatitis: a prospective randomized trial of the timing of surgery. Surg 1988;104:600–3.

101. Delorio AV Jr, Vitale GC, Reynolds M, et al. Acute biliary pancreatitis. The roles of laparoscopic cholecystectomy and endoscopic retrograde cholangiopancreatography. Surg Endosc 1995;9:392–6.

102. Brun A, Agarwal N, Pitchumoni CS. Fluid collections in and around the pancreas in acute pancreatitis. J Clin Gastroenterol 2011;45(7):614–25.

103. Nealon WH, Bawduniak J, Walser EM. Appropriate timing of cholecystectomy in patients who present with moderate to severe gallstone-associated acute pancreatitis with peripancreatic fluid collections. Ann Surg 2004;239(6): 741–51.

104. Martin RF, Hein AR. Operative management of acute pancreatitis. Surg Clin North Am 2013;93(3):595–610.

105. Johnson MD, Walsh RM, Henderson JM, et al. Surgical versus nonsurgical management of pancreatic pseudocysts. J Clin Gastroenterol 2009;43(6):586–90.

106. Beckingham IJ, Krige JEJ, Bornam PC, et al. Endoscopic management of pancreatic pseudocysts. Br J Surg 1997;84:1638–45.

107. Gumaste VV, Dave PB. Editorial: pancreatic pseudocyst—the needle or the scalpel? J Clin Gastroenterol 1991;13:500–5.

108. Samuelson AL, Shah RJ. Endoscopic management of pancreatic pseudocysts. Gastroenterol Clin North Am 2012;41(1):47–62.

109. Varadarajulu S, Lopes TL, Wilcox CM, et al. EUS versus surgical cystgastrostomy for management of pancreatic pseudocysts. Gastrointest Endosc 2008;68:649–55.

110. Melman L, Azar R, Beddow K, et al. Primary and overall success rates for clinical outcomes after laparoscopic, endoscopic, and open pancreatic cystogastrostomy for pancreatic pseudocysts. Surg Endosc 2009;23:267–71.

111. Kruger M, Schneider AS, Manns MP, et al. Endoscopic management of pseudocysts or abscesses after an EUS-guided 1-step procedure for initial access. Gastrointest Endosc 2006;63:409–16.

112. Adams DB, Anderson MC. Percutaneous catheter drainage compared with internal drainage in the management of pancreatic pseudocyst. Ann Surg 1992; 215:571–8.

113. Winbladh A, Gullstrand P, Svanvik J, et al. Systematic review of cholecystostomy as a treatment option in acute cholecystitis. HPB 2009;11(3):183–93.

114. Sheffield KM, Han Y, Kuo YF, et al. Variation in the use of intraoperative cholangiography during cholecystectomy. J Am Coll Surg 2012;214(4):668–79.

115. Griniatsos J, Karvounis E, Isla AM. Limitations of fluoroscopic intraoperative cholangiography in cases suggestive of choledocholithiasis. J Laparoendosc Adv Surg Tech A 2005;15:312–7.

116. Johnson PM, Walsh MJ. The impact of intraoperative cholangiography on recurrent pancreatitis and biliary complications in patients with gallstone pancreatitis. J Gastrointest Surg 2012;16(12):2220–4.

117. Ford JA, Soop M, Du J, et al. Systematic review of intraoperative cholangiography in cholecystectomy. Br J Surg 2012;99(2):160–7.

118. Tabone LE, Conlon M, Fernando E, et al. A practical cost-effective management strategy for gallstone pancreatitis. Am J Surg 2013;206(4):472–7.

119. Frossard JL, Hadengue A, Amouyal G, et al. Choledocholithiasis: a prospective study of spontaneous common bile duct stone migration. Gastrointest Endosc 2000;51(2):175–9.
120. Bennion RS, Wyatt LE, Thompson JE. Effect of intra-operative cholangiography during cholecystectomy on outcome after gallstone pancreatitis. J Gastrointest Surg 2002;6:575–81.
121. Ito K, Ito H, Tavakkolizadeh A, et al. Is ductal decompression always necessary before or during surgery for biliary pancreatitis? Am J Surg 2008;195:463–6.
122. Grubnik VV, Tkachenko AI, Ilyashenko VV, et al. Laparoscopic common bile duct exploration versus open surgery: comparative prospective randomized trial. Surg Endosc 2012;26(8):2165–71.
123. Koc B, Karahan S, Adas G, et al. Comparison of laparoscopic common bile duct exploration and endoscopic retrograde cholangiopancreatography plus laparoscopic cholecystectomy for choledocholithiasis: a prospective randomized study. Am J Surg 2013;206(4):457–63.
124. Jacobs M, Verdeja JC, Goldstein HS. Laparoscopic choledocholithotomy. J Laparoendosc Surg 1991;1:79–82.
125. Petelin J. Laparoscopic approach to common duct pathology. Surg Laparosc Endosc 1991;1:33–41.
126. Tokamura H, Umezawa A, Cao H, et al. Laparoscopic management of common bile duct stones: transcystic approach and choledochotomy. J Hepatobiliary Pancreat Surg 2002;9:206–12.
127. Rogers SJ, Cello JP, Horn JK, et al. Prospective randomized trial of LC + LCBDE vs ERCP/S + LC for common bile duct stone disease. Arch Surg 2010;145(1):28.
128. Sgourakis G, Karaliotas K. Laparoscopic common bile duct exploration and cholecystectomy versus endoscopic stone extraction and laparoscopic cholecystectomy for choledocholithiasis: a prospective randomized study. Minerva Chir 2002;57(4):467–74.
129. Paganini AM, Lezoche E. Follow-up of 161 unselected consecutive patients treated laparoscopically for common bile duct stones. Surg Endosc 1998;12:23–9.
130. Guruswamy KS, Samaraj K. Primer closure versus T-tube drainage after laparoscopic common bile duct exploration. Cochrane Database Syst Rev 2007;(1):CD005641.
131. Ebner S, Rechner J, Beller S. Laparoscopic management of common bile duct stones. Surg Endosc 2004;18:762–76.
132. Frey CF, Burbige EJ, Meinke WB, et al. Endoscopic retrograde cholangiopancreatography. Am J Surg 1982;144:109–14.
133. Moretti A, Papi C, Aratari A, et al. Is early endoscopic retrograde cholangiopancreatography useful in the management of acute biliary pancreatitis? Dig Liver Dis 2008;40(5):379–85.
134. Tse F, Yuan Y. Early routine endoscopic retrograde cholangiopancreatography strategy versus early conservative management strategy in acute gallstone pancreatitis. Cochrane Database Syst Rev 2012;(5):CD009779.
135. Van Santvoort HC, Besselink MG, de Vries AC, et al. Early endoscopic retrograde cholangiopancreatography in predicted severe acute biliary pancreatitis. Ann Surg 2009;250(1):68–75.
136. Fan ST, Lai E, Mok F, et al. Early treatment of acute biliary pancreatitis by endoscopic papillotomy. N Engl J Med 1993;328(4):228–32.

137. Cohen S, Bacon BR, Berlin JA. National Institutes of Health State-of-the-Sciences conference statement: ERCP for diagnosis and therapy. Gastrointest Endosc 2002;56(6):803–9.
138. Petrov MS, van Santvoort HC, Besselink MG, et al. Early endoscopic retrograde cholangiopancreatography versus conservative management in acute biliary pancreatitis without cholangitis: a meta-analysis of randomized trials. Ann Surg 2008;247(2):250–7.
139. Berci G, Morgenstern L. Laparoscopic management of common bile duct stones. A multi-institutional SAGES study. Society of American Gastrointestinal Endoscopic Surgeons. Surg Endosc 1994;8:1168–74.
140. Neoptolemos JP, Carr-Locke DL, London NJ, et al. Controlled trial of urgent endoscopic retrograde cholangiopancreatography and endoscopic sphincter-otomy versus conservative treatment for acute pancreatitis due to gallstones. Lancet 1988;2:979–83.
141. Folsch UR, Nitsche R, Ludtke R, et al. Early ERCP and papillotomy compared with conservative treatment for acute biliary pancreatitis. The German Study Group on Acute Biliary Pancreatitis. N Engl J Med 1997;336:237–42.
142. Baillie J. Does every patient with gallstone pancreatitis require ERCP? Curr Gastroenterol Rep 2008;10(2):147–9.
143. Acosta JM, Katkhouda N, Debian KA, et al. Early ductal decompression versus conservative management for gallstone pancreatitis with ampullary obstruction: a prospective randomized clinical trial. Ann Surg 2006;243:33–40.
144. van Geenen EJ, van der Peet DL, Mulder CJ, et al. Recurrent acute biliary pancreatitis: the protective role of cholecystectomy and endoscopic sphincter-otomy. Surg Endosc 2009;23:950–6.
145. Lau JY, Leow CK, Fung TM, et al. Cholecystectomy or gallbladder in situ after endoscopic sphincterotomy and bile duct stone removal in Chinese patients. Gastroenterol 2006;130:96–103.
146. Swanstrom LL, Marcus DR, Kenyon T. Laparoscopic treatment of known choledocholithiasis. Surg Endosc 1996;10(5):526–8.
147. Knott EM, Gasior AC, Bikhchandani J, et al. Surgical management of gallstone pancreatitis in children. J Laparoendosc Adv Surg Tech A 2012;22(5):501–4.
148. Chang YJ, Chao HC, Kong MS, et al. Acute pancreatitis in children. Acta Paediatr 2011;100:740–4.
149. Polydorou A, Karapanos K, Vezakis A, et al. A multimodal approach to acute biliary pancreatitis during pregnancy: a case series. Surg Laparosc Endosc Percutan Tech 2012;22(5):429–32.
150. Al-Hashem H, Muralidharan V, Cohen H, et al. Biliary disease in pregnancy with an emphasis on the role of ERCP. J Clin Gastroenterol 2009;43(1):58–62.
151. Ko CW, Beresford SA, Schulte SJ, et al. Incidence, natural history, and risk factors for biliary sludge and stones during pregnancy. Hepatology 2005;41(2):359–65.
152. Date RS, Kaushal M, Ramesh A. A review of the management of gallstone disease and its complications in pregnancy. Am J Surg 2008;196:599–608.
153. Pearl J, Price R, Richardson W, et al. Guidelines for diagnosis, treatment, and use of laparoscopy for surgical problems during pregnancy. Surg Endosc 2011;25(11):3479–92.
154. Lee A, Min SK, Park JJ, et al. Laparoscopic common bile duct exploration for elderly patients: as a first treatment strategy for common bile duct stones. J Korean Surg Soc 2011;81:128–33.
155. Schirmen BD, Winter KL, Edlich RF. Cholelithiasis and cholecystitis. J Long Term Eff Med Implants 2005;15:329–38.

156. Kaim A, Steinke K, Frank M, et al. Diameter of the common bile duct in the elderly patient: measurement by ultrasound. Eur Radiol 1998;8:1413–5.
157. Hazzan D, Geron N, Golijanin D, et al. Laparoscopic cholecystectomy in octogenarians. Surg Endosc 2003;17(5):773–6.
158. Marcari RS, Lupinacci RM, Nadal LR, et al. Outcomes of laparoscopic cholecystectomy in octogenarians. JSLS 2012;16(2):271–5.

Technical Aspects of Bile Duct Evaluation and Exploration

Sean B. Orenstein, MD, Jeffrey M. Marks, MD,
Jeffrey M. Hardacre, MD*

KEYWORDS

- Common bile duct exploration • Laparoscopic • Open • Cholangiogram • ERCP

KEY POINTS

- Choledocholithiasis is a common manifestation of biliary disease.
- Intraoperative cholangiography can be performed in a variety of ways.
- Common bile duct exploration can be safely performed but necessitates an advanced level of surgical experience to limit complications and improve success.
- An appropriate algorithm based on available resources and the physician skill set is vital for safe and effective management of choledocholithiasis.
- Endoscopic retrograde cholangiopancreatography requires the availability of an advanced endoscopist as well as significant equipment and resources.
- Current training of young surgeons is limited for open biliary procedures and common bile duct explorations. Educational guidelines are necessary to reduce this educational gap.

INTRODUCTION

More than 20 million Americans have some form of gallstone disease. Of these, 5% to 20% present with common bile duct (CBD) stones, with the elderly at greatest risk.[1–3] The presence of CBD stones can lead to a range of upstream and downstream effects throughout the biliary tract including obstructive jaundice, cholecystitis, cholangitis, and pancreatitis. The spectrum of morbidity from these diseases varies greatly, ranging from asymptomatic choledocholithiasis to critically ill cholangitis. Prompt identification and treatment are necessary to reduce the severity of illness caused by bile duct stones and subsequent biliary obstruction and ascending infection.

Managing choledocholithiasis can be challenging from an organizational standpoint. Method and timing of cholangiography, timing of operative intervention, potential need for bile duct exploration, and cooperation between surgery and gastroenterology all present challenges to the management of patients with choledocholithiasis.

Disclosure: The authors have no financial disclosures.
University Hospitals Case Medical Center, Cleveland, OH, USA
* Corresponding author. Department of Surgery, UH Case Medical Center, 11100 Euclid Avenue, Cleveland, OH 44106.
E-mail address: jeffrey.hardacre@uhhospitals.org

Surg Clin N Am 94 (2014) 281–296
http://dx.doi.org/10.1016/j.suc.2013.12.002
0039-6109/14/$ – see front matter © 2014 Elsevier Inc. All rights reserved.

surgical.theclinics.com

Often-overlooked critical aspects of bile duct stone management are resource use as well as availability of a skilled endoscopist. A separate endoscopy team with at least 1 or 2 nurses/technicians is typically necessary for endoscopic retrograde cholangio-pancreatography (ERCP), whether it be performed before, during, or after surgery. Specialized equipment is necessary for successful diagnostic and therapeutic endoscopic cholangiography. The experience of the endoscopist also affects the timing of cholangiography, because the clinician's skill set may dictate whether preoperative or postoperative cholangiography is warranted.

The skill level of the surgeon is another critical aspect affecting bile duct stone management. Although most surgeons complete residency with excellent training in laparoscopic cholecystectomy, most are inadequately trained for laparoscopic or open bile duct exploration. In addition, open cholecystectomies are also rarely performed in residency, with most chief residents having performed only 10 open cholecystectomies.[4]

PREOPERATIVE CHOLANGIOGRAPHY
Indications

There are a variety of scenarios in which preoperative cholangiography may be warranted. Such entities may overlap and include cholangitis, biliary pancreatitis, persistent jaundice, uncomplicated choledocholithiasis, benign stricture, and periampullary neoplasm. Of these, ascending cholangitis represents the most severe disease and warrants urgent biliary decompression, preferably by endoscopic means. However, if ERCP is not possible, percutaneous or open biliary decompression is indicated. Mild gallstone pancreatitis can typically be initially observed with trending of pancreatic enzymes; however, severe biliary pancreatitis with ductal disruption is another indication for urgent ERCP. Although variable, liver function tests can aid in diagnosing common duct disorders, but specific patterns and levels are debatable.[5–7]

The use of preoperative cholangiography may depend on the resources available in a particular health care setting. The absence of a skilled interventional endoscopist means that the surgeon is of the utmost importance in bile duct stone management. Not having the luxury of a skilled therapeutic endoscopist may encourage attempts at preoperative cholangiography. The finding of a bile duct stone may alter a surgeon's operative approach and provide for better preoperative counseling to the patient. Such a circumstance is preferable to finding a bile duct stone during surgery and deferring to a postoperative ERCP, only to have it fail. In addition, for patients presenting with biliary pancreatitis or choledocholithiasis who are unable to undergo cholecystectomy, dedicated ERCP for biliary sphincterotomy may be a viable option.

Magnetic Resonance Cholangiopancreatography Versus ERCP

With regard to the method of preoperative cholangiography, 2 common entities exist: magnetic resonance cholangiopancreatography (MRCP) and ERCP. Both are useful adjuncts in the diagnosis of biliary stone disease, and they each have appropriate indications. Although MRCP can provide anatomic detail of the biliary tract, it is only a diagnostic tool and, as such, cannot provide any direct therapeutic benefit.

ERCP is indicated when therapeutic interventions are needed, such as in acute cholangitis, biliary pancreatitis with ductal obstruction, and uncomplicated choledocholithiasis. However, ERCP should not be performed until a surgical plan is in place. This delay allows more efficient use of hospital resources, decreased hospital length of stay, and greater clarity for the patient as well as surgical/medical care providers. Often overlooked by nonendoscopists, ERCP uses significant resources and personnel to perform the procedure compared with MRCP. ERCP requires multiple pieces of equipment including a side-viewing endoscope, video and lighting equipment, CO_2 gas (if available) and connectors, guidewires, sphincterotomes, an electrical source such as ERBE or standard cautery, balloon catheters, lithotripsy devices, multiple sizes of stents, and fluoroscopic devices. Depending on the facility it may also require involvement of anesthesia, an endoscopic technician, nursing staff, and a radiology technician, in addition to the advanced endoscopist. A technical description of the ERCP procedure is given elsewhere in this issue.

However, MRCP can provide greater anatomic detail of surrounding organs and tissues, making MRCP more useful for evaluating persistent jaundice and diagnosing periampullary or biliary malignancies. Because many patients with biliary malignancies proceed to resection, ERCP may be more helpful in late-stage disease in which palliative biliary stenting is necessary, or if preoperative temporary stenting is required in earlier stage disease.

The risks of MRCP are minimal, with some restrictions for patients with implanted metallic objects or metallic foreign bodies that are not safe for magnetic resonance imaging (MRI). In addition, caution should be used when performing MRI with gadolinium on patients with severe renal disease, especially on dialysis, because there is a small risk of post-MRI nephrogenic fibrosing dermopathy.[8] In contrast, ERCP has a more extensive risk profile including acute pancreatitis (2.4%–4%), bleeding (0.3%–1.4%), ascending biliary infection (1.4%), perforation (0.6%), as well as a mortality of 0.2% to 0.9%.[9–11]

INTRAOPERATIVE CHOLANGIOGRAPHY

Cholangiography is a common adjunct to cholecystectomy, with approximately 30% of patients undergoing cholecystectomy receiving an intraoperative cholangiogram (IOC).[12,13] There are 3 principal goals with intraoperative cholangiography: identify ductal anatomy, confirm the presence or lack of stones, and education/training. Although some surgeons prefer to perform cholangiograms routinely, others are selective on which patients receive an IOC. When there is any doubt regarding ductal anatomy during dissection, a cholangiogram is warranted to further delineate cystic and/or common duct anatomy.

There are clear indications for intraoperative cholangiography based on preoperative data. Jaundice and increased liver function tests often indicate concurrent or recent choledocholithiasis. Persistent increased levels with or without accompanying jaundice should warrant an IOC.

Likewise, increased pancreatic enzymes in the setting of cholelithiasis indicate a passed or passing common duct stone. In our practice, surgical intervention for gallstone pancreatitis (cholecystectomy) is delayed until amylase and/or lipase levels are trending down, although complete normalization is not necessary as long as the patient's symptoms from pancreatitis are resolving. Although IOC should be considered for gallstone pancreatitis to ensure no remaining common duct stones persist, ERCP is typically not warranted, because the stone has likely passed into the duodenum.

Cholangiography is also indicated for radiographic evidence of biliary obstruction. Such obstruction can be manifested by a dilated biliary tree or the presence of common duct stones seen on ultrasonography, computed tomography, or MRI. However, ductal dilatation without the presence of gallstones should warrant further evaluation for a possible neoplastic source of biliary obstruction **Box 1**.

There is still debate about routine versus selective use of intraoperative cholangiography. Proponents of either method can cite numerous studies to justify their

Box 1
Indications for IOC
History of or current jaundice
Increased liver function tests
Increased pancreatic enzymes
Ductal dilatation on imaging
CBD stones seen on imaging

positions. For example, studies favoring routine use argue that IOC allows earlier detection of ductal injuries, stones, and other associated anomalies.[14,15] **Fig. 1** shows choledocholithiasis found incidentally on routine IOC during elective cholecystectomy. The earlier detection of common duct disorders may lead to quicker operative management with a reduced need for postoperative interventions, such as ERCP. In contrast, Horwood and colleagues[16] argue that selective use of IOC for only the indications listed earlier provide a more rational directed approach given the high positive predictive value for selective indications, as well as low rate of common duct disorders for asymptomatic patients not meeting selective criteria. A recent Medicare database study of elderly patients concluded that CBD injury rates were equivalent with or without IOC. Despite a significantly higher CBD injury rate without IOC on initial analysis, the investigators found no association between IOC and CBD injury after additional statistical analysis.[17] Others argue that even if the overall risk of CBD injury is not reduced with routine IOC, the severity of injury and resultant sequelae are mitigated with the use of IOC.[14,18]

In addition, some clinicians have questioned the routine use of IOC from a cost-analysis perspective. Studies have shown that the use of IOC adds more than the

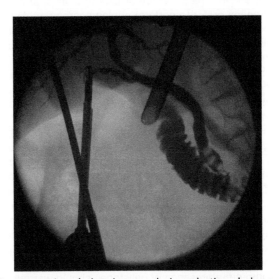

Fig. 1. Routine intraoperative cholangiogram during elective cholecystectomy showing multiple filling defects in the distal CBD. Note the normal CBD diameter and contrast flow into the duodenum. The patient underwent postoperative ERCP following cholecystectomy with drain placement.

average surgeon realizes, with an added approximately $700 to 900 or more per case.[12,13] However, there is still no definitive conclusion about whether routine or selective IOC provides the most effective and efficient treatment of patients with biliary disease. Regardless of cholangiography use, it is still vital to adhere to standards of biliary dissection, including obtaining the critical view of safety in order to limit misidentification of cystic duct anatomy and minimize biliary injury.[19,20]

Ultrasound Cholangiography

Ultrasonography-based techniques for cholangiography provide a safe and accurate method of detecting CBD stones with multiple benefits, including elimination of the radiation and contrast exposure associated with fluoroscopic cholangiography.[21–23] Compared with fluoroscopic cholangiography, ultrasonography is highly sensitive and specific in identifying CBD stones and ductal dilatation (83%–100% sensitivity and 98%–100% specificity).[21,24,25] Ductal diameter and thickness can be accurately measured, and adjacent anatomy, including vascular structures, bowel, and pancreas, can be visualized. In addition, compared with fluoroscopic cholangiography, ultrasonography is more cost effective, with an ultrasonography machine costing approximately US$40,000 to US$75,000 compared with a C-arm and supplies costing US$500,000 or more.[21,22,25] However, there are limitations to such a technique. First, ultrasonography is operator dependent with a large learning curve, and the use of ultrasonography is not frequently taught in residency. From an anatomic standpoint, difficulty can arise when differentiating structures such as the CBD from the cystic duct. Stones are typically well visualized, although they can display acoustic shadowing, which may, in turn, lead to difficulty in structural identification. In addition, the use of ultrasonography provides only diagnostic evaluation without any therapeutic benefits.

Ultrasonography technique

The camera should be moved to the epigastric port to allow introduction of the laparoscopic ultrasonography probe via the 12-mm umbilical port. Imaging quality may be improved with the placement of saline over the liver and porta hepatis. The liver is then retracted cephalad and the ultrasonography probe is placed over the porta hepatis; the probe is aimed toward the foramen of Winslow and perpendicular to the hepatoduodenal ligaments. As the probe is swept distally toward the duodenum, correct orientation is displayed as the so-called Mickey Mouse silhouette, with the head as the portal vein and the ears as the CBD and hepatic artery in cross section.[25] The probe is then swept proximally to visualize the common hepatic and left/right hepatic ducts and can be rotated 90° to view the ducts in cross section and longitudinally. In addition, the probe can be placed directly over the liver to visualize the left and right hepatic ducts and the confluence into the common hepatic duct. By sweeping along the CBD the takeoff of the cystic duct can be identified, ductal diameter can be measured, and the presence of stones can be visualized.[23,25]

Fluoroscopic Cholangiography

Although ultrasonography can diagnose CBD disorders, fluoroscopic cholangiography has the benefit of providing a route for therapeutic intervention. Using fluoroscopic IOC, stones can be identified with greater than 95% sensitivity and specificity, 5% false-positive, and 1% false-negative rate with some surgeons,[26] although these rates are highly variable depending on the study.[27] Because this technique is still widely used, many surgeons have acquired the required skill set for IOC in their residency training. However, compared with ultrasonography, more risks are present, including radiation and contrast exposure, as well as perforation or other injury to the duct.

Fluoroscopic technique

Before commencing cholangiography it is important that all supplies are available and ready. A C-arm, radiology technician, and radiation protective gear (lead gowns/aprons, thyroid shield) should be available at the start of the procedure. The operating table should be oriented in a way that allows the bottom component of the C-arm to move freely under the upper abdomen and lower thorax. The surgeon, resident(s) or assistant, and scrub technician should be knowledgeable about the cholangiogram catheters available at their institution. Once connected, the cholangiogram catheter system should be thoroughly flushed with saline; any air within the system can lead to false-positives during cholangiography. A 3-way stopcock can be set up with 1 syringe of saline and 1 of full-strength water-soluble contrast; this allows for limited exchanging of syringes and reduces air entry. The syringes should be labeled and clearly identified to ensure proper luminal contrast injection during fluoroscopy.

After cystic duct dissection and clear visualization of the critical view, a single metal clip is placed at the cystic duct–gallbladder junction. Using sharp laparoscopic scissors a small cystic ductotomy is made; this should be only large enough to allow the catheter to be inserted. One side of the Maryland grasper can be gently inserted as a guide. The cholangiogram catheter can be placed through various ports based on anatomic alignment with the cystic duct, or even a new port if all other ports are necessary for retraction. With gentle traction of the gallbladder neck inferiorly to straighten the cystic duct, the catheter is placed though the ductotomy and is secured in place with either an intraluminal balloon or laparoscopic cholangiogram grasper. The catheter is then flushed with saline to check the seal and flow. Although a minimal amount of saline extravasation is acceptable, a large rush of saline from the ductotomy should prompt replacement. Saline should flow easily without the need for excessive pressure on the syringe. If there is difficulty pushing the syringe without an active leak, the catheter may be against a spiral valve of Heister or the cholangiogram clamp may be on too tight, both of which warrant small incremental adjustments. Care is taken to remove all accessory instruments under direct visualization with gentle resting of the gallbladder down on the porta hepatis, followed by removal of the laparoscope.

The sterilely draped C-arm is brought in and spot radiographs are performed to check proper orientation and positioning, with the cholangiogram catheter slightly to the left and lower center of the screen. Using live fluoroscopy, contrast is rapidly injected. Cholangiography should not be considered complete until the entire biliary tree is visualized, including the cystic duct, the left and right hepatic ducts, and the common hepatic duct and CBD, and contrast is seen filling the duodenum (**Fig. 2**). Lack of filling of any of these structures should prompt reevaluation. Any filling defects warrant repeat cholangiogram after thoroughly flushing the system with saline to wash out any air or gas bubbles (see **Fig. 2**). At times, rapid filling into the duodenum can result in limited proximal duct filling. Placing the patient in Trendelenburg position can assist with gravity-induced proximal duct filling. Also, the administration of 1 to 2 mg of intravenous (IV) morphine can induce sphincter of Oddi contraction, thereby providing added back pressure for improve proximal filling. In contrast, if no duodenal filling is seen, 1 mg of IV glucagon can be administered for sphincter of Oddi relaxation. Confirmation of filling a defect such as a stone warrants CBD exploration (CBDE) or ERCP, as discussed later. Large-volume contrast extravasation may indicate ductal transection, and lack of proximal duct filling despite performing the aforementioned

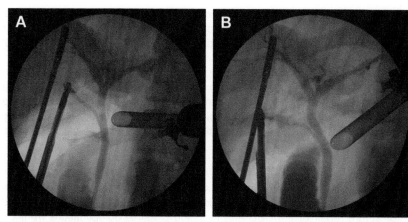

Fig. 2. (*A*) Intraoperative cholangiogram showing an air/gas bubble in the common hepatic duct just above the cystic duct–CBD junction. (*B*) Complete cholangiogram showing resolution of air/gas bubble after flushing system. The biliary tree is visualized including the cystic duct, the left and right hepatic ducts, and the common hepatic duct and CBD, and contrast is seen filling the duodenum.

maneuvers may indicate CBD ligation, both of which warrant urgent operative exploration. If normal, the cholangiogram catheter is removed and the cholecystectomy is completed per routine technique. If possible, confirmatory images showing completion cholangiogram with or without filling defects should be saved and sent to radiology for documentation purposes.

If cystic duct anatomy is not clearly identified or there is significant inflammation, it may be possible to perform the cholangiogram via the gallbladder. This procedure is performed in manner nearly identical to the transcystic technique, but it is initiated by making a small incision into the neck or body of the gallbladder. An endoloop can be placed around the cholangiogram catheter to help limit extravasation of bile around the catheter. If the gallbladder has significant edema and inflammation, an alternative approach involves partial dissection of the fundus followed by fundal cholecystotomy; this allows the endoloop to encircle the fundus and catheter for a tighter seal.

If the cholangiogram documents a common duct stone, therapeutic intervention is warranted. Management of CBD disorder, including CBDE performed laparoscopically or with conversion to open procedure, is discussed later. As an alternative, ERCP may play a role either during or after surgery to alleviate the obstruction and allow proper biliary drainage into the duodenum.

CBDE
Laparoscopic CBDE

Since the advent of laparoscopy, techniques have evolved to enhance or mirror those of the open counterpart. Although laparoscopic and open cholecystectomy differ significantly in procedural steps, laparoscopic CBDE uses virtually the same technique and steps as the open approach. Routes of entry into the biliary tract include transcystic, transcholecystic, or transcholedochal. Regardless of entry route, gallbladder dissection should be performed in standard fashion with the critical view obtained and clear visualization of biliary structures. Because of the technical challenges and time commitment with laparoscopic CBDE (LCBDE), the operating staff and anesthesia team should be apprised in order to prepare for a longer procedure and need for sedation/paralytics so that the laparoscopic working space is not reduced. Clinicians may also consider performing a complete cholecystectomy or near-complete dissection of the gallbladder so that there is limited manipulation of the gallbladder and cystic duct following completion of the CBDE.

It is of utmost importance to obtain the proper equipment and supplies in order to limit wasted time in setting up for the procedure. Some facilities have a designated CBDE cart or area in central supply to diminish delays and frustration as to necessary supplies.[28] In addition, all-in-one disposable kits are manufactured to reduce supply confusion. A supply list has been provided that contains the essential elements necessary for LCBDE (**Box 2**).

Transcystic technique

The principal benefits of transcystic CBDE are that access has already been achieved from the initial cholangiogram, and choledochotomy is avoided, thus eliminating the need for suture repair of the CBD and reducing possible complications from CBD manipulation (eg, leak or stricture). However, this technique is disadvantaged for proximal or multiple stones, stones larger than 5 to 7 mm, and tortuous or long cystic ducts. All steps should be performed under fluoroscopy in order to monitor wire and equipment location as well as to evaluate the progress of stone extraction.

1. Administer 1 mg of IV glucagon before the start of exploration.
2. Ensure that the cholangiogram catheter is well flushed with saline and all air bubbles have been evacuated.
3. Flush CBD with saline, which may be sufficient for small stones (<4 mm) to pass through the papilla. A follow-up cholangiogram may be performed to inspect for residual stones.
4. Advance flexible-tip guidewire into CBD.

Box 2
Supply list for laparoscopic CBDE

Glucagon, 1 mg

Additional 5-mm laparoscopic trocar

Fluoroscopy with C-arm

Radiation protective gear

Sharp laparoscopic scissors

Cholangiogram catheter

Guidewire

Saline

Water-soluble contrast

Fogarty balloon catheters, 4 or 5 Fr

Flexible choledochoscopes, 3 and 5 mm

Additional light and video source

Extraction basket

T tubes, 10 and 14 Fr

Resorbable monofilament suture (eg, 4-0 or 5-0 polydioxanone [PDS])

Laparoscopic suturing instruments

---

5. Using a balloon catheter, dilate the cystic duct to approximately 5 to 7 mm in a slow, controlled fashion, taking care to limit cystic duct dilatation to less than the CBD diameter.[28] This maneuver allows the passage of large instruments, such as a choledochoscope, into the CBD.

6. The stones can be extracted in one of 2 ways: retrograde with a wire basket or antegrade using a balloon catheter.

7. A basket retrieval system is used to extract the stones in a retrograde fashion through the cystic duct. Care needs to be taken to encompass the stone(s) with the basket and to avoid dragging stones or stone fragments higher into the hepatic biliary tree.

8. If an antegrade route is chosen, the first step should be to perform a dilation of the papilla to allow passage of stones and minimize tearing of the papillary tissue and adjacent ducts with the stones. However, the risks of bleeding, ductal trauma, and pancreatitis are still present with these maneuvers. After papillary dilatation, the balloon is inflated proximally in the duct and advanced in an antegrade direction to push the stones and debris into the duodenum.

9. Flushing with saline may assist clearing out residual fragments and debris.

10. If available, lithotripsy may be used to break up stones to allow easier retrieval and passage.

11. Endoscopic guidance may also be used to visualize papillary dilatation, confirm passage of stones, or assist with stone extraction by passing the wire through the papilla toward the endoscope. This rendezvous procedure should only be performed with the assistance of an advanced endoscopist to limit subsequent injuries.

12. As an option, a 3-mm or 5-mm choledochoscope is used to visualize the duct. Under direct visualization, wire basket retrieval, complete clearance of stones, and biliary injury can be evaluated. One drawback is its limited ability to visualize and clear proximal duct stones.

13. Additional saline flushing should be performed to clear out residual debris and stone fragments from catheter or equipment manipulation.

14. A completion cholangiogram should always be performed to document clearance of the biliary tract and to evaluate for ductal injury or leak.

15. Following removal of any catheters or scopes the cystic duct is ligated. We prefer to use an endoloop for ligation to reduce cystic stump leak, because ampullary spasm can lead to back pressure of bile.

16. Likewise, a Jackson-Pratt or Blake drain is left in place for a few days after surgery in case a leak should occur.

Transcholecystic technique

A transcholecystic approach may be attempted if transcystic approaches are unsuccessful, or in place of a transcystic approach. Such an approach may be warranted if the cystic duct is not clearly identified or the anatomy is distorted. This technique involves making a small incision into the neck or body of the gallbladder, or the fundus as described earlier. The use of an endoloop around the cholangiogram catheter may help limit extravasation of bile around the catheter. Through the cholecystotomy, the CBDE is performed in the manner described earlier for the transcystic approach.

Choledochotomy technique

If unsuccessful with transcystic or transcholecystic stone extraction, clinicians must proceed with either the choledochotomy technique or ERCP. Laparoscopic exploration via choledochotomy should only commence if the surgeon has had prior experience, because the potential for postoperative morbidity is severe if complications arise. The surgeon should be skilled with handling of the CBD and laparoscopic ductal suturing, as well as being knowledgeable about the necessary equipment.

Choledochotomy should only proceed if there is favorable anatomy and minimal inflammation. CBDE through this route requires a dilated duct of at least 8 to 10 mm, because smaller ducts have increased risk of iatrogenic injury including rupture and are more likely to stricture at the ductotomy site.[28,29] In addition, severely inflamed ducts may predispose the patient to greater perforation risk and/or persistent bile leak. Following a cholangiogram with identification of the biliary tree, CBDE is performed in a manner similar to the transcystic technique described earlier, but with significant differences in opening and closure of the duct.

1. Administer 1 mg of IV glucagon before the start of exploration.
2. The CBD is exposed by carefully dissecting the peritoneum overlying the porta hepatis.
3. Confirmation of the CBD can be achieved by either aspiration of bile with a fine-gauge needle, or with laparoscopic ultrasonography. The latter can also be of benefit by displaying CBD stones.
4. Using cold scissors an anterior longitudinal choledochotomy approximately 10 to 15 mm in length, or as big as the largest stone, is made. Care should be taken to avoid injury to the vascular supply of the CBD, which parallels the duct at the 3 and 9 o'clock positions, because subsequent vascular injury may lead to increased risk of stenosis and bile leak. Also, the ductotomy should be made as distal on the CBD as possible in order to preserve as much duct as possible in case a biliary-enteric anastomosis is necessary.
5. Although optional, stay sutures placed at both sides of the ductotomy using 4-0 or 5-0 PDS may assist in duct exposure and allow easier passage of catheters, baskets, stones, and so forth.
6. A catheter is then placed into the ductotomy through one of the laparoscopic ports that is most in line with the duct, typically one of the lateral ports. Although several CBDE catheters exist, some investigators advocate using a 14-Fr red rubber catheter, because this provides a semiflexible route for wire exchange and higher-pressure irrigation.[28]
7. The duct is then thoroughly flushed with hand-pressurized injections of saline because this may clear the duct. A follow-up cholangiogram can confirm the success of this maneuver.
8. If stones are still present, CBDE exploration is then performed as described earlier for the transcystic technique (steps 4 to 13).
9. If T-tube closure is chosen, the choledochotomy is then closed over a 10-Fr to 14-Fr T tube with the distal top portion of the T cut off to allow improved drainage around and through the tube, as well as to make it more pliable for ease of removal. The T tube can be gently pushed against the anteductomy side (intraluminally) while suturing the choledochotomy to avoid catching the tube with a suture. Running or interrupted resorbable sutures (eg, 4-0 or 5-0 PDS) are then placed proximal and distal to the tube; resorbable sutures are necessary to reduce stone formation at the suture sites. The T tube is then pulled back against the repair site while tying the final sutures close to the tube.
10. The T tube should be flushed with saline to assess for leakage around the tube, brought out through one of the lateral trocars, and secured to the skin. Care should be taken to position the tube intra-abdominally, allowing enough slack to avoid tension being placed at the CBD insertion site.

11. Before desufflation and trocar removal an optional drain is placed near the choledochotomy site and T tube in case of bile leakage around the tube during the immediate postoperative period.
12. A completion cholangiogram is then performed through the T tube, with documentation of ductal clearance.

Although once considered routine, placement of a T tube is now performed more selectively. Studies show comparable outcomes between routine and selective T-tube placement, but with longer operative times and length of stay when a T tube is placed.[30,31] Others show more complications with T-tube placement including bile leak and tube malfunction (slippage, entrapment).[32] However, we routinely close our defects over a T tube in order to adequately decompress the biliary system and provide access for further imaging. In addition, clinical staff members taking care of the patient on the ward should be educated as to proper T-tube care and maintenance. Staff members need to minimize exterior tension on the tube to ensure there is no pulling of the tube or accidental dislodgement. The tube should be flushed with sterile saline 2 to 3 times daily and placed to a gravity drainage bag for monitoring outputs.

If the surgeon is inexperienced in LCBDE and if an advanced endoscopist is available, an intraoperative ERCP with or without rendezvous procedure can be performed in which a guidewire is placed transcystically or transcholedochally through the papilla; the endoscope can grasp the guidewire for easier access to the biliary tree. Transcholedochal or other types of rendezvous procedures such as percutaneous and endoscopic ultrasonography–based wire placements aid in selective cannulation of the papilla, thus improving stone clearance rates when difficult anatomy is encountered. As an alternative, a postoperative ERCP can be performed after placing a drain near the cystic dump stump before closure. Because of increased intraluminal pressures from contrast injections and ductal manipulations, we advocate cystic stump closure using an endoloop for a more secure ligation. The biggest caveat is that if postoperative ERCP is unsuccessful, the patient has to return to the OR for an additional operative procedure for stone extraction.

Open CBDE

Although infrequently performed in surgical training programs, open common duct exploration still plays a role in ductal clearance of impacted stones. Patients already undergoing open procedures via midline or Kocher incisions, or conversions from laparoscopic to open procedures, undergo open CBDE (OCBDE), if warranted. In addition, OCBDE is indicated if unsuccessful with complete ductal clearance using any of the laparoscopic techniques, if the anatomy is distorted or too inflamed for safe access, or if the surgeon's experience is too limited to safely perform it laparoscopically. The OCBDE procedure mirrors that of the laparoscopic technique previously described, with some modifications. The CBD is opened in a similar fashion after aspirating bile to confirm biliary duct dissection. Again, the duct should be irrigated with saline to potentiate stone clearance; small stones may pass through the papilla or may float retrograde out through the choledochotomy. Papillary dilation with a balloon catheter should be attempted to allow efflux of larger stones. An open procedure has the benefit of direct manipulation and handling of the duct and catheters. The papilla can be identified using a combination of fluoroscopy and palpation of the catheter within the duodenum. Stone extraction and choledochoscopy should proceed as with a laparoscopic approach. A T tube with suture closure is likewise recommended, followed by flushing and a completion cholangiogram to confirm ductal clearance and show free flow of contrast.

Persistent biliary obstruction with impacted stones necessitates transduodenal exploration or, if severe enough, a biliary bypass procedure. Sphincterotomy can be performed open with a transduodenal approach, or endoscopically with an ERCP. For transduodenal sphincterotomy the duodenum is Kocherized followed by a 2-cm to 4-cm longitudinal incision on the anterior surface of the second portion of the duodenum. A catheter placed into the CBD from the choledochotomy helps identify the papilla. Traction sutures into the duodenal walls can be placed to improve exposure of the duodenal lumen and papilla.[29] A sphincterotomy is then performed in the biliary side of the papilla at 10 o'clock, opposite the pancreatic duct. The sphincterotomy may have to be extended over the stone if it is still impacted. Some surgeons prefer to mature the distal CBD mucosa with the duodenum using resorbable sutures to allow easier flow of stones and debris.[29] Following stone extraction and T-tube placement, the system should be flushed to clear debris and evaluate for leak at the sphincterotomy site or choledochotomy and a cholangiogram performed to confirm ductal clearance. The duodenotomy is then closed in 2 layers in a transverse manner. Before abdominal closure, 1 or 2 drains should be placed around the duodenotomy and choledochotomy until after adequate per oral intake, to rule out a duodenal or biliary leak. For severely dilated CBD (2 cm) or impacted stones not amenable to other extraction means, a biliary-enteric bypass procedure may be necessary, with either a choledochoduodenostomy or choledochojejunostomy.[33]

Intraoperative ERCP

Having an advanced endoscopist available to assist with ductal clearance in the operating room can be beneficial in the setting of preoperative liver function test (LFT) increase (ie, planned intraoperative ERCP), intraoperative discovery of ductal filling defects on cholangiogram, or inability to successfully clear the duct with CBDE. The principal advantages of intraoperative ERCP include a single, albeit longer, anesthetic exposure, the ability to identify complications from CBDE, and the ability to evaluate altered papillary anatomy intraluminally. The use of a rendezvous procedure may aid the endoscopist in accessing the papilla by placing a transcystic or transcholedochal guidewire through the papilla into the duodenum for easier CBD access. An important benefit of performing an ERCP intraoperatively is that, if the ERCP is unsuccessful, the patient and surgical team are already in the operating room and a laparoscopic or open CBDE can proceed without having the patient return for a subsequent procedure.

However, there are drawbacks to intraoperative ERCP beyond the logistical challenge of coordinating the surgeon and endoscopist schedules and managing resource use of the procedure. Adding ERCP increases the operative time and anesthetic time, especially for a difficult case. Difficulty might arise from the patient positioning, because ERCPs are typically performed with the patient in a prone position. Although supine-positioned ERCP is achievable it makes the procedure more challenging. There are independent risks of ERCP that potentially add to the surgical risks, including acute pancreatitis, bleeding, ascending biliary infection, and perforation.[9–11] Insufflation can cause bowel dilatation, which may reduce abdominal domain and operative working space. To compensate for this, clinicians may consider completing or nearly completing the cholecystectomy before starting the ERCP. In addition, the use of CO_2 gas instead of air may help reduce bowel distention as well as reduce postprocedure pain.[34]

Postoperative ERCP

There are several scenarios in which postoperative ERCP is warranted, including an unsuccessful LCBDE. In this setting, a transcystic stent can be placed for temporary biliary drainage, or a guidewire can be placed for easier endoscopic identification during ERCP. In general, if an OCBDE has been embarked on, the operation should not be terminated until stone clearance is complete and/or biliary drainage is achieved. If an IOC is positive for ductal stones, bile duct exploration is not technically feasible, and intraoperative ERCP is not available, the patient requires postoperative ERCP. It is also possible for a stone to be incidentally introduced into the CBD from the gallbladder or cystic duct during cholecystectomy following a negative cholangiogram. In addition, for an elderly or ill patient, ERCP may have to be deferred to a separate postoperative period in order to decrease the anesthetic risks of a longer single operative procedure, although the patient would be exposed to 2 separate anesthetic periods.

RESIDENT TRAINING IMPLICATIONS

There has been a significant paradigm shift over the last 2 decades with regard to resident and fellow training, because the advent of laparoscopy has shifted numerous procedures from traditional open operations to minimally invasive techniques such as laparoscopy or endoscopy. One of the most common situations in which this is seen is in biliary procedures. Although multiple benefits of laparoscopy are evident,[35–38] the risk of CBD injury remain higher for laparoscopic (0.2%–0.5%) versus open (0.2%)[39,40] cholecystectomy. This rate of CBD injury during laparoscopy has plateaued since resident and fellow trainees have become accustomed to the standard technique of hepatobiliary triangle dissection and obtaining a critical view in order to minimize CBD injury. In an effort to minimize and reduce CBD injury, Berci and colleagues[41] advocate not only standardization of biliary dissection for all practitioners but also intensive education of biliary surgical techniques for trainees. The investigators advocate specific educational components for cholangiography, simulation training, didactics, and routine use of cholangiography in order to gain an exacting description of biliary anatomy to minimize CBD injury.

The challenge of educating surgical trainees is to provide them with the fundamental knowledge to practice as general surgeons, despite a significant reduction in exposure to open biliary procedures and CBDE. This reduction has led to a growing trend of reliance on subspecialists and referrals to hepatobiliary-trained surgeons for management of what used to be in the realm of the general surgeon.[42,43] The number of open biliary operations has been greatly reduced over the last 2 decades, which has, in turn, led to reduced exposure to open procedures for trainees.[42] According to recent national case logs from the Accreditation Council for Graduate Medical Education (ACGME), the average surgical resident graduates with experience of only 10 open cholecystectomies performed compared with more than 100 laparoscopic cholecystectomies.[4] For CBDE, the average chief resident graduates having performed only 1 open and 1 laparoscopic CBDE, although this has not significantly changed over the last decade, with only 2.5 open and 1 laparoscopic CBDE reported on average from 1999 to 2002.[4] Residents' exposure to open and CBD procedures is too limited to make a graduate proficient at such procedures. Thus, further discussion and debate are necessary to determine effective and efficient methods for training residents and fellows for open and laparoscopic common duct explorations.

REFERENCES

1. Hunter JG. Laparoscopic transcystic common bile duct exploration. Am J Surg 1992;163(1):53–6 [discussion: 57–8].

2. Marks JM, Ponsky JL. Management of common bile duct stones. Gastroenterologist 1996;4(3):155–62.
3. Everhart JE, Khare M, Hill M, et al. Prevalence and ethnic differences in gallbladder disease in the United States. Gastroenterology 1999;117(3):632–9.
4. ACGME. General surgery case logs, national data reports: 2010–2012, 1999–2002. Available at: http://www.acgme.org/. Accessed August 30, 2013.
5. Padda MS, Singh S, Tang SJ, et al. Liver test patterns in patients with acute calculous cholecystitis and/or choledocholithiasis. Aliment Pharmacol Ther 2009;29(9): 1011–8.
6. Meroni E, Bisagni P, Bona S, et al. Pre-operative endoscopic ultrasonography can optimise the management of patients undergoing laparoscopic cholecystectomy with abnormal liver function tests as the sole risk factor for choledocholithiasis: a prospective study. Dig Liver Dis 2004;36(1):73–7.
7. Contractor QQ, Boujemla M, Contractor TQ, et al. Abnormal common bile duct sonography. The best predictor of choledocholithiasis before laparoscopic cholecystectomy. J Clin Gastroenterol 1997;25(2):429–32.
8. Grobner T. Gadolinium–a specific trigger for the development of nephrogenic fibrosing dermopathy and nephrogenic systemic fibrosis? Nephrol Dial Transplant 2006;21(4):1104–8.
9. Freeman ML, Nelson DB, Sherman S, et al. Complications of endoscopic biliary sphincterotomy. N Engl J Med 1996;335(13):909–18.
10. Andriulli A, Loperfido S, Napolitano G, et al. Incidence rates of post-ERCP complications: a systematic survey of prospective studies. Am J Gastroenterol 2007; 102(8):1781–8.
11. Coelho-Prabhu N, Shah ND, Van Houten H, et al. Endoscopic retrograde cholangiopancreatography: utilisation and outcomes in a 10-year population-based cohort. BMJ Open 2013;3(5).
12. Livingston EH, Miller JA, Coan B, et al. Costs and utilization of intraoperative cholangiography. J Gastrointest Surg 2007;11(9):1162–7.
13. Ragulin-Coyne E, Witkowski ER, Chau Z, et al. Is routine intraoperative cholangiogram necessary in the twenty-first century? A national view. J Gastrointest Surg 2013;17(3):434–42.
14. Nickkholgh A, Soltaniyekta S, Kalbasi H. Routine versus selective intraoperative cholangiography during laparoscopic cholecystectomy: a survey of 2,130 patients undergoing laparoscopic cholecystectomy. Surg Endosc 2006;20(6): 868–74.
15. Buddingh KT, Weersma RK, Savenije RA, et al. Lower rate of major bile duct injury and increased intraoperative management of common bile duct stones after implementation of routine intraoperative cholangiography. J Am Coll Surg 2011; 213(2):267–74.
16. Horwood J, Akbar F, Davis K, et al. Prospective evaluation of a selective approach to cholangiography for suspected common bile duct stones. Ann R Coll Surg Engl 2010;92(3):206–10.
17. Sheffield KM, Riall TS, Han Y, et al. Association between cholecystectomy with vs without intraoperative cholangiography and risk of common duct injury. JAMA 2013;310(8):812–20.
18. Ludwig K, Bernhardt J, Steffen H, et al. Contribution of intraoperative cholangiography to incidence and outcome of common bile duct injuries during laparoscopic cholecystectomy. Surg Endosc 2002;16(7):1098–104.
19. Strasberg SM, Hertl M, Soper NJ. An analysis of the problem of biliary injury during laparoscopic cholecystectomy. J Am Coll Surg 1995;180(1):101–25.

20. Strasberg SM, Brunt LM. Rationale and use of the critical view of safety in lapa-roscopic cholecystectomy. J Am Coll Surg 2010;211(1):132–8.
21. Thompson DM, Arregui ME, Tetik C, et al. A comparison of laparoscopic ultra-sound with digital fluorocholangiography for detecting choledocholithiasis during laparoscopic cholecystectomy. Surg Endosc 1998;12(7):929–32.
22. Falcone RA Jr, Fegelman EJ, Nussbaum MS, et al. A prospective comparison of laparoscopic ultrasound vs intraoperative cholangiogram during laparoscopic cholecystectomy. Surg Endosc 1999;13(8):784–8.
23. Patel AC, Arregui ME. Current status of laparoscopic ultrasound. Surg Technol Int 2006;15:23–31.
24. Tranter SE, Thompson MH. A prospective single-blinded controlled study comparing laparoscopic ultrasound of the common bile duct with operative chol-angiography. Surg Endosc 2003;17(2):216–9.
25. Onders RP. Ultrasound: the basics for laparoscopy. In: Talamini MA, editor. Advanced therapy in minimally invasive surgery. Oxford (United Kingdom): BC Decker; 2006. p. 53–8.
26. Videhult P, Sandblom G, Rasmussen IC. How reliable is intraoperative chol-angiography as a method for detecting common bile duct stones?: a pro-spective population-based study on 1171 patients. Surg Endosc 2009; 23(2):304–12.
27. Machi J, Tateishi T, Oishi AJ, et al. Laparoscopic ultrasonography versus opera-tive cholangiography during laparoscopic cholecystectomy: review of the litera-ture and a comparison with open intraoperative ultrasonography. J Am Coll Surg 1999;188(4):360–7.
28. Kroh M, Chand B. Choledocholithiasis, endoscopic retrograde cholangiopan-creatography, and laparoscopic common bile duct exploration. Surg Clin North Am 2008;88(5):1019–31, vii.
29. Verbesey JE, Birkett DH. Common bile duct exploration for choledocholithiasis. Surg Clin North Am 2008;88(6):1315–28, ix.
30. Gurusamy KS, Koti R, Davidson BR. T-tube drainage versus primary closure after laparoscopic common bile duct exploration. Cochrane Database Syst Rev 2013;(6):CD005641.
31. Yin Z, Xu K, Sun J, et al. Is the end of the T-tube drainage era in laparoscopic choledochotomy for common bile duct stones is coming? A systematic review and meta-analysis. Ann Surg 2013;257(1):54–66.
32. Ahmed I, Pradhan C, Beckingham IJ, et al. Is a T-tube necessary after common bile duct exploration? World J Surg 2008;32(7):1485–8.
33. Shojaiefard A, Esmaeilzadeh M, Ghafouri A, et al. Various techniques for the surgical treatment of common bile duct stones: a meta review. Gastroenterol Res Pract 2009;2009:840208.
34. Shi H, Chen S, Swar G, et al. Carbon dioxide insufflation during endoscopic retro-grade cholangiopancreatography: a review and meta-analysis. Pancreas 2013; 42(7):1093–100.
35. Pessaux P, Tuech JJ, Rouge C, et al. Laparoscopic cholecystectomy in acute cholecystitis. A prospective comparative study in patients with acute vs. chronic cholecystitis. Surg Endosc 2000;14(4):358–61.
36. Yetkin G, Uludag M, Oba S, et al. Laparoscopic cholecystectomy in elderly patients. JSLS 2009;13(4):587–91.
37. Dolan JP, Diggs BS, Sheppard BC, et al. The national mortality burden and significant factors associated with open and laparoscopic cholecystectomy: 1997-2006. J Gastrointest Surg 2009;13(12):2292–301.

38. Orenstein SB, Kaban GK, Litwin DE, et al. Evaluation of serum cytokine release in response to hand-assisted, laparoscopic, and open surgery in a porcine model. Am J Surg 2011;202(1):97–102.

39. Giger UF, Michel JM, Opitz I, et al. Risk factors for perioperative complications in patients undergoing laparoscopic cholecystectomy: analysis of 22,953 consecutive cases from the Swiss Association of Laparoscopic and Thoracoscopic Surgery database. J Am Coll Surg 2006;203(5):723–8.

40. Turner PL, Malangoni M. Cholecystectomy-surgical removal of the gallbladder (patient education). American College of Surgeons; 2013. Available at: http://www.facs.org/patienteducation. Accessed May 27, 2013.

41. Berci G, Hunter J, Morgenstern L, et al. Laparoscopic cholecystectomy: first, do no harm; second, take care of bile duct stones. Surg Endosc 2013;27(4):1051–4.

42. Chung RS, Ahmed N. The impact of minimally invasive surgery on residents' open operative experience: analysis of two decades of national data. Ann Surg 2010;251(2):205–12.

43. Eckert M, Cuadrado D, Steele S, et al. The changing face of the general surgeon: national and local trends in resident operative experience. Am J Surg 2010; 199(5):652–6.

Iatrogenic Biliary Injuries
Identification, Classification, and Management

Lygia Stewart, MD

KEYWORDS

- Bile duct injury • Biliary stricture • Laparoscopic cholecystectomy • Management
- Biliary-enteric anastomosis

KEY POINTS

- Laparoscopic bile duct injuries are more complex than those seen in the open era.
- The unique features of the laparoscopic environment facilitate these injuries; because of this, injuries involving misidentification of the common bile duct (CBD) for the cystic duct are the most common, resulting in a resectional injury of the main CBD and portions of the hepatic duct or ducts.
- The laparoscopic environment facilitates this illusion, so these injuries are generally not recognized intraoperatively. In addition, because many of these injuries present with a biliary fistula, as opposed to obstruction, clinical manifestations are often more subtle.
- The key to successful treatment is early recognition, control of intra-abdominal bile ascites and inflammation, nutritional repletion, and repair by a surgeon with expertise in biliary reconstruction. If these requirements are met, patients can have successful repair with long-term success in more than 90% of cases.

INTRODUCTION

More than 750,000 laparoscopic cholecystectomies are performed annually in the United States. Laparoscopic cholecystectomy offers several advantages over open cholecystectomy, including less pain, fewer wound infections, improved cosmesis, decreased activation of inflammatory mediators, and an earlier return to normal activities. Because of these advantages, laparoscopic cholecystectomy has largely replaced open cholecystectomy for the management of symptomatic gallstone disease. The only potential disadvantage to laparoscopic cholecystectomy is a higher incidence of major bile duct injury.[1–11] Several large population-based studies indicate that the incidence of major bile duct injury is 0.3% to 0.5%, which is higher than the 0.1% to 0.2% incidence reported with open cholecystectomy.[1–8] Some recent series[9,10] report a 0.2% incidence of bile duct injury with laparoscopic cholecystectomy, which approaches that seen in open series; however, single-incision laparoscopic cholecystectomy is associated with an even higher rate of bile duct injury (0.72%).[11]

Department of Surgery (112), University of California San Francisco and San Francisco VA Medical Center, San Francisco, CA 94121, USA
E-mail address: lygia.stewart@va.gov

Surg Clin N Am 94 (2014) 297–310
http://dx.doi.org/10.1016/j.suc.2014.01.008
0039-6109/14/$ – see front matter Published by Elsevier Inc.
surgical.theclinics.com

Obviously, prevention of these biliary injuries is ideal; however, when they do occur, early identification and appropriate treatment are critical to improving the outcomes of patients suffering a major bile duct injury. This report delineates the key factors in classification (and its relationship to mechanism and management), identification (intraoperative and postoperative), and management principles of these bile duct injuries.

CLASSIFICATION
Bismuth and Strasberg Classifications

Before the advent of laparoscopic cholecystectomy, biliary strictures were classified using the Bismuth classification (**Table 1**).[12,13] This useful classification delineated the severity of the biliary stricture based on the level of the biliary injury. The Strasberg classification[14] is similar to the Bismuth, but incorporates a few additional biliary injuries seen more commonly in the laparoscopic era (**Fig. 1**; see **Table 1**).

Stewart-Way Classification

The Stewart-Way classification incorporates the mechanism of the bile duct injury as well as its anatomy (**Table 2**). This approach is useful because it provides a means for the prevention of bile duct injury. The creators of this system found that an analysis of human error and cognitive processing provided considerable insight into the mechanisms of these bile duct injuries, the role of the laparoscopic environment in their facilitation, and improved means for their prevention.[15–19] This classification also differentiates between resectional injuries and strictures, a distinction useful in guiding preoperative evaluation and biliary reconstruction. The injury classification is as follows (**Fig. 2**A).

Class I injuries (6% of cases) involve an incision in the common bile duct (CBD) with no loss of duct. These injuries occur when the CBD is mistaken for the cystic duct, but the mistake is recognized during the initial operation (often with operative cholangiography); or when an incision in the cystic duct for a cholangiogram catheter is unintentionally extended into the CBD.

Class II injuries (24% of cases) consist of lateral damage to the hepatic duct with a resultant stenosis and/or fistula. These injuries result from unintended application of clips or cautery to the bile duct, usually during attempts to control bleeding in the triangle of Calot. For one reason or another the surgeon was working too deep in the triangle of Calot, unknowingly close to the common hepatic duct (CHD).

Class III injuries, the most common (60% of cases), involve transection and excision of a variable length of the duct, which always includes the cystic duct–common duct junction. Class III injuries result from a misperception error whereby the CBD is misidentified as the cystic duct. The surgeon transects the common duct (deliberately, thinking it is the cystic duct) early in the dissection and then transects the CHD (unknowingly) later in the process of separating the gallbladder from the liver bed. Consequently, the central portion of the extrahepatic bile duct is removed along with the gallbladder.

Class II and III injuries are subdivided based on the proximal extent of the injury as follows (see **Fig. 2**B). Class II/IIIA injuries spare the bifurcation with a remnant of CHD remaining. Class II/IIIB involves transection or stricture at the bifurcation of the CHD. Class II/IIIC results from extension of the stricture or duct excision above the bifurcation. Class IIID injuries (not seen with Class II) result from resection/transection above the first bifurcation of the lobar ducts. This last group (IIID) is uncommon and results from following the extrahepatic biliary tree into the porta with excision of all extrahepatic ducts.

Table 1
Bismuth and Strasberg classifications

Biliary Anatomy	Bismuth	Strasberg
Cystic duct leak or leak from small ducts in liver bed	—	A
Occlusion of an aberrant RHD	—	B
Transection without ligation of an aberrant RHD	—	C
Lateral injury to CBD (<50% circumference)	—	D
CHD stricture, stump >2 cm	Type 1	E1
CHD stricture, stump <2 cm	Type 2	E2
Hilar stricture, no residual CHD, confluence is preserved	Type 3	E3
Hilar stricture, involvement of confluence, loss of communication between RHD and LHD	Type 4	E4
Stricture of low-lying right sectorial duct (alone or with concomitant CHD stricture)	Type 5	—
Injury to an aberrant RHD plus injury in the hilum	Type 5	E5

Abbreviations: CBD, common bile duct; CHD, common hepatic duct; LHD, left hepatic duct; RHD, right hepatic duct.

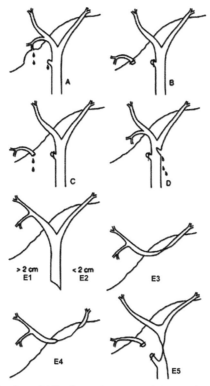

Fig. 1. Strasberg classification of bile duct injuries: injuries stratified from type A to type E. Type E injuries are further subdivided into E1 to E5 according to the Bismuth classification system. (*From* Strasberg SM, Hertl M, Soper NJ. An analysis of the problem of biliary injury during laparoscopic cholecystectomy. J Am Coll Surg 1995;180:105.)

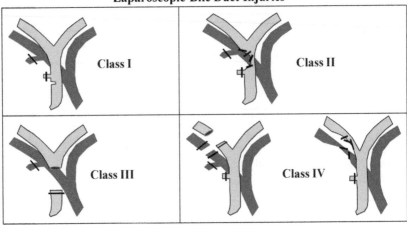

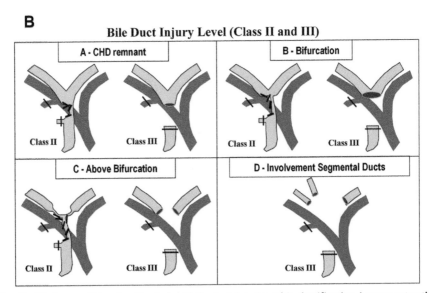

Fig. 2. (*A*) Stewart-Way classification of bile duct injuries. This classification incorporates the mechanism of injury as well as anatomic considerations. (*B*) Stewart-Way subclassification of levels of bile duct injury. This subclassification defines the levels of the Class II and Class III bile duct injuries, depending on the level of the injury. Note that the highest level, D, only occurs with Class III injuries (resectional injury with complete excision of the extrahepatic biliary tree). The Class III D injury pattern is not accounted for in the Bismuth and Strasberg classifications.

Class IV injuries (10% of cases) involve damage (transection or injury) of the right hepatic duct (RHD) (or a right sectoral duct), often (60%) combined with injury to the right hepatic artery (RHA). Class IV injuries are caused either by misidentifying the RHD (or a right sectoral duct) as the cystic duct and the RHA as the cystic artery; or from lateral injury to the RHD (or a right sectoral duct) during the dissection deep in the triangle of Calot.

Table 2
Stewart-Way classification: mechanism of major bile duct injury

Mechanism of Laparoscopic Bile Duct Injury	Associated RHA Injury (%)
Class I CBD mistaken for cystic duct, but recognized Cholangiogram incision in cystic duct extended into CBD	5
Class II Lateral damage to the CHD from cautery or clips placed on duct Associated bleeding, poor visibility	20
Class III CBD mistaken for cystic duct, not recognized CBD, CHD, RHD, LHD transected and/or resected	35

Class IV   RHD (or right sectoral duct) mistaken for cystic duct, RHA mistaken
     for cystic artery; RHD (or right sectoral duct) and RHA transected
     Lateral damage to the RHD (or right sectoral duct) from cautery or
     clips placed on duct
	60

Abbreviations: CBD, common bile duct; CHD, common hepatic duct; LHD, left hepatic duct; RHA, right hepatic artery; RHD, right hepatic duct.

Because the RHA lies posterior to the CBD, it can be injured or even transected in laparoscopic bile duct injuries.[18] This occurrence is particularly common in cases of resectional Class IV injury whereby the RHA is thought to be a large cystic artery and is consequently divided. The association between biliary injury and RHA injury is also shown in **Table 2**.

IDENTIFICATION OF BILE DUCT INJURY
Intraoperative Bile Duct Injury

A minority of bile duct injuries are recognized during the index cholecystectomy, only about 25% in most series. There are several factors that facilitate recognition of intraoperative injury, but the most important is a change in the surgeon's awareness to suspect and/or evaluate for a bile duct injury.[15] Several features of the gallbladder dissection might indicate the possibility of major bile duct injury. It is fundamental to remember that the CBD lies medial to the gallbladder and that the RHA passes behind the CBD in 80% to 90% of cases.

Analysis of operative reports among patients with bile duct injury[15,19] revealed several possible signs that might have indicated the dissection was in the wrong plane:

- Cholangiographic abnormalities with signs that the cholangiocatheter is unintentionally in the CBD
  - Failure to opacify the proximal hepatic ducts above the catheter balloon (**Fig. 3**A, compare with **Fig. 3**B)
  - Narrowing of the CBD at the site of the cholangiocatheter insertion
  - Failure to opacify a portion of the cystic duct
    - Can also occur when the incision for the cholangiocatheter is too close to the CBD (can result in a Class I injury)
- Bile drainage (obtain a cholangiogram)
  - Drainage of bile from a location other than a lacerated gallbladder
  - Bile draining from a tubular structure
- Second cystic artery or large artery posterior to what is perceived to be the cystic duct
  - This could be the RHA, which means that the CBD is being dissected

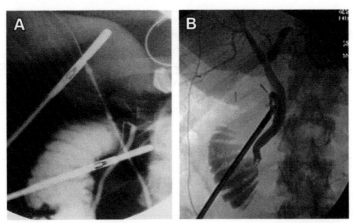

Fig. 3. (*A*) Intraoperative cholangiogram taken when the cholangiocatheter is in the common bile duct (CBD). Note that the proximal biliary radicles do not fill. In this case the CBD has been confused with the cystic duct. (*B*) Normal intraoperative cholangiogram showing opacification of the cystic duct, CBD, hepatic duct, right and left hepatic ducts, and the duodenum. Compare with panel *A*.

- Identification of an extra bile duct or tubular structure (obtain a cholangiogram)
  - This can be a sign that the CBD (rather than the cystic duct) is being dissected
  - It could be the proximal portion of a transected CHD
  - Have a high index of suspicion: resist the tendency to assign this as a second cystic artery, tubular structure, aberrant bile duct, or duct of Luschka
- Ductal abnormalities (obtain a cholangiogram)
  - Wide cystic duct: this may be the CBD
  - Accessory bile duct, duct of Luschka, second cystic duct: this may be the proximal CHD
  - Short cystic duct
    - This can be associated with bile duct injury
    - The tissue between the gallbladder infundibulum and CBD may have not been completely dissected, which can result in a bile duct injury
  - Bile duct can be traced to the duodenum: this is always the CBD
- Anomalous anatomy (obtain a cholangiogram)
  - Extra lymphatics or vessels around the cystic duct may indicate the CBD is being dissected
  - Abnormal gallbladder infundibulum may indicate the CBD is being dissected
    - Infundibulum goes deep toward the duodenum
    - Redundant infundibulum
  - Fibrous tissue in the gallbladder bed may indicate transection of the proximal CHD
  - Cystic duct structures seem more medial than usual
- Severe hemorrhage or inflammation (consider conversion to an open procedure)
  - Common mechanisms for Class II injuries

Surgeons who use clues, such as those listed, to consider the possibility of and search for a bile duct injury, can more commonly recognize the injury during the index operation.[15,19] This identification allows for prompt treatment of the injury. Recognition of a Class I injury with a cholangiogram also prevents it from being converted to a Class III injury.

Postoperative Bile Duct Injury

Unlike the open cholecystectomy era, during which patients with a biliary injury presented with the triad of jaundice, dilated bile ducts, and abdominal pain, most patients with a laparoscopic bile duct injury have an associated biliary fistula, are not jaundiced, and present in a more subtle fashion.[16,17] Most Class I and Class III injuries will have an associated biliary fistula, and about 50% of Class II and Class IV injuries also have an associated biliary fistula. Patients with a biliary fistula do not present with jaundice (liver function tests are minimally elevated) and their findings can be very subtle initially; for example, patients are sometimes treated for constipation when presenting to an emergency department. Despite large amounts of bile in the abdomen, most patients with bile collections do not present with bile peritonitis; instead they have bile ascites, with mild, relatively nonspecific symptoms including bloating and mild abdominal pain. Because of these vague symptoms, the presence of a bile collection and associated biliary injury can go unsuspected for some time. With a delay in diagnosis, bile peritonitis and serious illness can develop. In an analysis by the author's group, undrained bile for longer than 9 days was more often associated with bile peritonitis (and infected bile).[16] On the other hand, patients with biliary strictures are often recognized earlier because they present with the more classic presentation (jaundice, dilated ducts, and abdominal pain).

The key to early recognition is to suspect a problem in any patient who fails to do well following laparoscopic cholecystectomy. Because these patients usually do extremely well, any deviation from this should be recognized as a problem. A computed tomography (CT) scan should be obtained to look for bile. Ultrasonography can also be used, but is less sensitive and can lead to diagnostic delay. Cholescintigraphy scans should be avoided because they are much less reliable. In addition, nondilated bile ducts are the usual finding with laparoscopic biliary injuries, not dilated ducts. If a fluid collection is present, one should assume that it is bile and that there may be a bile duct injury, and the bile should be immediately drained percutaneously using interventional techniques.

There is no role for exploratory laparotomy, as this is associated with increased morbidity; in cases where this was used the diagnosis was often missed, and even if the injury was identified, the surgeon was generally not prepared to manage the complication.[17] In addition, patients with bile draining from an operatively placed drain should have complete evaluation for a possible biliary injury.

Complete cholangiography

Once the bile collection is drained, complete cholangiography of the biliary tree should be obtained. Complete cholangiography should also be obtained in patients with bile in an operative drain or obstructive jaundice. Cases with cystic duct leaks, Class I injuries, and most Class II injuries can generally be imaged with endoscopic retrograde cholangiopancreatography (ERCP). Both an ERCP and percutaneous transhepatic cholangiogram (PTC) are necessary to image the biliary tree in patients with Class III (**Fig. 4**) and most Class IV injuries. In all cases an ERCP should be obtained first, followed by a PTC if the entire biliary tree is not imaged.

Concomitant vascular injury

Some patients have associated injury to the RHA. These patients have a higher incidence of bleeding and hepatic abscess at presentation. Cases with an associated RHA injury more commonly have an associated hepatic abscess, bleeding, hemobilia, and right hepatic lobe ischemia.[18,20–30] As shown in **Table 2**, concurrent RHA injury was most common among patients with Class IV injuries, followed by those with Class

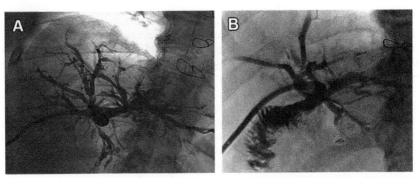

Fig. 4. (A) Percutaneous cholangiogram showing Class III injury. (B) Percutaneous cholangiogram of the patient in A, showing successful biliary reconstruction.

III injuries. It is important to consider this diagnosis in patients who have had a laparoscopic cholecystectomy and who present with significant hemorrhage, right hepatic ischemia, or hepatic abscess. Many of these patients require angioembolization for treatment of hemobilia and drainage of hepatic abscesses, and some require hepatectomy.[17,18,20–27] In rare cases, patients can also have associated injury to the portal vessels, and portal-vessel injury has also been reported to rarely occur following PTC.[18]

MANAGEMENT
Preoperative Evaluation

To guide surgical management, the full extent of the injury has to be defined. This evaluation requires complete cholangiography (as noted earlier). In addition, CT scan with intravenous contrast should be obtained to elucidate any evidence for vascular injuries, hepatic abscess, or presence of hepatic ischemia (generally right-sided if present).

Preoperative Patient Preparation

Before consideration of biliary injury repair, the patient needs to be stabilized and optimized for surgery. Control of intra-abdominal fluid collections, inflammation, and infection is essential, and is best achieved with percutaneous drainage. In addition, in some cases the patient presents in a debilitated state with poor nutritional status (manifested by decreased serum albumin and prealbumin) and poor functional status. Such patients require preoperative nutritional repletion and time to recover from the acute illness. Nutritional formulas that are associated with better outcomes in surgical patients can also be used preoperatively to optimize these patients.[31,32] Repair of the biliary injury is only performed once all intra-abdominal inflammation and infection has been controlled, the patient has regained functional status, and nutrition is restored. The time to achieve this depends largely on the patient's presentation and clinical course. By contrast, for patients referred early, with good control of intra-abdominal inflammation and normal nutritional state there is no need to delay operative repair.[33]

Surgical Management Principles

Bile duct injuries can be very serious complications that, if managed improperly, can result in life-threatening complications such as cholangitis, biliary cirrhosis, and portal hypertension. Even with successful management, quality of life may be diminished and survival may be impaired, especially in elderly patients.[34–37] In general, these injuries are less commonly managed successfully by the primary surgeon who performs the initial cholecystectomy. Biliary reconstruction by the primary surgeon results in success rates of between 17% and 30%.[33,38–40] There are very good data to suggest that these injuries are best managed by a surgeon with expertise in biliary reconstruction. If these biliary injuries are managed by such surgeons, outcomes can be excellent; many expert surgical series report long-term success rates of greater than 90%.[17,18,22,23,33,39,41–75] Given that the management of these injuries often requires an experienced multidisciplinary team (including interventional radiology, gastroenterology, and surgery), they are best managed in a tertiary referral center.

The tenets of a successful biliary surgical repair include:

- Eradication of all intra-abdominal infection and inflammation
- Anastomoses to healthy bile duct tissue
- Single-layer anastomoses using fine monofilament absorbable suture (Maxon or PDS)
- Tension-free anastomoses
- Roux-en-Y hepaticojejunostomy, in most cases
  - Retrocolic Roux limb
  - 40 to 60 cm length
- Experienced biliary surgeon
- Presence or absence of a biliary stent does not influence results

Specific Biliary Injuries

Cystic duct leaks

Cystic duct leaks are well managed with ERCP, stenting (with or without sphincterotomy), and drainage of intra-abdominal bile collections. Nearly all cystic duct leaks will close with this management scheme. It is crucial to drain bile collections; the stent only acts to decrease the pressure in the biliary tree, it does not cover the leak and prevent bile drainage.

Class I injuries

Class I injuries, which are recognized intraoperatively, can be immediately repaired using fine monofilament absorbable suture. These injuries are usually recognized with cholangiography, so only the small incision used to insert the cholangiocatheter needs to be repaired. There is no need to insert a T-tube. Extension of the laceration to facilitate T-tube insertion results in progression of the injury and an increased likelihood of stricture. The best approach is simple suture of the injury.

Bile duct injuries recognized intraoperatively

If bile duct injuries, other than Class I, are recognized intraoperatively, there are 2 options. If a biliary specialist is readily available he or she should be called for immediate reconstruction. If not, a drain can be placed (to evacuate bile) and the patient immediately referred to a biliary specialist for reconstruction. In general, repair by the primary surgeon is associated with less favorable outcomes, and sometimes the attempted repair can further damage the ducts and make subsequent reconstruction more difficult. Surgeons should take into consideration the magnitude of the injury and their own experience in biliary surgery when determining the best approach for management of these biliary injuries.

Class IV injuries

Class IV injuries that involve a sectoral bile duct and that do not include transection of the duct can often be managed nonoperatively. There is a growing body of literature in this area. Such patients can be treated with drainage and nonoperative stenting via either ERCP (preferred) or PTC, with good results in many cases.[75–78]

Class IV injuries involving transection of the bile ducts require reconstruction of the duct (either the RHD or a right sectoral duct) into a defunctionalized Roux limb. These ducts should not be sutured to the main hepatic duct, as this can increase the magnitude of the injury.

Timing of Biliary Reconstruction

Several studies reported that the timing of biliary reconstruction influences outcomes; these series reported worse outcomes for biliary reconstructions performed within 6 weeks of injury.[48,71,73] Stewart and Way[33] examined this question, using multivariate analysis, and noted that the timing of repair was not an independent predictor of successful biliary repair. Instead, success correlated with eradication of intra-abdominal infection, complete preoperative cholangiography, use of correct surgical technique, and repair by an experienced biliary surgeon. This timing issue most likely relates to the time required to eradicate intra-abdominal inflammation and to achieve nutritional repletion. In this series, good results were achieved with early biliary reconstruction in those patients with good nutrition, good functional status, and early control of intra-abdominal inflammation.[33]

SUMMARY

Laparoscopic bile duct injuries are more complex than those seen during the open era. The unique features of the laparoscopic environment facilitate these injuries and, because of this, injuries involving misidentification of the CBD for the cystic duct are the most common. This error results in a resectional injury of the main CBD and portions of the hepatic duct or ducts. The laparoscopic environment facilitates this illusion, so these injuries are generally not recognized intraoperatively. In addition, because many of these injuries present with a biliary fistula, as opposed to obstruction, clinical manifestations are often more subtle. The key to successful treatment is early recognition, control of intra-abdominal bile ascites and inflammation, nutritional repletion, and repair by a surgeon with expertise in biliary reconstruction. If these requirements are met, patients can have successful repair with long-term success in more than 90% of cases.

REFERENCES

1. Deziel DJ, Millikan KW, Economou SG, et al. Complications of laparoscopic cholecystectomy: a national survey of 4,292 hospitals and an analysis of 77,604 cases. Am J Surg 1993;165:9–14.
2. Vecchio R, MacFadyen BV, Latteri S. Laparoscopic cholecystectomy: an analysis on 114,005 cases of United States series. Int Surg 1998;83:215–9.
3. Adamsen S, Hansen OH, Funch-Jensen P, et al. Bile duct injury during laparoscopic cholecystectomy: a prospective nationwide series. J Am Coll Surg 1997; 184:571–8.
4. Nuzzo G, Giuliante F, Giovannini I, et al. Bile duct injury during laparoscopic cholecystectomy: results of an Italian national survey on 56,591 cholecystectomies. Arch Surg 2005;140:986–92.
5. Harboe KM, Bardram L. The quality of cholecystectomy in Denmark: outcome and risk factors for 20,307 patients from the national database. Surg Endosc 2011;25:1630–41.

6. Waage A, Nilsson M. Iatrogenic bile duct injury: a population-based study of 152 776 cholecystectomies in the Swedish Inpatient Registry. Arch Surg 2006; 141:1207–13.

7. A prospective analysis of 1518 laparoscopic cholecystectomies. The Southern Surgeons Club. N Engl J Med 1991;324:1073–8.

8. Tantia O, Jain M, Khanna S, et al. Iatrogenic biliary injury: 13,305 cholecystectomies experienced by a single surgical team over more than 13 years. Surg Endosc 2008;22:1077–86.

9. Ahmad J, McElvanna K, McKie L, et al. Biliary complications during a decade of increased cholecystectomy rate. Ulster Med J 2012;81:79–82.

10. Pekolj J, Alvarez FA, Palavecino M, et al. Intraoperative management and repair of bile duct injuries sustained during 10,123 laparoscopic cholecystectomies in a high-volume referral center. J Am Coll Surg 2013;216(5):894–901.

11. Joseph M, Phillips MR, Farrell TM, et al. Single incision laparoscopic cholecystectomy is associated with a higher bile duct injury rate: a review and a word of caution. Ann Surg 2012;256:1–6.

12. Bismuth H. Postoperative strictures of the bile ducts. In: Blumgart LH, editor. The biliary tract. 5th edition. Edinburgh: Churchill-Livingstone; 1982. p. 209–18.

13. Bismuth H, Majno PE. Biliary strictures: classification based on the principles of surgical treatment. World J Surg 2001;25:1241–4.

14. Strasberg SM, Hertl M, Soper NJ. An analysis of the problem of biliary injury during laparoscopic cholecystectomy. J Am Coll Surg 1995;180:101–25.

15. Stewart L, Dominguez CO, Way LW. A data/frame sensemaking analysis of operative reports. In: Mosier K, Fischer U, editors. Informed by knowledge: expert performance in complex situations. New York: Taylor & Francis; 2011. p. 329–38.

16. Lee CM, Stewart L, Way LW. Postcholecystectomy abdominal bile collections. Arch Surg 2000;135:538–44.

17. Stewart L. Treatment strategies for bile duct injury and Benign biliary stricture. In: Poston G, Blumgart L, editors. Hepatobiliary and pancreatic surgery. 1st edition. London: Martin Dunitz; 2002. p. 315–29.

18. Stewart L, Robinson TN, Lee CM, et al. Right hepatic artery injury associated with laparoscopic bile duct injury: incidence, mechanism, and consequences. J Gastrointest Surg 2004;8:523–30 [discussion: 530–1].

19. Way LW, Stewart L, Gantert W, et al. Causes and prevention of laparoscopic bile duct injuries: analysis of 252 cases from a human factors and cognitive psychology perspective. Ann Surg 2003;237:460–9.

20. Majno PE, Pretre R, Mentha G, et al. Operative injury to the hepatic artery. Consequences of a biliary-enteric anastomosis and principles for rational management. Arch Surg 1996;131:211–5.

21. Mathisen O, Soreide O, Bergan A. Laparoscopic cholecystectomy: bile duct and vascular injuries: management and outcome. Scand J Gastroenterol 2002;37:476–81.

22. Bachellier P, Nakano H, Weber JC, et al. Surgical repair after bile duct and vascular injuries during laparoscopic cholecystectomy: when and how? World J Surg 2001;25:1335–45.

23. Gupta N, Solomon H, Fairchild R, et al. Management and outcome of patients with combined bile duct and hepatic artery injuries. Arch Surg 1998;133:176–81.

24. Koffron A, Ferrario M, Parsons W, et al. Failed primary management of iatrogenic biliary injury: incidence and significance of concomitant hepatic arterial disruption. Surgery 2001;130:722–31.

25. Buell JF, Cronin DC, Funaki B, et al. Devastating and fatal complications associated with combined vascular and bile duct injuries during cholecystectomy. Arch Surg 2002;137:703–10.
26. Nishio H, Kamiya J, Nagino M, et al. Right hepatic lobectomy for bile duct injury associated with major vascular occlusion after laparoscopic cholecystectomy. J Hepatobiliary Pancreat Surg 1999;6:427–30.
27. Kayaalp C, Nessar G, Kaman S, et al. Right liver necrosis: complication of laparoscopic cholecystectomy. Hepatogastroenterology 2001;48:1727–9.
28. Laurent AM, Sauvanet AM, Farges OM, et al. Major hepatectomy for the treatment of complex bile duct injury. Ann Surg 2008;248(1):77–83.
29. Schmidt SC, Settmacher U, Langrehr JM, et al. Management and outcome of patients with combined bile duct and hepatic arterial injuries after laparoscopic cholecystectomy. Surgery 2004;135:613–8.
30. Li J, Frilling A, Nadalin S, et al. Management of concomitant hepatic artery injury in patients with iatrogenic major bile duct injury after laparoscopic cholecystectomy. Br J Surg 2008;95:460–5.
31. Heyland DK, Novak F, Drover JW, et al. Should immunonutrition become routine in critically ill patients? A systematic review of the evidence. JAMA 2001;286:944–53.
32. Kudsk KA. Immunonutrition in surgery and critical care. Annu Rev Nutr 2006;26: 463–79.
33. Stewart L, Way LW. Repair of laparoscopic bile duct injuries: timing of surgical repair does not influence success rate. HPB (Oxford) 2009;11:516–22.
34. Boerma D, Rauws EA, Keulemans YC, et al. Impaired quality of life 5 years after bile duct injury during laparoscopic cholecystectomy: a prospective analysis. Ann Surg 2001;234:750–7.
35. Moore DE, Feurer ID, Holzman MD, et al. Long-term detrimental effect of bile duct injury on health-related quality of life. Arch Surg 2004;139:476–81.
36. Flum DR, Cheadle A, Prela C, et al. Bile duct injury during cholecystectomy and survival in Medicare beneficiaries. JAMA 2003;290:2168–73.
37. Melton GB, Lillemoe KD, Cameron JL, et al. Major bile duct injuries associated with laparoscopic cholecystectomy: effect of surgical repair on quality of life. Ann Surg 2002;235:888–96.
38. Andrén Sandberg A, Johansson S, Bengmark S. Accidental lesions of the common bile duct at cholecystectomy. II. Results of treatment. Ann Surg 1985; 201(4):452–5.
39. Stewart L, Way LW. Bile duct injuries during laparoscopic cholecystectomy. Factors that influence the results of treatment. Arch Surg 1995;130:1123–8 [discussion: 1129].
40. Carroll BJ, Birth M, Phillips EH. Common bile duct injuries during laparoscopic cholecystectomy that result in litigation. Surg Endosc 1998;12:310–3 [discussion: 314].
41. Ahrendt AS, Pitt HA. Surgical therapy of iatrogenic lesions of biliary tract. World J Surg 2001;25:1360–5.
42. Bergman JJ, van den Brink GR, Rauws EA, et al. Treatment of bile duct lesions after laparoscopic cholecystectomy. Gut 1996;38:141–7.
43. Branum G, Schmitt C, Baillie J, et al. Management of major biliary complications after laparoscopic cholecystectomy. Ann Surg 1993;217:532–40 [discussion: 540–1].
44. Calvete J, Sabater L, Camps B, et al. Bile duct injury during laparoscopic cholecystectomy: myth or reality of the learning curve? Surg Endosc 2000;14: 608–11.

45. Chapman WC, Halevy A, Blumgart LH, et al. Postcholecystectomy bile duct strictures. Management and outcome in 130 patients. Arch Surg 1995;130: 597–602 [discussion: 602–4].
46. Csendes A, Navarrete C, Burdiles P, et al. Treatment of common bile duct injuries during laparoscopic cholecystectomy: endoscopic and surgical management. World J Surg 2001;25:1346–51.
47. Davids PH, Tanka AK, Rauws EA, et al. Benign biliary strictures. Surgery or endoscopy? Ann Surg 1993;217:237–43.
48. de Reuver PR, Grossmann I, Busch OR, et al. Referral pattern and timing of repair are risk factors for complications after reconstructive surgery for bile duct injury. Ann Surg 2007;245:763–70.
49. Frilling A, Li J, Weber F, et al. Major bile duct injuries after laparoscopic cholecystectomy: a tertiary center experience. J Gastrointest Surg 2004;8:679–85.
50. Gigot J, Etienne J, Aerts R, et al. The dramatic reality of biliary tract injury during laparoscopic cholecystectomy. An anonymous multicenter Belgian survey of 65 patients. Surg Endosc 1997;11:1171–8.
51. Innes JT, Ferrara JJ, Carey LC. Biliary reconstruction without transanastomotic stent. Am Surg 1988;54:27–30.
52. Johnson SR, Koehler A, Pennington LK, et al. Long-term results of surgical repair of bile duct injuries following laparoscopic cholecystectomy. Surgery 2000;128:668–77.
53. Lillemoe KD, Martin SA, Cameron JL, et al. Major bile duct injuries during laparoscopic cholecystectomy. Follow-up after combined surgical and radiologic management. Ann Surg 1997;225:459–68 [discussion: 468–71].
54. Lillemoe KD. Current management of bile duct injury. Br J Surg 2008;95:403–5.
55. Lillemoe KD, Melton GB, Cameron JL, et al. Postoperative bile duct strictures: management and outcome in the 1990s. Ann Surg 2000;232:430–41.
56. Lillemoe KD, Petrofski JA, Choti MA, et al. Isolated right segmental hepatic duct injury: a diagnostic and therapeutic challenge. J Gastrointest Surg 2000;4: 168–77.
57. McMahon AJ, Fullarton G, Baxter JN, et al. Bile duct injury and bile leakage in laparoscopic cholecystectomy. Br J Surg 1995;82:307–13.
58. Mercado MA. Early versus late repair of bile duct injuries. Surg Endosc 2006;20: 1644–7.
59. Mercado MA, Chan C, Orozco H, et al. Prognostic implications of preserved bile duct confluence after iatrogenic injury. Hepatogastroenterology 2005;52:40–4.
60. Mercado B, Franssen BI, Dominguez JC, et al. Transition from a low: to a high-volume centre for bile duct repair: changes in technique and improved outcome. HPB (Oxford) 2011;13:767–73.
61. Mirza DF, Narsimhan KL, Ferraz Neto BH, et al. Bile duct injury following laparoscopic cholecystectomy: referral pattern and management. Br J Surg 1997;84: 786–90.
62. Moraca RJ, Lee FT, Ryan JA, et al. Long-term biliary function after reconstruction of major bile duct injuries with hepaticoduodenostomy or hepaticojejunostomy. Arch Surg 2002;137:889–94.
63. Murr MM, Gigot JF, Nagorney DM, et al. Long-term results of biliary reconstruction after laparoscopic bile duct injuries. Arch Surg 1999;134:604–9 [discussion: 609–10].
64. Nordin A, Halme L, Makisalo H, et al. Management and outcome of major bile duct injuries after laparoscopic cholecystectomy: from therapeutic endoscopy to liver transplantation. Liver Transpl 2002;8:1036–43.

65. Ooi LL, Goh YC, Chew SP, et al. Bile duct injuries during laparoscopic cholecystectomy: a collective experience of four teaching hospitals and results of repair. Aust N Z J Surg 1999;69:844–6.

66. Pitt HA, Kaufman SL, Coleman J, et al. Benign postoperative biliary strictures: operate or dilate? Ann Surg 1989;210:417–27.

67. Ragozzino A, De Ritis R, Mosca A, et al. Value of MR cholangiography in patients with iatrogenic bile duct injury after cholecystectomy. Am J Roentgenol 2004;183:1567–72.

68. Savader SJ, Lillemoe KD, Prescott CA, et al. Laparoscopic cholecystectomy-related bile duct injuries: a health and financial disaster. Ann Surg 1997;225:268–73.

69. Schmidt SC, Langrehr JM, Hintze RE, et al. Long-term results and risk factors influencing outcome of major bile duct injuries following cholecystectomy. Br J Surg 2005;92:76–82.

70. Sicklick JK, Camp MS, Lillemoe KD, et al. Surgical management of bile duct injuries sustained during laparoscopic cholecystectomy: perioperative results in 200 patients. Ann Surg 2005;241:786–92 [discussion: 793–5].

71. Thomson BN, Parks RW, Madhavan KK, et al. Early specialist repair of biliary injury. Br J Surg 2006;93:216–20.

72. Walsh RM, Vogt DP, Ponsky JL, et al. Management of failed biliary repairs for major bile duct injuries after laparoscopic cholecystectomy. J Am Coll Surg 2004;199:192–7.

73. Walsh RM, Henderson JM, Vogt DP, et al. Long-term outcome of biliary reconstruction for bile duct injuries from laparoscopic cholecystectomies. Surgery 2007;142:450–6 [discussion: 456–7].

74. Xu XD, Zhang YC, Gao P, et al. Treatment of major laparoscopic bile duct injury: a long-term follow-up result. Am Surg 2011;77:1584–8.

75. Mazer LM, Tapper EB, Sarmiento JM. Non-operative management of right posterior sectoral duct injury following laparoscopic cholecystectomy. J Gastrointest Surg 2011;15:1237–42.

76. Perera MT, Monaco A, Silva MA, et al. Laparoscopic posterior sectoral bile duct injury: the emerging role of nonoperative management with improved long-term results after delayed diagnosis. Surg Endosc 2011;25:2684–91.

77. Perini RF, Uflacker R, Cunningham JT, et al. Isolated right segmental hepatic duct injury following laparoscopic cholecystectomy. Cardiovasc Intervent Radiol 2005;28(2):185–95.

78. Li J, Frilling A, Nadalin S, et al. Surgical management of segmental and sectoral bile duct injury after laparoscopic cholecystectomy: a challenging situation. J Gastrointest Surg 2010;14:344–51.

Proximal Biliary Tumors

Kimberly M. Brown, MD[a],*, David A. Geller, MD[b]

KEYWORDS

- Intra-hepatic cholangiocarcinoma • Peripheral cholangiocarcinoma
- Hilar cholangiocarcinoma • Klatskin tumor • Bile duct cancer

KEY POINTS

- For cholangiocarcinoma distribution, perihilar location is the most common, followed by distal; intrahepatic is the least common tumor location.
- Contrast-enhanced computed tomography or magnetic resonance imaging with delayed phase is recommended to assess tumor extent and determine resectability.
- Biliary decompression in the absence of cholangitis should only be performed under the direction of the multidisciplinary team that will be treating the patient.
- Complete surgical resection to negative margins is the only hope for long-term survival; highly selected patients with unresectable tumors or underlying liver disease such as primary sclerosing cholangitis may be considered for liver transplant.
- Untreated, unresectable disease portends a median survival of 4 to 5 months; following resection, 5-year survival ranges from 22% to 35%; R0 resection is associated with improved survival.
- Cisplatin-gemcitabine chemotherapy is associated with improved overall and progression-free survival in unresectable disease; a clear benefit in the adjuvant setting has not been established.

INTRODUCTION: NATURE OF THE PROBLEM

Cholangiocarcinoma is a tumor arising from the epithelium of the bile ducts and is further classified as intrahepatic, perihilar (also referred to as Klatskin tumor), or distal cholangiocarcinoma based on the tumor location (**Fig. 1**). Intrahepatic tumors arise from second-order bile ducts or more proximal, without involvement of the hepatic duct confluence; hilar tumors arise at or near the confluence of the right and left hepatic ducts, with further classification based on the extent of involvement (**Fig. 2**); distal tumors include any extrahepatic location beyond the common hepatic duct, although they essentially are periampullary tumors. Intrahepatic and hilar tumors together are referred to as proximal biliary tumors. Hilar and distal tumors are referred to as

a Department of Surgery, University of Texas Medical Branch, 301 University Boulevard, Galveston, TX 77555-0737, USA; b Liver Cancer Center, University of Pittsburgh Medical Center, 3459 Fifth Avenue, UPMC Montefiore, 7 South, Pittsburgh, PA 15213-2582, USA
* Corresponding author.
E-mail address: kim.brown@utmb.edu

Surg Clin N Am 94 (2014) 311–323
http://dx.doi.org/10.1016/j.suc.2013.12.003   surgical.theclinics.com

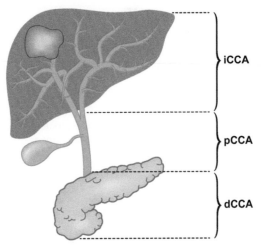

Fig. 1. Classification of cholangiocarcinoma based on the tumor's anatomic site of origin. Tumors located at or beyond the second-order bile ducts and not involving the hilum are classified as intrahepatic cholangiocarcinoma; tumors involving the hilum are hilar cholangiocarcinomas and tumors involving the distal common bile duct are referred to as distal cholangiocarcinomas.

extrahepatic cholangiocarcinomas. Important demographic aspects of cholangiocarcinomas include the following:

- Cholangiocarcinoma is a rare tumor.
- Approximately 5000 to 6000 new cases of cholangiocarcinoma are diagnosed in the United States every year.

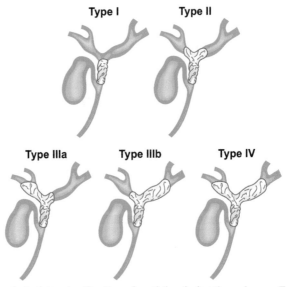

Fig. 2. The Bismuth-Corlette classification of perihilar cholangiocarcinoma. Type I tumors are below the confluence. Type II tumors involve the confluence of the left and right hepatic ducts. Type IIIa and IIIb tumors involve the confluence and the right and left hepatic ducts, respectively. Type IV tumors involve the confluence and extend into the second-order ducts on both sides.

- Intrahepatic, perihilar, and distal tumor locations are seen in approximately 10%, 50%, and 40% of cholangiocarcinomas, respectively.[1]

INTRAHEPATIC CHOLANGIOCARCINOMA

Intrahepatic cholangiocarcinoma (ICC) accounts for 10% to 20% of all primary liver malignancies and is the second most common primary liver tumor after hepatocellular carcinoma (HCC).[2] There are not any well-established risk factors for developing ICC. However, demographic and clinical factors associated with a higher risk of ICC include

- Male gender;
- Ethnicity—the incidence in Asians is twice that of Caucasians;
- Chronic biliary inflammation from hepatolithiasis, choledochal cysts, and liver fluke infestation; and
- Hepatitis B or C infection.

ICC forms several distinct macroscopic histologic subtypes: mass forming, periductal infiltrating, intraductal, and mixed mass forming-periductal infiltrating. Mass forming is the most common subtype in western series. The association of subtype and biologic behavior of the tumor is inconsistent.[3,4]

CLINICAL PRESENTATION AND WORKUP

ICC is initially asymptomatic. Patients most often present with nonspecific symptoms including abdominal pain, anorexia, or unexplained weight loss. Jaundice is uncommon. Physical examination findings are also nonspecific. Laboratory results may be normal or there may be elevations in liver transaminases, alkaline phosphatase, or bilirubin. Once a liver mass is identified, tumor markers including carcinoembryonic antigen (CEA), carbohydrate antigen (CA) 19-9, and alphafetoprotein should be checked, although these are also nonspecific.

Imaging

In a patient with right upper quadrant complaints, an ultrasound (US) is frequently the first imaging study ordered. On US, ICC may appear as a hypoechoic parenchymal mass or an irregular mass along an intra-hepatic duct. Multiphase cross-sectional imaging with either contrast-enhanced computed tomography (CT) or magnetic resonance imaging (MRI) will provide better anatomic detail of the mass and its relationship to internal hepatic structures. In addition, the presence of enlarged regional lymph nodes, peritoneal carcinomatosis, and distant metastatic disease can be assessed. Delayed-phase imaging is helpful, as these tumors will continue to enhance during the delayed phase. **Fig. 3** demonstrates a CT scan of an ICC.

Key factors to consider in the work up of a suspected ICC are the following:

- ICC does not have sensitive or specific imaging findings, unlike HCC.
- ICC is a diagnosis of exclusion—an intrahepatic mass may be an HCC or metastatic disease from an occult primary.
- Colonoscopy, upper endoscopy, chest CT, and mammography should be considered in evaluating for an occult primary.
- Biopsy is not necessary, but if performed, may show adenocarcinoma suggestive of pancreaticobiliary origin (CK-7+, CK20−, CDX2−) or may show poorly differentiated carcinoma that does not stain for any surface markers.

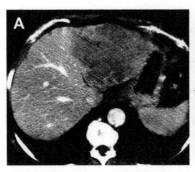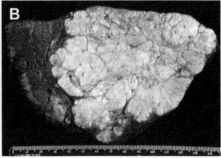

Fig. 3. (*A*) CT image of an ICC in the portal venous phase, demonstrating heterogeneous areas of enhancement and washout. These findings overlap with other solid lesions in the liver, making a preoperative workup for an occult primary tumor essential. (*B*) Gross specimen following resection of the same tumor.

Staging

The 7th edition of the American Joint Committee on Cancer (AJCC) Staging Manual was updated to include a staging system for ICC that is unique from HCC (**Table 1**). The tumor stage is based on prognostic factors identified by an analysis of data from the Survey, Epidemiology and End Results (SEER) database, including number of tumors, presence of vascular invasion, and direct extrahepatic tumor extension.[5]

THERAPEUTIC OPTIONS AND SURGICAL TECHNIQUES

Complete surgical resection offers the only hope of long-term survival. Preoperative planning assesses the suitability of the patient for resection, based on tumor factors and comorbidities. Surgery is reserved for the medically fit patient with no evidence of metastatic disease, including no lymph node involvement of the celiac or periaortic lymph nodes.

The goal of surgery is complete tumor removal to negative microscopic margins (R0 resection), and the extent of resection required depends on the tumor location. Up to 70% to 80% of a healthy liver can be resected, and the remaining liver will hypertrophy to the original volume and function. However, the future liver remnant needs to consist of at least 2 contiguous segments that have hepatic arterial and portal venous inflow, hepatic vein outflow, and biliary-enteric drainage. In cases of marginal future liver remnant, preoperative portal vein embolization of the tumor-bearing hemi-liver can induce contralateral lobar hypertrophy preoperatively, resulting in a larger future liver remnant and potentially less risk of postoperative hepatic insufficiency.[6]

Regional lymph node involvement portends a poor prognosis; for this reason, routine regional lymphadenectomy is performed at some centers. However, based on the paucity of evidence to suggest that lymphadenectomy influences survival, many Western centers remove only suspicious lymph nodes.[7]

Orthotopic liver transplantation (OLT) has been described for ICC, but tumor recurrence is high and survival is not improved compared to resection.[8,9] Clinical factors such as multifocal disease, perineural or lymphovascular invasion, or history of primary sclerosing cholangitis (PSC) may help predict which patients will benefit from OLT.[9] However, OLT for ICC should only be performed in the context of a clinical trial.

Systemic chemotherapy may be used in an adjuvant setting or as palliative treatment of patients with unresectable or recurrent disease. Historically, 5-fluoro-uracil

Table 1
American Joint Commission on Cancer (AJCC) 7th edition staging classification for ICC

Primary tumor (T) staging			
TX	Primary tumor can not be assessed		
T1	Solitary tumor, no vascular invasion		
T2a	Solitary tumor, vascular invasion present		
T2b	Multiple tumors, with or without vascular invasion		
T3	Tumor directly invades local extrahepatic structures or perforates visceral peritoneum		
T4	Tumor with periductal invasion		
Regional lymph node (N) staging			
Nx	Regional lymph nodes can not be assessed		
N1	No regional lymph node metastasis		
N2	Regional lymph node metastasis present		
Distant metastasis (M) staging			
MX	Distant metastasis can not be assessed		
M0	No distant metastasis		
M1	Distant metastatic disease present		
Stage groupings			
Stage 1	T1	N0	M0
Stage II	T2	N0	M0
Stage III	T3	N0	M0
Stage IVA	T4	N0	M0
	Any T	N1	M0
Stage IVB	Any T	Any N	M1

Used with the permission of the American Joint Committee on Cancer (AJCC), Chicago, Illinois. The original source for this material is the AJCC Cancer Staging Manual, Seventh Edition (2010) published by Springer Science and Business Media LLC, www.springer.com.

was the only agent available, and outcomes were poor.[10,11] Gemcitabine, as a single agent, first demonstrated activity against advanced biliary tract cancers with a reasonable safety profile.[12,13] Subsequently, gemcitabine-cisplatin systemic chemotherapy was shown to improve overall survival in patients with unresectable biliary tract cancers, compared to single-agent gemcitabine (11.7 months vs 8.1 months).[14] There are no randomized studies of adjuvant chemotherapy in ICC; one retrospective study of 157 patients with cancer arising from the biliary tract, of whom 54 had ICC, found that neither adjuvant nor neoadjuvant treatment was associated with improved survival.[15]

Transcatheter arterial chemoembolization (TACE) with gemcitabine alone or in combination with cisplatin or oxaliplatin is an option for patients with unresectable ICC. With a median of 3.5 TACE treatments, gemcitabine-cisplatin was associated with the longest median survival at 9.1 months, compared to 6.3 months with single-agent gemcitabine.[16]

CLINICAL OUTCOMES

- In experienced centers, surgical resection of ICC can be performed with less than 3% mortality.[4,17–21]
- Complication rates range from 6% to 38%.[1,3,17,18,21–24]

- Morbidity and mortality are influenced by the extent of liver resection and the need for vascular or biliary reconstruction.
- 5-year overall survival after resection ranges from 20% to 40%.[1,3–5,17,19–22,25,26]
- Median survival after resection is 19 to 53 months.[1,3–5,17,19–22,25,26]
- Overall survival in unresectable disease is less than 1 year.[12,13,27]

HILAR CHOLANGIOCARCINOMA

Hilar cholangiocarcinoma most commonly develops in the absence of risk factors but may be associated with inflammatory conditions of bile ducts, including PSC, ulcerative colitis, or parasitic infestation. These tumors tend to be locally invasive and slow growing, with spread to locoregional lymph nodes, liver, or peritoneum; systemic metastasis occurs late in the disease process. Hilar tumors may be characterized by macroscopic subtype, although the location and extent of involvement are more commonly used to classify tumors for staging and treatment purposes (see **Fig. 2**).

CLINICAL PRESENTATION AND WORKUP

- Early signs and symptoms are most commonly nonspecific.
- One-third of patients will have weight loss, abdominal pain, jaundice, or pruritus.
- Physical examination may show hepatomegaly or skin excoriations from pruritus.
- Most common laboratory abnormalities are elevated bilirubin and alkaline phosphatase levels; aspartate aminotransferase/alanine aminotransferase may also be elevated.
- CEA and CA 19-9 are often ordered but are nonspecific; IgG4 can help distinguish malignancy from IgG4-associated inflammatory disease.
- Cholangitis is a very rare presentation in the absence of instrumentation of biliary tree.
- An alternative diagnosis is seen in 10% to 15% of patients with focal strictures of proximal biliary tree, including gallbladder cancer, Mirizzi syndrome, benign stricture, benign fibrosing disease, hepatic pseudotumors, and iatrogenic injury.

Imaging

Ultrasound is often the first imaging study performed for nonspecific abdominal symptoms or jaundice. US will show unilateral or bilateral intrahepatic biliary ductal dilatation with decompressed extrahepatic ducts. US may show a mass, invasion of liver parenchyma, or portal vein involvement with loss of vascular flow. Cross-sectional imaging is necessary for precise staging. Contrast-enhanced CT will show the level of biliary obstruction, the presence of atrophy, and may show a mass, or vascular involvement. Delayed-phase imaging is recommended for cholangiocarcinoma, as enhancement will persist (contrast retention) in the delayed phase. Although CT may allow determination of resectability, it is not always helpful in demonstrating the proximal extent of ductal involvement, which is a key feature for determining resectability.

Historically, direct imaging of the bile ducts with percutaneous transhepatic cholangiography (PTC) or endoscopic retrograde cholangiography (ERCP) was used to determine the extent of biliary involvement and to perform preoperative decompression. However, ERCP is often unable to traverse strictures and risks contamination of otherwise sterile bile in the obstructed ducts. In both procedures, decompression of the hemiliver that would ultimately be removed during surgery reverses the natural atrophy that occurs in a chronically obstructed hemiliver, as well as the compensatory hypertrophy of the future liver remnant. This works against the usual preoperative strategy of maximizing the future liver remnant. Thus, ERCP and PTC are no longer routinely used in the preoperative imaging of hilar cholangiocarcinoma.

MRI with magnetic resonance cholangiopancreatography (MRCP) is a more sensitive noninvasive modality for the preoperative assessment of a hilar cholangiocarcinoma.[28] MRI/MRCP is able to image obstructed or isolated ducts; better determine the level of ductal involvement; and assess vascular invasion, nodal involvement, and distant metastases (**Fig. 4**A).

Tissue Diagnosis

The need for preoperative tissue diagnosis in a patient with a potentially resectable proximal biliary stricture is somewhat controversial. Although a negative or nondiagnostic biopsy does not exclude a cancer, and therefore surgical resection may still be performed, tissue confirmation is sometimes necessary for treatment plans that include preoperative chemotherapy or radiation therapy and may be helpful in preoperative patient counseling.

- ERCP with brushings may be used to establish a tissue diagnosis—30% sensitivity; risks include cholangitis (see **Fig. 4**B).
- PTC can be performed with blind brushings.
- SpyGlass Direct Visualization System is a new endoscopic technology allowing visualization of the bile duct and thus more focused, directed biopsy; sensitivity is higher than blind brushings.
- Endoscopic ultrasound (EUS) directs US beams from the lumen of the stomach or duodenum; EUS-directed needle biopsy requires passage through peritoneum, with concerns for tumor seeding; this modality is not often used for hilar tumors.
- Invasive procedures for diagnostics should only be performed under the direction of the multidisciplinary team that will be providing treatment of the patient.

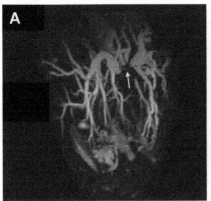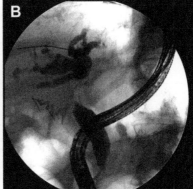

Fig. 4. Imaging studies used to assess extent of tumor in hilar cholangiocarcinoma. (*A*) MRCP image showing dilated intrahepatic bile ducts that abruptly terminate just proximal to the confluence of the right and left hepatic ducts (*arrow*). (*B*) ERCP image of a hilar cholangiocarcinoma, showing dilated intrahepatic ducts and an absence of contrast material throughout the malignant stricture.

Staging

Preoperative staging of hilar cholangiocarcinoma requires

- Precise knowledge of the proximal extent of tumor on the left and right side;
- Assessment of presence or absence and extent of vascular invasion; and
- Evaluation for distant metastases—abdomen and chest.

The current AJCC staging classification is inadequate for surgical planning, as it does not incorporate resectability criteria for the tumor. The Blumgart staging system takes resectability factors into consideration and has been shown to correlate with survival.[29–31] Both systems are presented in **Table 2**. A recent international collaborative proposed a new staging system that takes into account the degree of bile duct involvement, tumor size, macroscopic histologic subtype, degree of portal vein and hepatic artery involvement, future liver remnant volume, underlying liver disease, as well as the presence of lymph node or distant metastasis.[32] The correlation between this staging system and prognosis remains to be determined.

THERAPEUTIC OPTIONS AND SURGICAL TECHNIQUES
Surgical Resection

As with ICC, complete surgical resection is the only potentially curative treatment available for hilar cholangiocarcinoma and is possible in 30% to 40% of patients.[31,33] Resection of the involved extrahepatic bile ducts, en bloc liver resection of the hemiliver with most extensive tumor involvement, and lymphadenectomy are the standard operations. The extent of liver resection depends on the tumor location, as demonstrated in **Fig. 5**. Caudate lobe resection is recommended based on evidence for increased rates of R0 resection compared to cases where caudate resection is omitted.[34] Biliary-enteric continuity is reestablished via Roux-en-Y hepaticojejunostomy.

Potential surgical candidates need careful assessment of their fitness for surgery. Given the complexity of these cases, correction of malnutrition and coagulopathy

	AJCC	**MSKCC**
T1	Confined to the bile duct	Tumor involves biliary confluence +/– extension to secondary bile duct unilaterally
T2	Invades beyond the wall of the bile duct to adjacent adipose (a) or hepatic parenchyma (b)	Same criteria as T1 AND ipsilateral PV involvement and/or ipsilateral hepatic lobar atrophy
T3	Invades unilateral PV or HA branches	
T4	Invades main PV or bilateral PV branches or CHA or secondary bile ducts bilaterally, OR unilateral secondary bile duct involvement with contralateral PV or HA involvement	

Table 2
AJCC and Memorial-Sloan Kettering T-Stage criteria for hilar cholangiocarcinoma

Abbreviations: CHA, common hepatic artery; HA, hepatic artery; PV, portal vein.
Data from Jarnagin W, Winston C. Hilar cholangiocarcinoma: diagnosis and staging. HPB (Oxford) 2005;7:244–51; and Edge SB, Byrd D, Compton CC, et al, editors. American Joint Committee on Cancer Staging Manual. 7th Edition. New York: Springer; 2010.

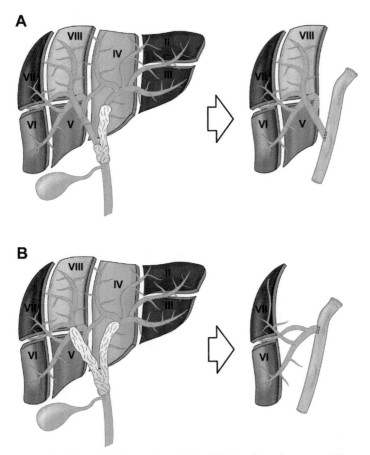

Fig. 5. Cartoon depiction of (*A*) resection of the left hemiliver for a type IIIb tumor, with biliary-enteric anastomosis to the right hepatic duct, and (*B*) extended left hepatectomy for a type IIIa tumor that involves the right anterior sectoral duct, requiring resection of segments I-IV, V and VIII and a biliary-enteric anastomosis to the right posterior sectoral duct draining segments VI and VII.

should be undertaken. The multidisciplinary team may consider preoperative stenting of the future liver remnant if the patient is severely jaundiced or if there is evidence of infection, but this is not routine practice. Ideally, time should be given for jaundice to resolve before resection if stenting is used. The future liver remnant should be calculated to be at least 30% to 35% of liver volume in a patient with no underlying liver disease; in cases of borderline remnant volume, portal vein embolization of the hemiliver to be removed can be used to induce hypertrophy of the future liver remnant.

The following factors should be considered when selecting a patient for surgical resection of ICC:[35]

- Patient factors
  - No significant comorbidities—cardiopulmonary, cirrhosis
  - Optimized nutritional, coagulation status
  - Reasonable age and functional status
  - Bilirubin level less than or equal to 10 mg/dL

- Tumor factors
  - No encasement or occlusion of main portal vein or hepatic artery (bilateral arterial involvement or arterial involvement proximal to the bifurcation)
  - No involvement of bilateral secondary (sectoral) ducts or unilateral ductal involvement with contralateral vascular involvement or compromise
  - No atrophy of one hemiliver with contralateral secondary ductal or portal venous involvement
  - No metastatic disease beyond regional (hepatoduodenal ligament) lymph nodes

Transplantation

Complete resection of the liver and biliary tree with OLT has been used in the treatment of highly selected patients with unresectable hilar cholangiocarcinoma or patients with an underlying liver condition such as PSC that precludes surgical resection.[36,37] Centers offering this treatment use preoperative chemotherapy and radiation therapy and a staging laparotomy. For patients who do not progress while waiting for transplantation, post-transplant overall 5-year survival is as high as 70%, and 20% to 44% of patients will have tumor recurrence.[36,37]

Adjuvant Therapy

Studies evaluating systemic chemotherapy in the adjuvant setting are lacking; local recurrence is the more common pattern of failure, which indicates a possible role for adjuvant radiotherapy.[38] However, an analysis of SEER data from 1973 to 2005 found no survival difference at 5 years between patients treated with and without adjuvant radiotherapy.[39] Given the paucity of data to support adjuvant treatment, chemotherapy and/or radiation should only be given in the context of a clinical trial.

Palliative Treatment

Patients who are not appropriate for surgical resection or transplantation may be treated with systemic chemotherapy with or without radiation, with phase III evidence to support the use of gemcitabine and cisplatin over single-agent gemcitabine (overall survival 11.7 vs 8.1 months).[14] Transcatheter arterial chemoembolization is another option, with single-agent gemcitabine or gemcitabine-containing regimens.[16] Biliary obstruction is the most common symptom considered for palliative treatment. Indications for intervention include cholangitis, intractable pruritus, and the need to normalize bilirubin to deliver chemotherapy. Percutaneous drainage is more effective than endoscopic approaches due to technical and mechanical limitations of the latter; initial percutaneous drainage can be followed by self-expanding metallic stent placement. Although 2 or 3 stents may be necessary to drain all ducts, partial decompression can offer symptom relief. As many as 50% of patients explored for potentially resectable hilar cholangiocarcinoma will be unresectable, usually due to metastatic disease discovered at laparotomy[35]; these patients may benefit from an intrahepatic biliary-enteric bypass, the most common of which is a segment III hepaticojejunostomy at the umbilical fissure.[40]

CLINICAL OUTCOMES

- Patients with unresectable tumors have a median survival of 4 to 5 months.[41,42]
- Treatment with gemcitabine-cisplatin can prolong median overall survival to approximately 12 months.[14]

- Surgical resection is associated with a mortality of 2% to 10% and 25% to 44% rate of morbidity.[30,33,35,41–44]
- Five-year overall survival following resection is 20% to 35%.[35,41–44]
- Median overall survival is approximately 40 months.[33,35,41,43]
- Factors associated with improved survival include
  - Complete (R0) resection[35,44];
  - Concomitant liver resection versus bile duct resection only[35];
  - Well-differentiated histology[35]; and
  - No lymph node metastases[42,44]
- Patients undergoing resection for hilar cholangiocarcinoma have a higher likelihood of a complete (R0) resection when en bloc liver resection is performed with the bile duct resection.[42]
- Five-year overall survival following transplant is approximately 65% to 70%.[36]

SUMMARY

Proximal biliary tumors are relatively uncommon; hilar tumors are more common than ICC. Both are associated with a poor prognosis, and complete surgical resection offers the only hope of long-term survival. Contrast-enhanced imaging with delayed phase is the most effective modality for preoperative staging and treatment planning. For perihilar tumors, precise identification of the proximal and distal extent of tumor involvement bilaterally is necessary for determining eligibility for resection. Transplant is an option for highly selected patients as part of established protocols including preoperative chemoradiation, chemotherapy, and operative staging. Overall survival after resection is low, although patients with R0 resections have improved prognosis. Gemcitabine-cisplatin is offered to medically fit patients with preserved organ function and unresectable tumors.

REFERENCES

1. DeOliveira ML, Cunningham SC, Cameron JL, et al. Cholangiocarcinoma: thirty-one-year experience with 564 patients at a single institution. Ann Surg 2007; 245(5):755–62.
2. Sia D, Tovar V, Moeini A, et al. Intrahepatic cholangiocarcinoma: pathogenesis and rationale for molecular therapies. Oncogene 2013;32(41):4861–70.
3. de Jong MC, Nathan H, Sotiropoulos GC, et al. Intrahepatic cholangiocarcinoma: an international multi-institutional analysis of prognostic factors and lymph node assessment. J Clin Oncol 2011;29(23):3140–5.
4. Shimada K, Sano T, Sakamoto Y, et al. Surgical outcomes of the mass-forming plus periductal infiltrating types of intrahepatic cholangiocarcinoma: a comparative study with the typical mass-forming type of intrahepatic cholangiocarcinoma. World J Surg 2007;31(10):2016–22.
5. Nathan H, Aloia TA, Vauthey JN, et al. A proposed staging system for intrahepatic cholangiocarcinoma. Ann Surg Oncol 2009;16(1):14–22.
6. Ebata T, Yokoyama Y, Igami T, et al. Portal vein embolization before extended hepatectomy for biliary cancer: current technique and review of 494 consecutive embolizations. Dig Surg 2012;29(1):23–9.
7. Morine Y, Shimada M, Utsunomiya T, et al. Clinical impact of lymph node dissection in surgery for peripheral-type intrahepatic cholangiocarcinoma. Surg Today 2012;42(2):147–51.

8. Hong JC, Jones CM, Duffy JP, et al. Comparative analysis of resection and liver transplantation for intrahepatic and hilar cholangiocarcinoma: a 24-year experience in a single center. Arch Surg 2011;146(6):683–9.

9. Hong JC, Petrowsky H, Kaldas FM, et al. Predictive index for tumor recurrence after liver transplantation for locally advanced intrahepatic and hilar cholangiocarcinoma. J Am Coll Surg 2011;212(4):514–20 [discussion: 520–1].

10. Choi CW, Choi IK, Seo JH, et al. Effects of 5-fluorouracil and leucovorin in the treatment of pancreatic-biliary tract adenocarcinomas. Am J Clin Oncol 2000; 23(4):425–8.

11. Ducreux M, Van Cutsem E, Van Laethem JL, et al. A randomised phase II trial of weekly high-dose 5-fluorouracil with and without folinic acid and cisplatin in patients with advanced biliary tract carcinoma: results of the 40955 EORTC trial. Eur J Cancer 2005;41(3):398–403.

12. Tsavaris N, Kosmas C, Gouveris P, et al. Weekly gemcitabine for the treatment of biliary tract and gallbladder cancer. Invest New Drugs 2004;22(2):193–8.

13. Lin MH, Chen JS, Chen HH, et al. A phase II trial of gemcitabine in the treatment of advanced bile duct and periampullary carcinomas. Chemotherapy 2003;49(3): 154–8.

14. Valle J, Wasan H, Palmer DH, et al. Cisplatin plus gemcitabine versus gemcitabine for biliary tract cancer. N Engl J Med 2010;362(14):1273–81.

15. Glazer ES, Liu P, Abdalla EK, et al. Neither neoadjuvant nor adjuvant therapy increases survival after biliary tract cancer resection with wide negative margins. J Gastrointest Surg 2012;16(9):1666–71.

16. Gusani NJ, Balaa FK, Steel JL, et al. Treatment of unresectable cholangiocarcinoma with gemcitabine-based transcatheter arterial chemoembolization (TACE): a single-institution experience. J Gastrointest Surg 2008;12(1):129–37.

17. Ali SM, Clark CJ, Zaydfudim VM, et al. Role of major vascular resection in patients with intrahepatic cholangiocarcinoma. Ann Surg Oncol 2013;20(6):2023–8.

18. Endo I, Gonen M, Yopp AC, et al. Intrahepatic cholangiocarcinoma: rising frequency, improved survival, and determinants of outcome after resection. Ann Surg 2008;248(1):84–96.

19. Paik KY, Jung JC, Heo JS, et al. What prognostic factors are important for resected intrahepatic cholangiocarcinoma? J Gastroenterol Hepatol 2008;23(5): 766–70.

20. Shen WF, Zhong W, Xu F, et al. Clinicopathological and prognostic analysis of 429 patients with intrahepatic cholangiocarcinoma. World J Gastroenterol 2009; 15(47):5976–82.

21. Weber SM, Jarnagin WR, Klimstra D, et al. Intrahepatic cholangiocarcinoma: resectability, recurrence pattern, and outcomes. J Am Coll Surg 2001;193(4): 384–91.

22. Konstadoulakis MM, Roayaie S, Gomatos IP, et al. Fifteen-year, single-center experience with the surgical management of intrahepatic cholangiocarcinoma: operative results and long-term outcome. Surgery 2008;143(3):366–74.

23. Lang H, Sotiropoulos GC, Fruhauf NR, et al. Extended hepatectomy for intrahepatic cholangiocellular carcinoma (ICC): when is it worthwhile? Single center experience with 27 resections in 50 patients over a 5-year period. Ann Surg 2005;241(1):134–43.

24. Madariaga JR, Iwatsuki S, Todo S, et al. Liver resection for hilar and peripheral cholangiocarcinomas: a study of 62 cases. Ann Surg 1998;227(1):70–9.

25. Guglielmi A, Ruzzenente A, Campagnaro T, et al. Intrahepatic cholangiocarcinoma: prognostic factors after surgical resection. World J Surg 2009;33(6):1247–54.

26. Lang H, Sotiropoulos GC, Sgourakis G, et al. Operations for intrahepatic cholangiocarcinoma: single-institution experience of 158 patients. J Am Coll Surg 2009; 208(2):218–28.
27. Raderer M, Hejna MH, Valencak JB, et al. Two consecutive phase II studies of 5-fluorouracil/leucovorin/mitomycin C and of gemcitabine in patients with advanced biliary cancer. Oncology 1999;56(3):177–80.
28. Clary B, Jarnigan W, Pitt H, et al. Hilar cholangiocarcinoma. J Gastrointest Surg 2004;8(3):298–302.
29. Jarnagin WR, Fong Y, DeMatteo RP, et al. Staging, resectability, and outcome in 225 patients with hilar cholangiocarcinoma. Ann Surg 2001;234(4):507–17 [discussion: 517–9].
30. Zaydfudim VM, Clark CJ, Kendrick ML, et al. Correlation of staging systems to survival in patients with resected hilar cholangiocarcinoma. Am J Surg 2013; 206(2):159–65.
31. Matsuo K, Rocha FG, Ito K, et al. The Blumgart preoperative staging system for hilar cholangiocarcinoma: analysis of resectability and outcomes in 380 patients. J Am Coll Surg 2012;215(3):343–55.
32. Deoliveira ML, Schulick RD, Nimura Y, et al. New staging system and a registry for perihilar cholangiocarcinoma. Hepatology 2011;53(4):1363–71.
33. Hemming AW, Reed AI, Fujita S, et al. Surgical management of hilar cholangiocarcinoma. Ann Surg 2005;241(5):693–9 [discussion: 699–702].
34. Dinant S, Gerhards MF, Busch OR, et al. The importance of complete excision of the caudate lobe in resection of hilar cholangiocarcinoma. HPB (Oxford) 2005; 7(4):263–7.
35. Jarnagin WR, Bowne W, Klimstra DS, et al. Papillary phenotype confers improved survival after resection of hilar cholangiocarcinoma. Ann Surg 2005;241(5): 703–12 [discussion: 712–4].
36. Gores GJ, Darwish Murad S, Heimbach JK, et al. Liver transplantation for perihilar cholangiocarcinoma. Dig Dis 2013;31(1):126–9.
37. Duignan S, Maguire D, Ravichand CS, et al. Neoadjuvant chemoradiotherapy followed by liver transplantation for unresectable cholangiocarcinoma: a single-centre national experience. HPB (Oxford) 2013;16(1):91–8.
38. Jarnagin WR, Ruo L, Little SA, et al. Patterns of initial disease recurrence after resection of gallbladder carcinoma and hilar cholangiocarcinoma: implications for adjuvant therapeutic strategies. Cancer 2003;98(8):1689–700.
39. Fuller CD, Wang SJ, Choi M, et al. Multimodality therapy for locoregional extrahepatic cholangiocarcinoma: a population-based analysis. Cancer 2009;115(22): 5175–83.
40. Jarnagin WR, Burke E, Powers C, et al. Intrahepatic biliary enteric bypass provides effective palliation in selected patients with malignant obstruction at the hepatic duct confluence. Am J Surg 1998;175(6):453–60.
41. Saxena A, Chua TC, Chu FC, et al. Improved outcomes after aggressive surgical resection of hilar cholangiocarcinoma: a critical analysis of recurrence and survival. Am J Surg 2011;202(3):310–20.
42. Ito F, Agni R, Rettammel RJ, et al. Resection of hilar cholangiocarcinoma: concomitant liver resection decreases hepatic recurrence. Ann Surg 2008;248(2):273–9.
43. Neuhaus P, Jonas S, Bechstein WO, et al. Extended resections for hilar cholangiocarcinoma. Ann Surg 1999;230(6):808–18 [discussion: 819].
44. de Jong MC, Marques H, Clary BM, et al. The impact of portal vein resection on outcomes for hilar cholangiocarcinoma: a multi-institutional analysis of 305 cases. Cancer 2012;118(19):4737–47.

Distal Cholangiocarcinoma

Paxton V. Dickson, MD, Stephen W. Behrman, MD*

KEYWORDS

- Cholangiocarcinoma • Pathophysiology • Surgery • Adjuvant therapy

KEY POINTS

- Cancer of the distal common bile duct (distal cholangiocarcinoma) is a rare malignancy that often clinically presents similar to pancreatic cancer; however, it has a distinct set of risk factors indicating a unique pathophysiology relative to other periampullary neoplasms.
- Patients with primary sclerosing cholangitis (PSC) have a markedly increased risk for cholangiocarcinoma (CC) and should undergo rigorous surveillance to preempt malignant transformation.
- Patients with imaging and endoscopy suggesting only locoregional disease, and of adequate performance status, should undergo exploration for possible pancreaticoduodenectomy.
- Once resected, surgeons and pathologists should work together to mark the critical margins of the surgical specimen. Positive resection margins and lymph node metastases have consistently been shown to lead toward poor prognosis after pancreaticoduodenectomy.
- There are limited data to support adjuvant chemotherapy after potentially curative resection for distal cholangiocarcinoma. Institutional series suggest a potential benefit from postoperative chemoradiation, particularly in patients with R1 resection or positive nodes.
- For patients with unresectable or metastatic disease, palliative systemic chemotherapy usually includes gemcitabine and cisplatin; however, median survival in these patients is less than 1 year.

Cholangiocarcinoma (CC) involving the distal common bile duct (distal cholangiocarcinoma [DCC]) is a periampullary neoplasm less common than, but often difficult to distinguish from, pancreatic adenocarcinoma (PDA). Although the prognosis and cure rate of DCC is improved over that of PDA, it remains a highly lethal disease. Although the diagnostic and therapeutic management of DCC is not dissimilar from PDA, the pathophysiology is, in many instances, distinctly different. Certain patient populations demand close surveillance for the development of DCC and, in some instances, preemptive surgical extirpation of a diseased biliary tree before the development of frank carcinoma is necessary. Furthermore, recent work has elucidated aberrant molecular and inflammatory mediators that might predispose to the development of DCC and offer the potential

Division of Surgical Oncology, Department of Surgery, University of Tennessee Health Science Center, 910 Madison Avenue, Suite 329, Memphis, TN 38163, USA
* Corresponding author.
E-mail address: sbehrman@uthsc.edu

Surg Clin N Am 94 (2014) 325–342
http://dx.doi.org/10.1016/j.suc.2013.12.004
0039-6109/14/$ – see front matter © 2014 Elsevier Inc. All rights reserved.

for a more targeted approach toward this challenging disease. Current neo/adjuvant management schemes are suboptimal, and in many instances extrapolated from those of intrahepatic and hilar CC, and PDA and other periampullary neoplasms.

EPIDEMIOLOGY

It is difficult to determine the exact incidence of DCC because studies often collectively include intrahepatic, hilar, and distal CC, and gallbladder carcinoma. However, trends in the United States and other countries indicate the incidence of extrahepatic CC (hilar and distal) is stable or in some instances decreasing. This is in contradistinction to intra-hepatic CC, which is rising in incidence worldwide. These epidemiologic trends suggest a biologic difference relative to the anatomic location of these tumors.[1,2] Although there have been no epidemiologic studies specifically analyzing the incidence of distal disease, this is important going forward because DCC is, in many aspects, a vastly different disorder than hilar CC and gallbladder carcinoma. CC, regardless of anatomic location, is more common in Asia than in Western countries.[3]

RISK FACTORS FOR DCC

Approximately 80% of all patients diagnosed with CC in any anatomic location have no identifiable risk factor for the development of the disease. In contrast, there are well-described conditions leading to chronic biliary inflammation that have a clear association with the development of CC. Recent work has accelerated knowledge of the molecular pathways and genetic aberrations that may contribute toward the development of cholangiocarcinogenesis. For the purposes of this discussion, only the pathophysiology most often encountered specific to DCC is presented.

Clinical: Social

Although population-based analyses have found smoking and alcohol consumption common among patients with CC, there are no data to clearly link these factors with disease development. Interestingly, a recent meta-analysis suggests that diabetes may significantly increase the risk of CC including extrahepatic CC.[4,5]

Clinical: Disease Specific

Primary sclerosing cholangitis
Primary sclerosing cholangitis (PSC) is an autoimmune disease that can affect the entire biliary tree. PSC confers a lifetime risk for the development of CC of 9% to 31% or a 1500-fold increase over that of the general population. Moreover, the risk of PSC-associated CC increases in those with concomitant ulcerative colitis.[6] PSC is isolated to the extrahepatic biliary tree in 10% to 20% of patients, frequently presents as an isolated high-grade stricture, and has been demonstrated on pathologic examination of Whipple specimens performed for suspected malignant disease.[7,8] Furthermore, the development of CC in the residual native bile duct has been described following orthotopic hepatic transplantation for PSC.[9,10] Currently, there is no single test identifying CC in the setting of PSC; therefore, an aggressive surveillance program for these individuals is mandatory. Findings that may indicate the development of CC in a patient with PSC include a rising carbohydrate antigen (CA) 19-9 and/or carcinoembryonic antigen (CEA), the emergence of a dominant stricture, clinical and biochemical deterioration of liver function, weight loss, jaundice, and the presence of bile duct dysplasia on brush cytology. Diagnostically, endoscopic retro-grade cholangiopancreatography (ERCP) in conjunction with endoscopic intraductal ultrasound and cholangioscopic biopsy has proved most accurate in establishing

the diagnosis of CC in the setting of PSC.[11] Resected CC for a dominant stricture resulting from unsuspected PSC in the absence of other objective criteria for the diagnosis remains exceptional.[8]

Choledochal cyst

Choledochal cysts are congenital cystic dilations of the intrahepatic and/or extrahepatic biliary tree. Although this disorder is most commonly recognized in infancy, the disease may go unrecognized until adulthood. Patients may present with symptoms related to associated choledocholithiasis, such as nausea, vomiting, and epigastric pain. Elevated liver function tests and jaundice are not uncommon. The pathophysiology of extrahepatic cysts is believed to result from an anomalous junction of the pancreatic and biliary ducts resulting in a long common channel thereby allowing reflux of pancreatic enzymes into the biliary tree with resultant cystic degeneration from chronic inflammation. Type I (solitary extrahepatic) and type IV (extrahepatic and intrahepatic dilation involving the bile duct confluence) cysts have the highest lifetime risk of CC with an incidence up to 30%.[12] When discovered, types I and IV choledochal cysts, even if asymptomatic, should be resected as a measure of prophylaxis against malignant degeneration. This typically involves resection of the extrahepatic biliary tree to the level of the ductal confluence and reconstruction with Roux-en-Y hepaticojejunostomy. Even after resection, this population remains at higher risk for the development of CC relative to the general population, especially if the entirety of the biliary tree at risk is not removed.[4,13]

Parasitic Infections

Biliary infestation with the liver flukes *Opisthorchis viverrini* and *Clonorchis sinensis*, both of which are prevalent in Southeast Asia, is associated with the development of CC. Chronic inflammation of the biliary epithelium by these parasites is believed to increase the susceptibility to cholangiocarcinogenesis.[14] Both hospital- and population-based case-control studies from Thailand and Korea examining infection with liver flukes by *O viverrini* antibody titers and the presence of *C sinensis* in stool have noted a strong association with the development of CC, irrespective of anatomic location within the biliary tree.[15–17] Limited data suggest that all areas of the biliary tree including extrahepatic locations are prone to carcinoma.[17] Because infestation is linked to poor sanitation, therapeutic intervention has focused on prevention. Treatment with anthelmintic agents is important if infection is documented.

BIOLOGIC BASIS OF CHOLANGIOCARCINOGENESIS
Inflammatory Mediators

Cholestasis, regardless of cause, results in abnormal exposure of the biliary epithelium to bile acids. Deoxycholic acid, a derivative of bile acids, has been shown to activate epidermal growth factor receptor and serve as a neoplastic stimulus by promoting cellular proliferation and attenuating apoptosis in cholangiocytes.[18,19] The cytokine interleukin-6 is upregulated in CC relative to normal biliary tract cells and is regarded as a growth factor for its propagation.[20] Interleukin-6 has also been shown to desensitize CC to normal apoptotic cell death.[21] Furthermore, interleukin-6 induces increased expression of progranulin in CC in contrast to nonmalignant cholangiocytes. Progranulin expression is found in multiple tumor types and is associated with high tumorigenecity.[22] Cyclooxygenase-2, a prostaglandin, is overexpressed in CC and premalignant conditions, such as PSC. Cyclooxygenase-2 accumulation results in cellular proliferation and inhibition of apoptosis in CC, a process reversed by the administration of the cyclooxygenase-2 inhibitor celecoxib.[5,23]

Growth Factors

Human CC cell lines express high levels of vascular endothelial growth factor leading to angiogenesis and cancer growth. Inhibition of vascular endothelial growth factor reduces cell proliferation and leads to apoptosis in tumor tissue.[7,24] Epidermal growth factor receptor is a mediator of cholangiocarcinogenesis as previously noted. Epidermal growth factor receptor has been detected in more than one-third of samples obtained from patients with CC.[25]

Stromal Alterations

In common with pancreatic carcinoma, CC exhibits an epithelial-mesenchymal transition that results in a desmoplastic stroma predominantly composed of cancer-associated fibroblasts surrounding glandular structures. As opposed to tumors with epithelial expression, those exhibiting the mesenchymal phenotype have been associated with the development of chemoresistance in pancreatic cancer and tumor progression in CC.[26,27] Furthermore, CC is associated with increased levels of matrix metalloproteinases, which break down the extracellular matrix to allow tumor spread.[28]

Genetic Aberrations

A mutation of the p53 tumor suppressor gene is seen in 20% to 61% of patients with CC, resulting in inhibition of the normal cellular apoptotic response.[29] Mutations of many other genes in CC have been identified and offer the potential for future targeted therapy.[30] miRNAs are single-strand noncoding RNA products that may have tumor suppressor or oncogenic activity. Aberrant regulation of miRNA has been described in CC resulting in cancer cell proliferation and survival.[31] Manipulation of dysregulated miRNA may offer a potential avenue for CC treatment.

CLINICAL PRESENTATION AND EVALUATION

Patients with DCC typically present with painless jaundice and experience pruritus, clay colored stools, and tea-colored urine, similar to patients with PDA or other periampullary malignancies. Although biliary obstruction rarely results in cholangitis, patients may begin to experience right upper quadrant discomfort and a bloating sensation. Laboratory assessment most frequently reveals elevated bilirubin, alkaline phosphatase, γ-glutamyl transpeptidase, and the eventual elevation of hepatic transaminases.

The diagnostic evaluation of a patient with suspected DCC or periampullary neoplasm generally involves a combination of radiographic and endoscopic studies aimed at trying to define the local extent of disease, evaluate for potential metastases, and obtain tissue confirmation if the diagnosis is unclear. For patients who present with jaundice, transabdominal ultrasound is often the initial imaging modality and is very sensitive for identifying intrahepatic and extrahepatic ductal dilation, the presence of a choledochal cyst, cholelithiasis or choledocholithiasis, and potential mass lesions.[32,33] This is often followed by cross-sectional imaging with either computed tomography or magnetic resonance imaging. Patients with DCC (and other periampullary neoplasms) often have a finding of a distended gallbladder with dilated extrahepatic and intrahepatic ducts. Conversely, perihilar CC has dilated intrahepatic ducts with a normal-sized common bile duct and possibly a contracted gallbladder. A mass lesion may or may not be identified on computed tomography or magnetic resonance imaging but both studies are helpful in identifying a choledochal cyst. Contrast-enhanced triple-phase computed tomography allows for evaluation of critical vascular anatomy, regional lymph node basins, and potentially identifies distant metastases.[34] DCC may result in biliary dilation alone but not uncommonly results in the classic double-duct sign found with PDA.

When imaging findings are suggestive of a periampullary mass or distal bile duct stricture, endoscopic evaluation is usually the most appropriate next step if the diagnosis is uncertain, the lesion appears borderline resectable, metastatic disease is suggested, or deep jaundice is present requiring preoperative surgical decompression.[35] This may include ERCP, endoscopic ultrasound (EUS), and/or cholangioscopy. ERCP permits accurate visualization of the biliary tree, allows for tissue sampling for possible diagnosis, and placement of preoperative or palliative endobiliary stents. When a tissue diagnosis is necessary for treatment planning, transampullary biopsy has been shown to have a higher sensitivity than bile sampling or brush cytology.[36–38] EUS with fine-needle aspiration biopsy is another modality useful in evaluation and potential diagnosis of biliary malignancy and, unlike ERCP, does not require cannulation of the biliary tree.[39] EUS not only allows for biopsy of biliary strictures or masses, but also permits evaluation of regional lymph nodes and vascular structures. Recently, peroral cholangioscopy has evolved as a technique that allows direct visualization of biliary epithelium and accurate targeting for biopsies.[40] The combined ability to visualize mucosal abnormalities and obtain directed biopsies potentially offers improved diagnostic yield over ERCP or EUS[41] and is most helpful in those with PSC. Certainly, the endoscopic modality of choice is largely driven by institutional expertise and the nature of individual cases.

The tumor markers CA 19-9 and CEA have been used in patients with biliary tract malignancies.[42,43] These markers have marginal sensitivity in diagnosing CC, and may often be elevated in benign inflammatory or stricturing processes of the biliary tree. For patients with PSC, serial measurements of CA 19-9 and/or CEA should be a component of surveillance for possible malignant transformation.[44] Another use of these markers is for monitoring of possible recurrence or response to therapy in patients with a confirmed diagnosis of CC.

PRINCIPLES OF SURGICAL TECHNIQUE

The diagnosis of DCC cannot always be definitively ascertained either preoperatively or intraoperatively because the tumor may infiltrate the pancreatic head and lead to a desmoplastic reaction often difficult to distinguish from PDA. Similar to other periampullary neoplasms, it is imperative that surgical extirpation of DCC focus on the achievement of R0 resection because margin positivity is associated with poor long-term survival.[45] Pancreaticoduodenectomy for DCC must focus on meticulous medial perivascular dissection of tissue off the superior mesenteric artery (SMA) and vein and a careful regional lymphadenectomy.

Medial dissection of the pancreatic head/uncinate process is crucial because this margin is typically closest to the epicenter of the tumor and most difficult to maximize. Adequate extirpation requires completely skeletonizing the right anterolateral aspect of the SMA down to the level of the adventitia and mobilization of the uncinate process off this vessel. This enhances pancreatic tissue yield while broadening the medial (retroperitoneal) margin relative to the carcinoma (**Fig. 1**). As detailed next, portal or superior mesenteric vein resection or reconstruction is occasionally required.[46,47]

The liberal use of partial or complete vein resection when tumor infiltration is suspected during pancreaticoduodenectomy has been extensively studied with respect to PDA and it would be reasonable to extrapolate these findings to DCC.[48–50] On evaluation of excised specimens in patients undergoing vein resection, only 60% to 70%

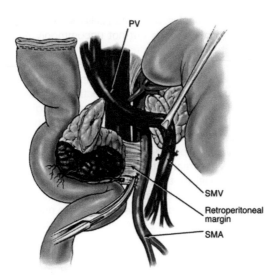

Fig. 1. Complete mobilization of the superior mesenteric (SMV) and portal veins, and separation of the specimen from the right lateral border of the superior mesenteric artery (SMA). PV, portal vein. (*From* Wayne JD, Abdalla EK, Wolff RA, et al. Localized adenocarcinoma of the pancreas: the rationale for preoperative chemoradiation. Oncologist 2002;7(1):34–45.)

had histologic evidence of frank tumor involvement and R0 resections were still not obtainable in 10% to 30%. However, if an R0 resection is obtained with vein excision, longevity seems similar to those with R0 resections without venous involvement, with no significant increase in morbidity and mortality. These data support an aggressive approach to partial or complete vein excision if tumor infiltration is suspected, although acceptance of this concept is not universal. Although the numbers are more limited, similar findings have been noted with respect to arterial resection and reconstruction and judicious use of this technique seems to be reasonable in select populations.[50,51] A recent meta-analysis reviewing vascular resection suggests that the safety and survival outcome of patients having vascular resection during a Whipple procedure is equivalent to those having standard resection alone if performed at high-volume centers.[52]

Lymphadenectomy should include a thorough dissection of regional nodes. Specific to DCC, all nodes surrounding the common bile duct and porta hepatis should be carefully excised as potential draining basins from distal common bile duct cancers. Hepatic artery nodes should be considered for resection if there is clinical suspicion of involvement because these basins have been shown to have prognostic implications in PDA and possibly also could in CC.[53]

PATHOLOGIC ANALYSIS
Specimen Orientation and Margin Assessment

The primary purpose of pathologic analysis of the Whipple specimen is to determine the pathologic stage of the tumor by evaluating the type, grade, size, and extent of the cancer. The National Comprehensive Cancer Network® (NCCN®) panel for pancreatic adenocarcinoma has proposed guidelines for pathologic analysis to bring uniformity to reporting to allow consistent interpretation from institution to institution.[54] These recommendations are most appropriate for DCC.

Specimen orientation, margin identification, and inking should involve pathologist and surgeon because this helps ensure accurate assessment of the size and extent of the tumor and proximity concerns of the malignancy to the margins assessed. One of the impediments to comparison of data across institutions is the variability in the names given to various margins. Definitions of the margins and uniformity of nomenclature are critical to ensure accurate reporting. The NCCN® recommends the following margins be inked and assessed separately (**Fig. 2**).[54]

SMA (Retroperitoneal/Uncinate) Margin

The most important margin is the ragged, soft tissue directly adjacent to the proximal 3 to 4 cm of the SMA. In common with other margins assessed, radial rather than en face sections are recommended and more clearly demonstrate how closely this margin is approached by tumor. The simple step of palpating the specimen can help guide the pathologist as to the best location along the SMA margin to select for sampling.

Posterior (Retroperitoneal) Margin

This margin is from the posterior caudad aspect of the pancreatic head that merges with the uncinate margin and that appears to be covered by loose connective tissue.

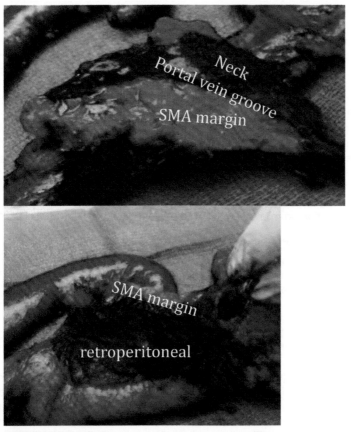

Fig. 2. The surgeon and pathologist should collaborate to appropriately mark/ink the critical margins including the pancreatic neck, superior mesenteric, and portal vein groove.

In some instances this margin can be included in the same section as the SMA margin section.

Portal Vein Groove Margin

This is the smooth-surfaced groove on the posterior surface of the pancreatic head that rests over the portal vein. As is true for the posterior margin, in some instances this margin can be included in the same section as the SMA section.

Pancreatic Neck (Transection) Margin

This is the en face section of the transected pancreatic neck. The section should be placed into the cassette with true margin facing up so that the initial section into the block represents the true surgical margin. For purposes of frozen section analysis in the operating room, the authors recommend assessment 5 mm from the transected pancreatic neck. This eliminates any cautery artifact that may impede the pathologist's assessment for cancer on frozen section. Furthermore, this ensures a minimum of a 5-mm clearance of tumor from this particular margin. If tumor is found on microscopic assessment, resection of further pancreas to achieve an R0 resection can be easily accomplished.

Bile Duct Margin

In common with the pancreatic neck and particularly relevant to DCC the authors recommend assessment of the entirety of the portion of bile duct submitted for frozen section analysis intraoperatively because further excision of the extrahepatic biliary tree can be accomplished readily to maximize tumor clearance. Moreover, when there is clinical suspicion or pathologic confirmation of DCC, the stump of the distal common bile duct demands specific scrutiny. Specifically, the circumferential soft tissue sheath or radial periductal margin around the distal common bile duct should be assessed.[55]

Other margins analyzed in Whipple specimens include the proximal and distal enteric margins (en face sections) and anterior surface (closest representative). The anterior surface is not a true margin, but identification and reporting of this surface when positive may portend a risk of local recurrence, and so should be reported in all cases.[56] Collectively, these pancreatic tissue surfaces constitute the circumferential radial margin. Designating the various specific margins with different colored inks allows recognition on microscopy.

Specimen Grossing Technique and Extent of Tissue Sampling

The approach to histologic sectioning of a Whipple specimen has unfortunately been based on institutional or pathologist preference and experience and has not been uniformly applied between centers of excellence. Options include (1) axial slicing through a plane perpendicular to the second portion of the duodenum; (2) bivalve or multivalve sectioning, bisecting the pancreas along probes placed in the bile and pancreatic ducts and then serially section along each half of the pancreas; or (3) breadloafing technique whereby the specimen is sectioned perpendicular to the neck of the pancreas (**Fig. 3**).[56]

The bivalve technique does not allow a satisfactory three-dimensional perspective of the carcinoma relative to the entire specimen. The breadloafing technique becomes difficult in the region of the duodenum and may distort the relationship of the tumor to the ampulla and the insertion of the pancreatic and bile ducts. In contrast to other techniques, axial slicing (**Fig. 4**) provides an overall assessment of the epicenter of the tumor relative to the ampulla, bile duct, duodenum, and pancreas, and all of the

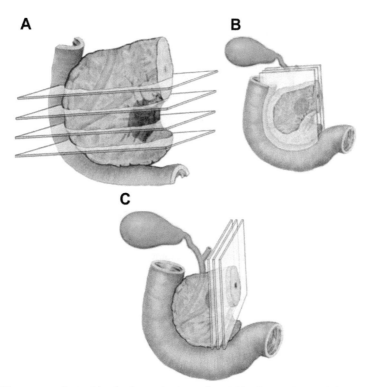

Fig. 3. The approach to histologic sectioning of a Whipple specimen. (*A*) Axial slicing through a plane perpendicular to the second portion of the duodenum. (*B*) Bivalve or multivalve sectioning, bisecting the pancreas along probes placed in the bile and pancreatic ducts and then serially sectioning along each half of the pancreas. (*C*) Bread loafing technique whereby the specimen is sectioned perpendicular to the neck of the pancreas. (*From* Verbeke CS. Resection margins and R1 rates in pancreatic cancer: are we there yet? Histopathology 2008;52(7):787–96; with permission.)

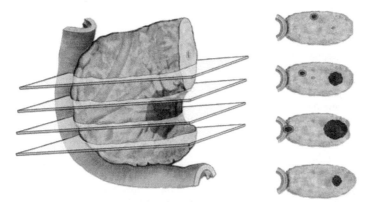

Fig. 4. Axial slicing of the Whipple specimen provides an overall assessment of the epicenter of the tumor relative to the ampulla of Vater, bile duct, duodenum, and pancreas, and all pancreatic circumferential tissue margins. (*From* Verbeke CS. Resection margins and R1 rates in pancreatic cancer: are we there yet? Histopathology 2008;52(7):787–96; with permission.)

pancreatic circumferential tissue margins mentioned previously. In addition, axial slicing correlates with preoperative computed tomography or magnetic resonance imaging. Achievement of a large number of thin slices (>12) is possible by this technique allowing a dogmatic assessment of the primary tumor relative to the margins of resection.[55]

Although the NCCN favors axial slicing there is no one correct way to dissect a Whipple specimen. The most important aspects of dissection are clear and accurate assessment of the margins.[54] It is currently unknown what constitutes an adequate margin in DCC resection specimens. The authors strongly recommend reporting tumor clearance in millimeters for all pertinent margins described previously to allow prospective accumulation of these important data for future analysis.

The NCCN Pancreatic Adenocarcinoma Panel currently supports pathology synoptic reports from the College of American Pathologists.[57] The proposal included herein is an abbreviated *minimum* analysis of pancreatic cancer specimens from the College of American Pathologists recommendations that we believe should be used for DCC (**Table 1**). In addition to the standard TNM staging, other variables are included, all of

---

Table 1
Proposed pathologic analysis of DCC

Tumor size (obtained from careful gross measurement of the largest dimension of the tumor in
    centimeters)
Histologic grade (G [x-4])
Primary tumor extent of invasion (T [x-4])
Regional lymph nodes (N [x-1])
    Number of nodes recovered
    Number of nodes involved
Metastases (M [0-1])
Margins (involvement should be defined and surgical clearance measured in millimeters)
    Whipple resection
        SMA (retroperitoneal/uncinate) margin
        Posterior margin
        Portal vein groove margin
        Pancreatic neck (transection) margin
        Bile duct margin
        Enteric margins
        Anterior surface
    Distal pancreatectomy
        Proximal pancreatic (transection) margin
        Anterior (cephalad) peripancreatic (peripheral) surface (optional)
        Posterior (caudad) peripancreatic (peripheral) margin
Lymphatic (small vessel) invasion (L)
Vascular (large vessel) invasion (V)
Perineural invasion (P)
Additional pathologic findings
    Pancreatic intraepithelial neoplasia
    Chronic pancreatitis
Final Stage: G, T, N, M, L, V, P.

which have prognostic implications in the evolution of pancreatic carcinoma that might be important in DCC.[58,59]

STAGING AND PROGNOSIS

The median survival of patients who undergo resection for DCC is approximately 2 years with a 5-year survival of 20% to 40% depending on the extent of disease.[60] Several institutional series have identified prognostic factors for patients who undergo resection for DCC, helping to form the framework for the current staging classification. In the seventh edition of the American Joint Commission on Cancer Staging Manual, distal bile tumors are classified as lesions arising between the junction of the cystic duct–common bile duct and the ampulla of Vater and are staged separately from perihilar and intrahepatic CC (previous editions had staged perihilar and distal CCs together).[60] The current staging classification schema is shown in **Table 2**.

DeOliveira and colleagues[61] reported on more than 500 patients with CC treated at the Johns Hopkins hospital, including 239 individuals with distal tumors. In this series,

Table 2			
Seventh edition American Joint Commission on Cancer staging for distal bile duct tumors			
Primary Tumor			
Tx Primary tumor cannot be assessed			
T0 No evidence of primary tumor			
Tis Carcinoma in situ			
T1 Tumor confined to the bile duct histologically			
T2 Tumor invades beyond the wall of the bile duct			
T3 Tumor invades the gallbladder, pancreas, duodenum, or other adjacent organs without involvement of the celiac axis, or the superior mesenteric artery			
T4 Tumor involves the celiac axis, or the superior mesenteric artery			
Regional Lymph Nodes			
NX Regional lymph nodes not assessed			
N1 No regional lymph node metastases			
N2 Regional lymph node metastases			
Distant Metastasis			
M0 No distant metastases			
M1 Distant metastases			
Staging Classification			
Stage 0	Tis	N0	M0
Stage IA	T1	N0	M0
Stage IB	T2	N0	M0
Stage IIA	T3	N0	M0
Stage IIB	T1	N1	M0
	T2	N1	M0
	T3	N1	M0
Stage III	T4	Any N	M0
Stage IV	Any T	Any N	M1

Used with the permission of the American Joint Committee on Cancer (AJCC), Chicago, Illinois. The original source for this material is the AJCC Cancer Staging Manual, Seventh Edition (2010) published by Springer Science and Business Media LLC, www.springer.com.

5-year overall survival for patients with DCC was 23%. On multivariate analysis, resection margin status (R0 vs R1/R2), lymph node status (positive vs negative), tumor size (< or >2 cm), and degree of tumor differentiation were all found to significantly impact survival among this group of patients. Similarly, Murakami and colleagues[62] found margin status and lymph node status to significantly impact survival in patients who underwent resection for CC. In a follow-up series from this same institution, specifically examining 43 patients with distal bile duct tumors, resection margin status and lymph node status were again identified as important prognostic factors for survival[63] with 5-year survivals of 8% and 60% for patients with positive and negative margins, respectively, and 5-year survivals of 18% and 46% for patients with positive and negative nodes, respectively. Other factors shown to be predictive of poor prognosis include perineural invasion, lymphovascular invasion, pancreatic invasion, and depth of tumor invasion.[64,65]

POSTOPERATIVE THERAPY FOR LOCOREGIONAL DISEASE

The role of adjuvant therapy in patients with DCC after potentially curative resection is ill defined. Data evaluating the use of adjuvant chemotherapy for CC are limited, and for the most part, combine patients with intrahepatic and extrahepatic CC, gallbladder cancer, and ampullary and pancreatic cancer. In a phase III trial evaluating surgery followed by treatment with 5-FU and mitomycin-C versus surgery alone in patients with bile duct, gallbladder, pancreatic, or ampullary cancer, postoperative chemotherapy offered no benefit in overall or disease-free survival in patients with bile duct carcinoma, regardless of resection margin status.[66] The European Study Group for Pancreatic Cancer-3 periampullary trial, which randomized patients to postoperative observation or 6 months of chemotherapy with either 5-FU/leucovorin or gemcitabine, included 96 patients with bile duct carcinoma.[67] Subset analysis of this group did not demonstrate any improvement in median survival between those randomized to 5-FU/leucovorin (18.3 months) or gemcitabine (19.5 months) versus observation (27.2 months). Given results observed in these trials, there is a general lack of support for the use of adjuvant chemotherapy after R0 resection of bile duct carcinoma.

Because local recurrence presents an obstacle in curing patients with DCC, several investigators have examined the use of radiation therapy in the adjuvant setting. Hughes and colleagues[68] reported on 34 patients with DCC treated with pancreaticoduodenectomy and adjuvant chemoradiation at the Johns Hopkins Hospital. Actuarial 5-year overall survival was 35% and local control was 70%. When compared with historical control subjects from the same institution (patients managed with surgery alone)[69] the addition of chemoradiation seemed to confer a survival benefit (36.9 vs 22 months; $P<.05$). Nelson and colleagues[70] reported similar 5-year actuarial survival (33%) and local control rates (78%) among 45 patients with extrahepatic CC treated at Duke University with surgery and either neoadjuvant or adjuvant chemoradiation. In each of these institutional reviews, most patients had disease recurrence at distant sites, leading investigators to conclude that chemoradiation offers a local control benefit for resected extrahepatic CC. In a retrospective review of 65 patients from the M.D. Anderson Cancer Center with extrahepatic CC, there was no difference in locoregional recurrence or 5-year survival rates between patients who underwent R0 resection and had negative nodes (N0) and received no adjuvant therapy and patients who had either R1 resection and/or positive nodes (N1) and were treated with postoperative chemoradiation.[71] These results suggest a benefit of postoperative chemoradiation in individuals with features that place them at high risk of recurrence.

Finally, Lim and colleagues[72] examined outcomes in 120 patients with extrahepatic bile duct carcinoma treated with radical resection followed by chemoradiation or chemoradiation and subsequent systemic chemotherapy. In this study, postoperative chemoradiation followed by systemic chemotherapy resulted in significantly improved 3-year disease-free and overall survival compared with patients treated with postoperative chemoradiation alone. Although limited by small sample size and their retrospective nature, collectively these data suggest that postoperative chemoradiation with or without systemic chemotherapy may offer improved local control and possible survival benefit after resection for extrahepatic CC, particularly in patients with R1 resection and/or node-positive disease. For patients who undergo R0 resection and have node-negative disease, current NCCN Clinical Practice Guidelines in Oncology (NCCN Guidelines®) recommend observation, enrollment in a clinical trial, consideration of chemoradiation, or consideration of fluoropyrimidine or gemcitabine chemotherapy.[35] For patients with positive resection margins and/or node-positive disease these guidelines recommend consideration of chemoradiation followed by chemotherapy or chemotherapy alone. Clearly, there is a need for randomized prospective trials to better define the appropriate adjuvant therapy in patients who undergo potentially curative resection for DCC.

PALLIATION FOR PATIENTS WITH UNRESECTABLE DISEASE AND/OR DISTANT METASTASES

For patients who have locally advanced, unresectable disease or distant metastases, the prognosis is very poor. Several chemotherapy regimens have been evaluated in the management of these patients.[73] An analysis of clinical trials evaluating chemotherapy for patients with advanced biliary tract cancer suggested that a combination of gemcitabine and platinum-based agents confers the greatest survival benefit.[74] The Advanced Biliary Cancer 02 Trial was a randomized, controlled, phase 3 study comparing cisplatin plus gemcitabine with gemcitabine alone in patients with metastatic or locally advanced biliary tract malignancy.[75] Patients randomized to receive cisplatin-gemcitabine demonstrated a significant improvement in median overall (11.7 vs 8.1 months; $P<.0001$) and progression-free (8 vs 5 months) survival. Based on these data, doublet chemotherapy with cisplatin-gemcitabine is considered standard first-line chemotherapy for patients with locally advanced unresectable or metastatic CC (NCCN Guidelines®). Before initiation of systemic therapy, a definitive tissue diagnosis should be confirmed, and adequate biliary drainage should be achieved.

SUMMARY

DCC is a rare malignancy that often clinically presents similar to pancreatic cancer; however, it has a distinct set of risk factors indicating a unique pathophysiology relative to other periampullary neoplasms. In particular, patients with PSC have a markedly increased risk for CC and should undergo rigorous surveillance to preempt malignant transformation. Patients with imaging and endoscopy suggesting only locoregional disease, and of adequate performance status, should undergo exploration for possible pancreaticoduodenectomy. Once resected, surgeons and pathologists should work together to mark the critical margins of the surgical specimen. Positive resection margins and lymph node metastases have consistently been shown to lead toward poor prognosis after pancreaticoduodenectomy. There are limited data to support adjuvant chemotherapy after potentially curative resection for DCC. Institutional series suggest a potential benefit from postoperative chemoradiation, particularly in patients with R1 resection or positive nodes. For patients with unresectable or metastatic disease, palliative systemic chemotherapy usually includes gemcitabine and cisplatin; however, median survival in these patients is less than 1 year. It is hoped that investigation into the biologic and genetic basis of this disease will lead toward a targeted approach to treatment that might offer improved survival.

REFERENCES

1. Welzel TM, McGlynn KA, Hsing AW, et al. Impact of classification of hilar chol-angiocarcinomas (Klatskin tumors) on the incidence of intra- and extrahepatic cholangiocarcinoma in the United States. J Natl Cancer Inst 2006;98(12): 873–5.
2. Cardinale V, Semeraro R, Torrice A, et al. Intra-hepatic and extra-hepatic chol-angiocarcinoma: new insight into epidemiology and risk factors. World J Gastro-intest Oncol 2010;2(11):407–16.
3. Shaib Y, El-Serag HB. The epidemiology of cholangiocarcinoma. Semin Liver Dis 2004;24(2):115–25.
4. Tyson GL, El-Serag HB. Risk factors for cholangiocarcinoma. Hepatology 2011; 54(1):173–84.
5. Jing W, Jin G, Zhou X, et al. Diabetes mellitus and increased risk of cholangio-carcinoma: a meta-analysis. Eur J Cancer Prev 2012;21(1):24–31.
6. Claessen MM, Vleggaar FP, Tytgat KM, et al. High lifetime risk of cancer in pri-mary sclerosing cholangitis. J Hepatol 2009;50(1):158–64.
7. Bjornsson E, Lindqvist-Ottosson J, Asztely M, et al. Dominant strictures in pa-tients with primary sclerosing cholangitis. Am J Gastroenterol 2004;99(3):502–8.
8. Abraham SC, Wilentz RE, Yeo CJ, et al. Pancreaticoduodenectomy (Whipple resections) in patients without malignancy: are they all 'chronic pancreatitis'? Am J Surg Pathol 2003;27(1):110–20.
9. Sutcliffe RP, Lam W, O'Sullivan A, et al. Pancreaticoduodenectomy after liver transplantation in patients with primary sclerosing cholangitis complicated by distal pancreatobiliary malignancy. World J Surg 2010;34(9):2128–32.
10. Landaverde C, Ng V, Sato A, et al. De-novo cholangiocarcinoma in native com-mon bile duct remnant following OLT for primary sclerosing cholangitis. Ann Hepatol 2009;8(4):379–83.
11. Aljiffry M, Renfrew PD, Walsh MJ, et al. Analytical review of diagnosis and treat-ment strategies for dominant bile duct strictures in patients with primary scle-rosing cholangitis. HPB (Oxford) 2011;13(2):79–90.
12. Soreide K, Korner H, Havnen J, et al. Bile duct cysts in adults. Br J Surg 2004; 91(12):1538–48.
13. Dong JH, Yang SZ, Xia HT, et al. Aggressive hepatectomy for the curative treat-ment of bilobar involvement of type IV-A bile duct cyst. Ann Surg 2013;258(1): 122–8.
14. Kaewpitoon N, Kaewpitoon SJ, Pengsaa P, et al. Opisthorchis viverrini: the carcinogenic human liver fluke. World J Gastroenterol 2008;14(5):666–74.
15. Parkin DM, Srivatanakul P, Khlat M, et al. Liver cancer in Thailand. I. A case-control study of cholangiocarcinoma. Int J Cancer 1991;48(3):323–8.
16. Honjo S, Srivatanakul P, Sriplung H, et al. Genetic and environmental determinants of risk for cholangiocarcinoma via Opisthorchis viverrini in a densely infested area in Nakhon Phanom, northeast Thailand. Int J Cancer 2005;117(5):854–60.
17. Shin HR, Lee CU, Park HJ, et al. Hepatitis B and C virus, Clonorchis sinensis for the risk of liver cancer: a case-control study in Pusan, Korea. Int J Epidemiol 1996;25(5):933–40.

18. Yoon HA, Noh MH, Kim BG, et al. Clinicopathological significance of altered Notch signaling in extrahepatic cholangiocarcinoma and gallbladder carcinoma. World J Gastroenterol 2011;17(35):4023–30.

19. Werneburg NW, Yoon JH, Higuchi H, et al. Bile acids activate EGF receptor via a TGF-alpha-dependent mechanism in human cholangiocyte cell lines. Am J Physiol Gastrointest Liver Physiol 2003;285(1):G31–6.

20. Isomoto H, Kobayashi S, Werneburg NW, et al. Interleukin 6 upregulates myeloid cell leukemia-1 expression through a STAT3 pathway in cholangiocarcinoma cells. Hepatology 2005;42(6):1329–38.

21. Kobayashi S, Werneburg NW, Bronk SF, et al. Interleukin-6 contributes to Mcl-1 up-regulation and TRAIL resistance via an Akt-signaling pathway in cholangiocarcinoma cells. Gastroenterology 2005;128(7):2054–65.

22. Frampton G, Invernizzi P, Bernuzzi F, et al. Interleukin-6-driven progranulin expression increases cholangiocarcinoma growth by an Akt-dependent mechanism. Gut 2012;61(2):268–77.

23. Yoon JH, Canbay AE, Werneburg NW, et al. Oxysterols induce cyclooxygenase-2 expression in cholangiocytes: implications for biliary tract carcinogenesis. Hepatology 2004;39(3):732–8.

24. Ogasawara S, Yano H, Higaki K, et al. Expression of angiogenic factors, basic fibroblast growth factor and vascular endothelial growth factor, in human biliary tract carcinoma cell lines. Hepatol Res 2001;20(1):97–113.

25. Nonomura A, Ohta G, Nakanuma Y, et al. Simultaneous detection of epidermal growth factor receptor (EGF-R), epidermal growth factor (EGF) and ras p21 in cholangiocarcinoma by an immunocytochemical method. Liver 1988;8(3):157–66.

26. Arumugam T, Ramachandran V, Fournier KF, et al. Epithelial to mesenchymal transition contributes to drug resistance in pancreatic cancer. Cancer Res 2009;69(14):5820–8.

27. Yao X, Wang X, Wang Z, et al. Clinicopathological and prognostic significance of epithelial mesenchymal transition-related protein expression in intrahepatic cholangiocarcinoma. Onco Targets Ther 2012;5:255–61.

28. Itatsu K, Sasaki M, Yamaguchi J, et al. Cyclooxygenase-2 is involved in the up-regulation of matrix metalloproteinase-9 in cholangiocarcinoma induced by tumor necrosis factor-alpha. Am J Pathol 2009;174(3):829–41.

29. Nault JC, Zucman-Rossi J. Genetics of hepatobiliary carcinogenesis. Semin Liver Dis 2011;31(2):173–87.

30. Voss JS, Holtegaard LM, Kerr SE, et al. Molecular profiling of cholangiocarcinoma shows potential for targeted therapy treatment decisions. Hum Pathol 2013;44(7):1216–22.

31. Papaconstantinou I, Karakatsanis A, Gazouli M, et al. The role of microRNAs in liver cancer. Eur J Gastroenterol Hepatol 2012;24(3):223–8.

32. Corazziari E. Biliary tract imaging. Curr Gastroenterol Rep 1999;1(2):123–31.

33. Sharma MP, Ahuja V. Aetiological spectrum of obstructive jaundice and diagnostic ability of ultrasonography: a clinician's perspective. Trop Gastroenterol 1999;20(4):167–9.

34. Slattery JM, Sahani DV. What is the current state-of-the-art imaging for detection and staging of cholangiocarcinoma? Oncologist 2006;11(8):913–22.

35. Benson AB 3rd, Abrams TA, Ben-Josef E, et al. NCCN Clinical Practice Guidelines in Oncology (NCCN Guidelines®). Hepatobiliary Cancers. Version 1.2014. © 2014 National Comprehensive Cancer Network, Inc. Available at: NCCN.org. Accessed February 27, 2014.

36. Kubota Y, Takaoka M, Tani K, et al. Endoscopic transpapillary biopsy for diagnosis of patients with pancreaticobiliary ductal strictures. Am J Gastroenterol 1993;88(10):1700–4.

37. Ponchon T, Gagnon P, Berger F, et al. Value of endobiliary brush cytology and biopsies for the diagnosis of malignant bile duct stenosis: results of a prospective study. Gastrointest Endosc 1995;42(6):565–72.

38. Sugiyama M, Atomi Y, Wada N, et al. Endoscopic transpapillary bile duct biopsy without sphincterotomy for diagnosing biliary strictures: a prospective comparative study with bile and brush cytology. Am J Gastroenterol 1996; 91(3):465–7.

39. Wu LM, Jiang XX, Gu HY, et al. Endoscopic ultrasound-guided fine-needle aspiration biopsy in the evaluation of bile duct strictures and gallbladder masses: a systematic review and meta-analysis. Eur J Gastroenterol Hepatol 2011;23(2): 113–20.

40. Gabbert C, Warndorf M, Easler J, et al. Advanced techniques for endoscopic biliary imaging: cholangioscopy, endoscopic ultrasonography, confocal, and beyond. Gastrointest Endosc Clin N Am 2013;23(3):625–46.

41. Osanai M, Itoi T, Igarashi Y, et al. Peroral video cholangioscopy to evaluate indeterminate bile duct lesions and preoperative mucosal cancerous extension: a prospective multicenter study. Endoscopy 2013;45(8):635–42.

42. Malaguarnera G, Paladina I, Giordano M, et al. Serum markers of intrahepatic cholangiocarcinoma. Dis Markers 2013;34(4):219–28.

43. Alvaro D. Serum and bile biomarkers for cholangiocarcinoma. Curr Opin Gastroenterol 2009;25(3):279–84.

44. Jesudian AB, Jacobson IM. Screening and diagnosis of cholangiocarcinoma in patients with primary sclerosing cholangitis. Rev Gastroenterol Disord 2009; 9(2):E41–7.

45. Konishi M, Iwasaki M, Ochiai A, et al. Clinical impact of intraoperative histological examination of the ductal resection margin in extrahepatic cholangiocarcinoma. Br J Surg 2010;97(9):1363–8.

46. Yeo TP, Hruban RH, Leach SD, et al. Pancreatic cancer. Curr Probl Cancer 2002; 26(4):176–275.

47. Nakeeb A, Lillemoe KD, Grosfeld JL. Surgical techniques for pancreatic cancer. Minerva Chir 2004;59(2):151–63.

48. Riediger H, Makowiec F, Fischer E, et al. Postoperative morbidity and long-term survival after pancreaticoduodenectomy with superior mesenterico-portal vein resection. J Gastrointest Surg 2006;10(8):1106–15.

49. Harrison LE, Klimstra DS, Brennan MF. Isolated portal vein involvement in pancreatic adenocarcinoma. A contraindication for resection? Ann Surg 1996; 224(3):342–7 [discussion: 347–9].

50. Tseng JF, Raut CP, Lee JE, et al. Pancreaticoduodenectomy with vascular resection: margin status and survival duration. J Gastrointest Surg 2004;8(8):935–49 [discussion: 949–50].

51. Stitzenberg KB, Watson JC, Roberts A, et al. Survival after pancreatectomy with major arterial resection and reconstruction. Ann Surg Oncol 2008;15(5):1399–406.

52. Chua TC, Saxena A. Extended pancreaticoduodenectomy with vascular resection for pancreatic cancer: a systematic review. J Gastrointest Surg 2010;14(9): 1442–52.

53. LaFemina J, Chou JF, Gonen M, et al. Hepatic arterial nodal metastases in pancreatic cancer: is this the node of importance? J Gastrointest Surg 2013; 17(6):1092–7.

54. Tempero MA, Arnoletti JP, Behrman SW, et al. NCCN Clinical Practice Guidelines in Oncology (NCCN Guidelines®). Pancreatic Adenocarcinoma. Version 1.2014. © 2013 National Comprehensive Cancer Network, Inc. Available at: NCCN.org. Accessed February 27, 2014.

55. Verbeke CS. Resection margins in pancreatic cancer. Surg Clin North Am 2013; 93(3):647–62.

56. Verbeke CS. Resection margins and R1 rates in pancreatic cancer: are we there yet? Histopathology 2008;52(7):787–96.

57. Washington K, et al. Protocol for the Examination of Specimens From Patients With Carcinoma of the Exocrine Pancreas. College of American Pathologists (CAP). Available at: cap.org. Accessed February 28, 2014.

58. Mitsunaga S, Hasebe T, Iwasaki M, et al. Important prognostic histological parameters for patients with invasive ductal carcinoma of the pancreas. Cancer Sci 2005;96(12):858–65.

59. Gebhardt C, Meyer W, Reichel M, et al. Prognostic factors in the operative treatment of ductal pancreatic carcinoma. Langenbecks Arch Surg 2000;385(1): 14–20.

60. Distal bile duct. In: Edge SB, Byrd DR, editors. AJCC cancer staging manual. 7th edition. New York: Springer; 2010. p. 227–33.

61. DeOliveira ML, Cunningham SC, Cameron JL, et al. Cholangiocarcinoma: thirty-one-year experience with 564 patients at a single institution. Ann Surg 2007; 245(5):755–62.

62. Murakami Y, Uemura K, Sudo T, et al. Prognostic factors after surgical resection for intrahepatic, hilar, and distal cholangiocarcinoma. Ann Surg Oncol 2011; 18(3):651–8.

63. Murakami Y, Uemura K, Hayashidani Y, et al. Prognostic significance of lymph node metastasis and surgical margin status for distal cholangiocarcinoma. J Surg Oncol 2007;95(3):207–12.

64. He P, Shi JS, Chen WK, et al. Multivariate statistical analysis of clinicopathologic factors influencing survival of patients with bile duct carcinoma. World J Gastroenterol 2002;8(5):943–6.

65. Hong SM, Pawlik TM, Cho H, et al. Depth of tumor invasion better predicts prognosis than the current American Joint Committee on Cancer T classification for distal bile duct carcinoma. Surgery 2009;146(2):250–7.

66. Takada T, Amano H, Yasuda H, et al. Is postoperative adjuvant chemotherapy useful for gallbladder carcinoma? A phase III multicenter prospective randomized controlled trial in patients with resected pancreaticobiliary carcinoma. Cancer 2002;95(8):1685–95.

67. Neoptolemos JP, Stocken DD, Bassi C, et al. Adjuvant chemotherapy with fluorouracil plus folinic acid vs gemcitabine following pancreatic cancer resection: a randomized controlled trial. JAMA 2010;304(10):1073–81.

68. Hughes MA, Frassica DA, Yeo CJ, et al. Adjuvant concurrent chemoradiation for adenocarcinoma of the distal common bile duct. Int J Radiat Oncol Biol Phys 2007;68(1):178–82.

69. Yeo CJ, Sohn TA, Cameron JL, et al. Periampullary adenocarcinoma: analysis of 5-year survivors. Ann Surg 1998;227(6):821–31.

70. Nelson JW, Ghafoori AP, Willett CG, et al. Concurrent chemoradiotherapy in resected extrahepatic cholangiocarcinoma. Int J Radiat Oncol Biol Phys 2009; 73(1):148–53.

71. Borghero Y, Crane CH, Szklaruk J, et al. Extrahepatic bile duct adenocarcinoma: patients at high-risk for local recurrence treated with surgery and

adjuvant chemoradiation have an equivalent overall survival to patients with standard-risk treated with surgery alone. Ann Surg Oncol 2008;15(11): 3147–56.

72. Lim KH, Oh DY, Chie EK, et al. Adjuvant concurrent chemoradiation therapy (CCRT) alone versus CCRT followed by adjuvant chemotherapy: which is better in patients with radically resected extrahepatic biliary tract cancer? A non-randomized, single center study. BMC Cancer 2009;9:345.

73. Hezel AF, Zhu AX. Systemic therapy for biliary tract cancers. Oncologist 2008; 13(4):415–23.

74. Eckel F, Schmid RM. Chemotherapy in advanced biliary tract carcinoma: a pooled analysis of clinical trials. Br J Cancer 2007;96(6):896–902.

75. Valle J, Wasan H, Palmer DH, et al. Cisplatin plus gemcitabine versus gemcitabine for biliary tract cancer. N Engl J Med 2010;362(14):1273–81.

Gallbladder Cancer

Jessica A. Wernberg, MD*, Dustin D. Lucarelli, MD

KEYWORDS

- Gallbladder cancer • Radical cholecystectomy • Port site recurrence
- Biliary tract malignancy • Incidental gallbladder cancer

KEY POINTS

- Gallbladder cancer remains a disease with poor overall prognosis.
- Chronic inflammatory conditions of the gallbladder are associated with gallbladder cancer.
- T stage translates into the likelihood of identifying residual disease at reoperation for incidental gallbladder cancer, and residual disease negatively impacts survival.
- In select patients with radical operative intervention, there is an improvement in survival if R0 (margin negative) resection is achieved.
- There is no difference in survival in patients undergoing staged curative resection versus single-stage radical operation.
- Port site involvement of disease is predictive of poor outcome, often correlating with the presence of carcinomatosis.
- Improved systemic therapy is paramount to improving the overall survival in patients with gallbladder cancer.

INTRODUCTION

Gallbladder cancer remains a relatively rare malignancy with a highly variable presentation. Gallbladder cancer is the most common biliary tract malignancy with the worst overall prognosis. With the advent of the laparoscope, in comparison with historical controls, this disease is now more commonly diagnosed incidentally and at an earlier stage.[1–4] However, when symptoms of jaundice and pain are present, the prognosis remains dismal.[5] From a surgical perspective, gallbladder cancer can be suspected preoperatively, identified intraoperatively, or discovered incidentally on final surgical pathology.

INCIDENCE AND EPIDEMIOLOGY

Biliary tract cancers include intrahepatic bile duct cancers, extrahepatic bile duct cancers, and gallbladder cancers. These adenocarcinomas all arise from the biliary

There are no conflicts of interest to disclose for either author.
Department of General Surgery, Marshfield Clinic, 1000 North Oak Avenue, Marshfield, WI 54449, USA
* Corresponding author.
E-mail address: wernberg.jessica@marshfieldclinic.org

Surg Clin N Am 94 (2014) 343–360
http://dx.doi.org/10.1016/j.suc.2014.01.009
0039-6109/14/$ – see front matter © 2014 Elsevier Inc. All rights reserved.

epithelium, with gallbladder cancer being the most common.[6] There will be an estimated 10,310 new cases of gallbladder and extrahepatic biliary tract cancers diagnosed in 2013. This subset is the sixth most common gastrointestinal malignancy, with gallbladder carcinomas composing most of this group.[6]

Worldwide, there are regional variations in the incidence of gallbladder cancer. Central and Northern European, Indian, and Chilean populations have a higher incidence of gallbladder cancer when compared with the overall US population. The incidence rates of gallbladder cancer in Chile are more than 25 per 100,000 females and 9 per 100,000 males. These rates far exceed those that are found in the United States. The US incidence rates for gallbladder cancer are 0.9 and 0.5 per 100,000 females and males, respectively.[7] Racial discrepancies are also found with gallbladder cancer in the United States. American Indians, Alaskan natives, Asian Pacific/Islanders, blacks, and Hispanics all have a higher incidence when compared with non-Hispanic whites.[8–10]

As with most malignancies, the incidence of gallbladder cancer increases with age. The mean age at diagnosis is 65 years.[11] There is a strong predilection for gallbladder cancer among women, with female-to-male ratios varying from 1.3 to 3.5:1.0.[8,11–13] Sex and ethnicity are further discussed later as they relate to risk factors for this disease.

RISK FACTORS

Most gallbladder cancers are adenocarcinomas arising from the gallbladder mucosa. It is thought that chronic inflammation of the gallbladder mucosa may trigger progression from dysplasia to carcinoma in susceptible patients. Most of the known risk factors associated with gallbladder cancer are related to inflammation.[14]

Gallstones

The development of cholelithiasis is multifactorial in nature. Some of the risk factors for the development of cholelithiasis include age, sex, race, parity, and rapid weight loss.[15] Within the United States, cholesterol stones are the predominant stone type and are formed as a result of cholesterol supersaturation of bile, accelerated cholesterol crystal nucleation, and impaired gallbladder motility.[16] As discussed later, there is a potential genetic association that independently increases the risk of cholelithiasis and, thus, gallbladder cancer.[17,18]

There is clearly an association between benign gallstones and gallbladder cancer.[19–22] Piehler and Crichlow's[23] review of more than 2000 patients with gallbladder cancer found that 73.9% of patients had stones present. Other investigators have found similar results. Most patients (70%–88%) who present with gallbladder cancer have a history or presence of stones, but the incidence of gallbladder cancer among patients with stones is only 0.3% to 3.0%.[4,13,19,24] Diehl[24] showed that there is an increased association with gallbladder cancer as the size of gallstone increases. Although this is a graded phenomenon, stone size greater than 3 cm is thought to confer an up to 10 times increased risk of gallbladder cancer.[24] Roa and colleagues[25] showed that patients with gallbladder cancer will have an increased volume, weight, and density of their gallstones. Gallstone volume is associated with increased relative risk (RR) for developing gallbladder carcinoma, with volumes of 6 mL and 10 mL having RRs of 4.92 and 11.0, respectively.[25]

Gallbladder Polyps

Most polyps are not adenomatous, and most gallbladder cancers do not arise from polyps; however, removal of gallbladders containing polyps greater than 10 mm is recommended for cancer risk reduction.[26,27]

Polypoid lesions of the gallbladder greater than 10 mm, or those showing rapid growth, have classically been associated with gallbladder cancer.[22,28–31] An association between patient age and polypoid lesions containing malignancy has been shown. There is an increased risk for cancer with patients older than 50 years and polyps larger than 10 mm; thus, many surgeons will recommend elective cholecystectomy for this population.[30,32–34] Gallbladder polyps greater than 10 mm in patients older than 60 years and associated with gallstones were shown by Terzi and colleagues[34] to have an increased risk of being malignant in nature. In patients with polyps greater than 10 mm, 88% were found to harbor malignancy and 15% were thought to be benign.[34]

Infection

Bacterial-induced chronic inflammation has also been implicated as a risk factor for gallbladder cancer. Hepatobiliary cancers have been linked to specific bacterial infections, most notably *Salmonella typhi*.[21,22,35,36] Caygill and colleagues[35] demonstrated that chronic typhoid or paratyphoid carriers will have a significantly elevated risk (167 times observed/expected) of gallbladder cancer. Bile acid analysis demonstrated *Salmonella typhi* in 40% of patients with gallbladder cancer compared with 8% of patients with simple cholelithiasis, thus, suggesting that typhoid infection carries a stronger correlation with gallbladder cancer than simple cholelithiasis.[37] Typhoid-endemic areas, such as Chile, have an increased risk of gallbladder cancer.[18] Additionally, previous reports from India have shown an association with chronic typhoid carriage and gallbladder cancer.[38]

Anomalous Junction

Anomalous junction of the pancreaticobiliary ductal system (AJPBDS) has also been implicated as a potential risk factor for gallbladder cancer.[21] This anomaly will typically allow reflux of pancreatic fluid into the common bile duct and bile reflux into the pancreatic duct. The act of regurgitation can lead to inflammation and metaplasia within the gallbladder, thus, presenting a potential mechanism for adenocarcinoma pathogenesis.[39] The bile duct has a lower hydrostatic pressure than that found in the pancreatic duct; therefore, patients with AJPBDS have an increased propensity of flow from the pancreatic duct into the bile duct. Tanaka and colleagues[40] found that 17.8% of patients with AJPBDS developed a coexistent carcinoma, concluding that AJPBDS increases the risk of malignancy, including gallbladder cancer. Kang and colleagues[41] demonstrated that not only is there an increased incidence of gallbladder cancer with AJPBDS but that adenocarcinoma in this population tends to present at a younger age.

Porcelain Gallbladder

Porcelain gallbladder was once thought to significantly increase the risk of gallbladder cancer, as published by Etala[42] in 1962. In that study, there was a 12% to 61% incidence of gallbladder cancer among those patients with a calcified gallbladder. In the past 15 years, this has been refuted with studies showing a much lower incidence (5%–6%) of cancer associated with a calcified gallbladder.[43,44] Towfigh and colleagues[45] looked at 10,741 cholecystectomy patients, 15 of whom had a porcelain gallbladder. Of those 15 patients, none had evidence of gallbladder carcinoma. Stephen and Berger[43] found that the pattern of gallbladder wall calcification can depict its malignant potential. Although they showed an overall incidence of 5% malignancy associated with calcified gallbladder, a pattern of nondiffuse mucosal calcification carried an increased risk of malignancy. There continues to be a risk associated with calcified gallbladders, but the risk is more likely related to the inflammatory condition resulting in the porcelain gallbladder as opposed to the porcelain gallbladder itself. Porcelain gallbladder is minimally a surrogate for inflammation; given that gallbladder mucosal inflammation is a risk factor for gallbladder cancer, porcelain gallbladder remains an indication for cholecystectomy in appropriate patients.

Genetics

Given the epidemiology with known high-risk populations, a specific genetic link has been sought. Miguel and colleagues[17] showed a specific genetic link between cholesterol-laden bile and specific populations. Even without the typical lithogenic risk factor of obesity, specific ethnic groups with Amerindian maternal lineage in the Chilean population have an increased prevalence of gallstone formation thought to be associated with mtDNA polymorphisms. These factors support the theory of a genetic predisposition found within specific ethnic populations.[17,18] With previous work showing that cholelithiasis carries an increased risk of gallbladder cancer, and now a genetic link with lithogenic bile in specific populations, it may be inferred that there is a genetic risk for the development of gallbladder cancer.

There also seems to be a familial component that carries an increased risk for gallbladder cancer.[46,47] The Swedish Family Cancer Database has shown there is a 5.1-fold increased risk for developing gallbladder carcinoma when a parent had a diagnosis of gallbladder cancer.[47] An Italian case report found an RR of 13.9 for gallbladder cancer among first-degree relatives.[46] A cohort study from the United States found an association among first-degree relatives with an RR of 2.1,[48] although it is unclear whether this is genetic or environmentally based.

Sex

Worldwide, the incidence of gallbladder cancer is generally about double in females versus males. Norway, with an overall low incidence, has a female-to-male ratio of 2.0, 0.4 per 100,000 versus 0.2 per 100,000, respectively. In Chile, with a comparatively high incidence, the female-to-male ratio is 2.7, 25.3 per 100,000 versus 9.3 per 100,000, respectively. In the United States, the ratio across all ethnic groups is 1.8, female to male.[2,7,49] Although female sex is a risk factor for the development of gallbladder cancer, it has generally been thought to be related to the increased incidence of gallstones in women. That said, a recent study published in *Gene* suggests a sex-specific link to a genetic variant in the prostate stem cell antigen gene associated with gallbladder cancer.[50]

Others

Environmental risks have been demonstrated with specific occupations. The Cancer-Environment Registry study from Sweden found that there is an increased risk of gallbladder cancer in patients who work in the petroleum refining, textile, paper mill, and shoemaking industries.[51,52] There was an increased incidence of gallbladder cancer by 3.8 with petroleum refining workers, and a 1.8 increased incidence with paper mill workers compared with control cohorts.[51] Female workers in the textile industry have an increased RR of gallbladder cancer of 3.19.[52] Rubber industry workers are also thought to have a higher incidence of gallbladder cancer.[23]

Additional associated risk factors include cigarette smoking, drugs, chemical exposure, postmenopausal state, autoimmune disorders, and inflammatory bowel

disease.[2,53,54] Most of the nonepidemiologic risk factors seem to be related to the potential for mucosal inflammation and dysplasia.

ANATOMY

The anatomy of the gallbladder is relatively straightforward, with the gallbladder adherent to the undersurface of the liver along liver segments IV and V. Of course, cystic duct and cystic artery anatomy can be aberrant; but typically the cystic duct joins the main bile ducts defining the junction of the common hepatic and common bile ducts, and the cystic artery is generally a branch of the right hepatic artery. The venous drainage of the gallbladder is predominantly via the liver bed.[55]

The wall of the gallbladder, unless diseased, is thinner than that of other hollow viscus organs because there is no submucosa. The wall of the gallbladder is composed of mucosa, a muscular layer, perimuscular connective tissue, and serosa on the peritoneal surface. The T stage of a gallbladder cancer is anatomically related to the depth of invasion through the wall of the gallbladder. T1a tumors demonstrate invasion of the lamina propria; T1b tumors invade the muscular layer; T2 tumors invade perimuscular connective tissue without extension beyond the serosa or into the liver; and T3 perforates the serosa and/or directly penetrates the liver and/or one other adjacent organ (**Figs. 1** and **2**).[56]

PATHOLOGY

The standards for the evaluation of a cholecystectomy specimen vary. Generally, the specimen is inspected grossly by the pathologist or pathology assistant. If there are no obvious findings, or if clinical history is only that of benign disease, 3 slides are submitted for review: one from the fundus, one from the body, and one from the neck.[57] If a tumor is grossly identified or identified microscopically, additional sections are submitted. A European review that looked at incidental gallbladder cancer noted 13 cases identified only after port site or distant metastatic disease was detected in the face of negative initial surgical pathology from the gallbladder

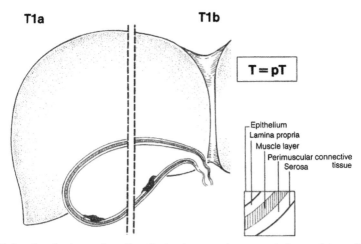

Fig. 1. T1 showing the tumor invading the lamina propria or muscle layer of the gallbladder. (Used with the permission of the American Joint Committee on Cancer (AJCC), Chicago, Illinois. The original source for this material is the AJCC Cancer Staging Manual, Seventh Edition (2010) published by Springer Science and Business Media LLC, www.springer.com.)

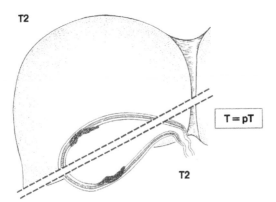

Fig. 2. T2 showing the tumor invading perimuscular connective tissue of the gallbladder with no extension of the tumor beyond serosa or into the liver. (Used with the permission of the American Joint Committee on Cancer (AJCC), Chicago, Illinois. The original source for this material is the AJCC Cancer Staging Manual, Seventh Edition (2010) published by Springer Science and Business Media LLC, www.springer.com.)

specimen.[55,58] If untoward pathologic conditions are suspected by the operating surgeon, a full histologic review of the specimen may be warranted.

STAGING/PROGNOSIS

In 1976, Nevin and colleagues[59] proposed a method that used histologic grading along with staging to determine the prognosis of gallbladder cancer. They stated that stage I and stage II cancers could be cured by simple cholecystectomy with a 5-year survival of 100%. Both stage III and stage IV had a poor prognosis; the 5-year survival rates were 6% and 3%, respectively.[59] In 1978, Piehler and Crichlow[23] reported a 4.1% 5-year survival for all patients and a 16.5% 5-year survival for those who were aggressively surgically resected. Currently, as with most other cancers, the American Joint Committee on Cancer (AJCC) uses the TNM staging system whereby T describes the tumor growth within the gallbladder or into adjacent organs, N describes lymphatic spread, and M indicates any evidence of metastases (**Table 1**).[56]

The seventh edition of the AJCC staging system was released in 2009 and incorporated into practice in 2010. As the stage of gallbladder cancer increases, the prognosis worsens precipitously as depicted in the survival curves (**Fig. 3**,[56] p. 212, **Table 2**). With the most current edition of the TNM staging system, nodal status seems to be the most suggestive of overall prognosis.[56,60] Earlier studies indicated that tumor status was inversely correlated with prognosis.[61,62] Oh and colleagues[60] found that as nodal status increased, regardless of T stage, there was a decrease in 3-year survival rates. Based on a single-center review of patients with gallbladder cancer, the median survival for stages I to III was 12 months, with median survival for stage IV patients being only 5.8 months.[63,64]

As more patients undergo laparoscopic cholecystectomy, the incidence of incidental gallbladder cancer will continue to increase. Proper staging workup is necessary in these patients to help guide treatment recommendations.

PREOPERATIVE IMAGING

Early gallbladder cancer is often associated with sonographic findings mistakable for cholecystitis; however, when more ominous features of malignancy exist, additional

Table 1
American Joint Committee on cancer 7th edition TNM staging for gallbladder cancer

Primary Tumor

TX	Primary tumor cannot be assessed
T0	No evidence of primary tumor
Tis	Carcinoma in situ
T1	Tumor invades lamina propria or muscular layer
T1a	Tumor invades lamina propria
T1b	Tumor invades muscular layer
T2	Tumor invades perimuscular connective tissue; no extension beyond serosa or into liver
T3	Tumor perforates the serosa (visceral peritoneum) and/or directly invades the liver and/or one other adjacent organ or structure, such as the stomach, duodenum, colon, pancreas, omentum, or extrahepatic bile ducts
T4	Tumor invades main portal vein or hepatic artery or invades at least 2 extrahepatic organs or structures

Regional Lymph Nodes

NX	Regional lymph nodes cannot be assessed
N0	No regional lymph node metastasis
N1	Metastases to nodes along the cystic duct, common bile duct, hepatic artery, and/or portal vein
N2	Metastases to periaortic, pericaval, superior mesenteric artery, and/or celiac artery lymph nodes

Distant Metastasis

M0	No distant metastasis
M1	Distant metastasis

Anatomic Stage/Prognostic Groups			
Stage	**T**	**N**	**M**
0	Tis	N0	M0
I	T1	N0	M0
II	T2	N0	M0
IIIA	T3	N0	M0
IIIB	T1–3	N1	M0
IVA	T4	N0–1	M0
IVB	Any T	N2	M0
	Any T	Any N	M1

Used with the permission of the American Joint Committee on Cancer (AJCC), Chicago, Illinois. The original source for this material is the AJCC Cancer Staging Manual, Seventh Edition (2010) published by Springer Science and Business Media LLC, www.springer.com.

imaging is warranted. Specifically, evidence of a lesion, as opposed to simple wall thickening, especially if associated with invasion, vascularity, sessile shape, or adenopathy, should increase the index of suspicion.[26] High-resolution computed tomography (CT) or magnetic resonance imaging may be helpful in determining resectability and ruling out distant disease. Additionally, ^{18}F-fluorodeoxyglucose (FDG) positron emission tomography (PET) CT may be appropriate for preoperative evaluation. Gallbladder cancer is thought to be highly FDG avid, with PET changing management in almost a quarter of patients in some series.[2,65,66] That said, negative PET imaging does not preclude reresection of incidentally found cancers,

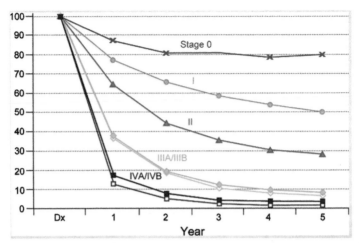

Fig. 3. Observed survival rates for 10,705 gallbladder cancers. Dx, diagnosis. Data from the National Cancer Data Base (Commission on Cancer of the American College of Surgeons and the American Cancer Society) diagnosed in years 1989 to 1996. (Used with the permission of the American Joint Committee on Cancer (AJCC), Chicago, Illinois. The original source for this material is the AJCC Cancer Staging Manual, Seventh Edition (2010) published by Springer Science and Business Media LLC, www.springer.com.)

because clearly small-volume disease or non–FDG-avid disease can be missed on PET.

Although asymptomatic gallbladder cancer discovered on imaging done for other reasons is truly incidental, the diagnosis is known, or at least suspected, by the surgeon preoperatively, thereby allowing additional preoperative evaluation. Whether initial imaging is done for gallbladder-related symptoms or for completely unrelated reasons, an abnormal appearance to the gallbladder may trigger more complex imagining to better define the extent of the disease. Biopsy of distant disease may be warranted for diagnostic purposes, generally to help guide palliative treatment. Biopsy of suspicious but presumably resectable disease is generally unnecessary.

INCIDENTALLY IDENTIFIED GALLBLADDER CANCER

Gallbladder cancer that is unsuspected preoperatively and subsequently discovered either at the time of cholecystectomy or on receipt of surgical pathology is referred to as *incidentally discovered* or *incidental gallbladder cancer*. With the advent of

Table 2	
5-year survival rates as depicted in Fig. 3	
Stage	**5-y Survival Rate (%)**
0	80
I	50
II	28
IIIA	8
IIIB	7
IVA	4
IVB	2

laparoscopy and the dramatic increase in the number of cholecystectomies performed, there has been an increase in the number of incidentally discovered gallbladder carcinomas.[1–3,55]

Most cholecystectomies performed in the United States are done laparoscopically. Gallbladder cancer is diagnosed during laparoscopic cholecystectomy or histologically on review of surgical pathology 0.2% to 2.0% of the time.[3,55,67–69] Most patients with gallbladder cancer also have gallstones, making a preoperative diagnosis of stone disease typical. Although the prognosis in this group is highly variable and based on overall staging, patients with incidentally discovered disease have improved survival versus those presenting nonincidentally, despite most patients having residual disease at reoperation.[2,3] Worse prognosis in the non-incidental group likely reflects an increased disease burden in those presenting with a more obvious carcinoma.

OPERATIVE MANAGEMENT

Up to half of all gallbladder cancers are diagnosed pathologically after cholecystectomy for presumed benign disease.[56] It is well recognized that T1a tumors require no further management beyond simple cholecystectomy, assuming negative resection margins.[63] The prognosis for Tis and T1a tumors is good, with 85% to 100% cured after simple cholecystectomy.[70]

In most patients presenting with symptoms from gallbladder cancer, the disease is advanced. The most common presenting symptoms are right upper quadrant pain and jaundice, with jaundice being an independent indicator of poor prognosis.[5,71] More than two-thirds of patients presenting to a tertiary cancer center without prior operation were found, either by imaging or at time of laparotomy, to have unresectable disease.[71]

Clearly, whether disease is incidental or known preoperatively, complete resection of all known disease is the objective of any oncologic procedure. Unfortunately, even with aggressive resectional therapy, R0 resection rates remain suboptimal. Shih and colleagues[1] reported R0 resection rates of 85% in patients with reexplored, incidentally discovered gallbladder cancer and only 25% in patients with primarily explored, nonincidentally discovered gallbladder cancer. Patients who are reexplored in the setting of incidentally discovered gallbladder cancer are a highly selected group, generally with lower tumor burden, likely explaining the improved R0 resection rates. This correlates with improved survival rates in those with incidentally discovered disease.[3]

There has been no difference in survival in patients undergoing staged curative resection (simple cholecystectomy followed by radical reresection) versus single-stage operation for gallbladder cancer. This fact would imply that for surgeons making intraoperative diagnoses of gallbladder cancer, closure and referral to a tertiary center does not adversely impact patient outcomes. This practice is the standard recommendation if the primary surgeon is not comfortable with the management of more complex hepatobiliary disease.[1,71]

Primary Operation (Known or Suspected Malignancy)

Patients presenting with incidentally discovered disease have a better median survival versus those presenting with known disease. Intuitively, patients presenting with symptoms or findings that suggest malignancy, either on history, examination, or imaging, are likely to have more advanced disease at presentation. Regardless, the goal of operative intervention is the same as for those with incidentally discovered disease: achieve an R0 resection. Thorough staging workup is appropriate to rule out distant metastatic disease or locally unresectable disease before proceeding with operative intervention. Diagnostic laparoscopy is also appropriate in this group, given the significant potential for peritoneal disease.[72] Assuming patients are reasonable operative candidates and that there is no evidence of distant disease or unresectability, proceeding with cholecystectomy, en block liver resection, lymphadenectomy, and bile duct resection, as necessary, is appropriate.[63]

Secondary Operation (After Incidental Discovery of Malignancy)

Repeat operative intervention is often indicated for incidentally discovered gallbladder carcinoma. In patients with margin negative T1a disease (invasion of lamina propria), locally unresectable disease, or distant metastases, there is no role for additional operative intervention.[63]

The National Comprehensive Cancer Network's (NCCN) guidelines recommend reoperation for T1b (invasion into muscular layer), T2 (invasion into perimuscular connective tissue), and T3 (perforates the serosa and/or directly penetrates the liver and/or one other adjacent organ) tumors (see **Figs. 1** and **2**).[56,63] There has been some controversy over the role of aggressive operative intervention in T1b disease; however, a Surveillance, Epidemiology, and End Results (SEER) registry review by Hari and colleagues[73] published in 2012 showed differential survival in patients with T1a versus T1b tumors treated with cholecystectomy alone, further supporting the NCCN's guidelines.

The NCCN's guideline surrounding T2 tumors is based on several reports showing improved survival in patients with T2 tumors undergoing radical cholecystectomy versus cholecystectomy alone.[74,75] A SEER review published in 2007 found that less than 10% of patients with T2 gallbladder cancer were treated based on these recommendations. There are, of course, intrinsic concerns with a retrospective database review; however, these results are concerning and may warrant further investigation.[74]

Residual Disease

In 2007, Pawlik and colleagues[3] published a multicenter review evaluating the likelihood of finding residual disease in patients undergoing reresection for incidental gallbladder cancer. There were 225 patients from 6 international centers included; 148 (65.8%) had incidental gallbladder cancer and 77 (34.2%) had nonincidental disease. The overall median survival of the cohort was 18 months. Of the 148 with incidental disease, 115 had staged operations and 33 had a definitive operation or were determined to be unresectable at the initial intervention. At the time of reoperation, 70 of 115 (60.8%) patients had residual or metastatic disease. Even in patients deemed appropriate for reresection, more than 40% had residual disease after initial cholecystectomy. The T stage correlated with the risk of finding residual disease. Patients with T1, T2, and T3 disease had a 37.5%, 56.7%, and 77.3% chance of having additional disease, respectively. Patients with no residual disease at reoperation had a 5-year survival of 84.8% versus 36.9% (P = .01) for those with residual disease.[3]

In a French database review of patients with incidental gallbladder cancer, those patients undergoing reexcision had a better overall survival at 1 year: 76% in the reresection group (n = 148) and 52% (n = 70) in the no reresection group.[76] Of those undergoing reresection, 56% were found to have residual disease. In this retrospective review, reasons for not undergoing reresection included age and T stage; specifically, no T1a patients underwent reresection.[76] One of the limitations with this and other similar studies is the difficulty in knowing the true stage of the unresected group. Clearly, there are patients who are thought clinically to be T2 who actually have peritoneal disease, possibly skewing the data in favor of the reresection group.[76]

Management of the Liver Bed

Gallbladder cancer has the potential to spread via direct extension into the liver, along the ducts, or into adjacent organs. Metastatic disease can also be disseminated via the peritoneum, the lymphatic system, and/or hematogenously. The gallbladder lies anatomically along the caudal aspect of the liver at the junction of the left and right lobes, allowing for direct invasion into the liver at this site.

Some have advocated radical liver resection for gallbladder cancer. Dixon and colleagues[77] compared 2 time periods, with the more contemporary time period representing more radical liver resection based on a change in disease management strategy. There was improved overall survival in the contemporary group undergoing more radical liver resection versus the earlier group. Survival rates in both periods were similar in the R0 and R1 resection groups; however, more R0 resections were achieved in the period of radical resection. They concluded that R0 resection improves overall survival in patients undergoing curative resection for gallbladder cancer and that radical resection improves the likelihood of obtaining a negative resection margin.[77] In that series, radical resection (2 to 6 liver segments) was associated with a complication rate of 49% (major complications requiring intervention in 29%) and a mortality rate of 2%.[77]

Pawlik and colleagues[3] reviewed 97 patients undergoing hepatic resection (wedge resection vs formal segmentectomy vs hemihepatectomy) at the time of reoperation for incidental gallbladder cancer and found that the extent of hepatic resection was not associated with a survival benefit. The likelihood of finding additional disease in the liver correlated with the T stage, with 0%, 10.4%, and 36.4% having hepatic disease at the time of reresection for incidentally identified T1, T2, and T3 gallbladder cancer, respectively.[3]

Other studies have also shown that the extent of liver resection and bile duct resection did not impact survival and that more extensive resections may instead only increase morbidity.[1,70,76,78] In most cases, extended hepatectomy is unnecessary. Although there are clearly large variations in extent of liver resection performed for curative intent, the inability to achieve an R0 resection may be an indicator of aggressive biology and, as such, a marker of poor prognosis.

Management of the Cystic Duct Stump and Extrahepatic Bile Ducts

Some surgeons perform extrahepatic bile duct resection as part of a standard radical resection for gallbladder cancer; others advocate this approach to facilitate nodal dissection; and some selectively perform bile duct resection only for a positive cystic duct margin.

As with residual liver disease, cystic duct margin positivity correlates with the likelihood of finding residual ductal disease at reresection. Residual ductal disease was identified in only 4.3% (1 of 23) of patients with pathologically negative cystic duct margins but was found in 42.1% (8 of 19) of those with positive cystic duct margins. In all reresected patients with incidental gallbladder cancer, residual disease was identified in the bile ducts in about 20%.[3] Although bile duct resection was not found to improve lymph node yield for lymphadenectomy, R0 resection rates are thought to be improved in patients undergoing common duct resection in the setting of an initially positive cystic duct margin.[3] Multiple studies have failed to show a survival benefit with extended biliary resection, and the NCCN's guidelines do not routinely advocate bile duct resection in the setting of a negative cystic duct margin.[1,3,63,76]

Role of Lymphadenectomy

The seventh edition of the AJCC staging manual defines N1 disease as nodal involvement of the cystic duct, common bile duct, portal vein, and/or hepatic artery nodes.[56] N2 disease involves periaortic, pericaval, celiac, and/or superior mesenteric artery lymph nodes (see **Table 1**). N2 disease is stage IVB disease, and there is no role for aggressive resection.

T stage is thought to correlate with the likelihood of regional nodal metastases at reresection in patients with incidentally discovered gall bladder cancer: T1 (12.5%), T2 (31.2%), and T3 (45.5%).[3] Although there is no proven survival benefit to lymphadenectomy, nodal status is an important prognostic feature; therefore, routine lymphadenectomy is recommended in T1b and higher resectable gallbladder cancers with clinical N0 or N1 disease.[63,79]

In a retrospective review of patients undergoing reoperation for incidentally discovered gallbladder cancer, Pawlik and colleagues[3] found pathologic evidence of nodal metastases in 16 of 24 patients, with at least one cystic duct node evaluated with the initial cholecystectomy specimen. In those undergoing subsequent lymphadenectomy, a median of 3 nodes was resected, regardless of whether the lymphadenectomy was done in conjunction with a common bile duct resection.[3] This finding suggests that, despite some proponents of common duct resection for facilitation of lymphadenectomy, the yield of the nodal harvest may not be improved despite a more radical approach and associated increased morbidity.[3,70,78]

Diagnostic Laparoscopy

Gallbladder cancer has a high rate of peritoneal disease, with carcinomatosis identified in 30% to 75% of patients.[2] In 2002, Weber and colleagues[72] published a prospective series of 100 patients evaluating the use of diagnostic laparoscopy for biliary tract malignancy. Of the 100 eligible patients, 44 had a primary gallbladder cancer, with 21 of 44 having disease identified at time of laparoscopy that precluded laparotomy. Of those with disease identified at the time of laparoscopy, 15 had peritoneal metastases and 6 had previously undiscovered liver metastases. The other 23 patients went on to laparotomy, with 15 of those subsequently determined to be unresectable because of peritoneal disease in one patient, liver disease in 2 patients, extensive nodal disease in 3 patients, and locally advanced unresectable disease in 9 patients. Although laparoscopy did not prevent nontherapeutic laparotomy in all cases, 48% of patients were spared more extensive operative exploration with presumably faster recovery and shorter time to the onset of palliative treatments.[72] In a disease with a median survival of only about 5 months in the setting of unresectable disease, extended surgical recovery is potentially unwarranted. That said, without laparotomy, it is difficult to determine local resectability.

In another series evaluating cases of suspected gallbladder cancer, 5 of 54 were unresectable by preoperative imaging, 1 refused further surgery, and 48 of 54 underwent surgical exploration.[1] Of the 48 explored patients, 15 (31%) were deemed unresectable at laparotomy, 5 (10%) were deemed unresectable at laparoscopy, and 28 (58%) went on to have resectional therapy.[1]

The yield of staging laparoscopy decreases in patients with incidentally discovered gallbladder cancer likely because of decreased disease burden or identification of metastatic disease at the initial operation making them ineligible to present for subsequent laparoscopy. As few as 20% of patients will be found to have advanced disease in the subgroup of incidentally discovered gallbladder cancer,[72] possibly limiting the utility of laparoscopy in those patients having undergone a recent laparoscopic cholecystectomy.

Port Site Management

In the modern era, most gallbladder cancers are identified incidentally after laparoscopic cholecystectomy done for presumed stone-related symptoms. Because gallbladder cancer has a high propensity for peritoneal seeding and carcinomatosis, port site recurrence is a relatively common phenomenon after laparoscopic cholecystectomy in the setting of incidentally discovered gallbladder cancer. In some series, subsequent port site tumoral involvement can be as much as 10%, with a range from 1% to 40%.[1,3,76,80]

Maker and colleagues[80] reviewed their data on port site involvement in 69 patients having T1b, T2, or T3 disease who had port sites resected at the time of radical resection. They reported that 19% of patients (13 of 69) with port site resection had pathologic involvement; however, this was only seen in patients with T2 and T3 disease. Although port site resection was not associated with improved survival, patients with port site involvement had a worse prognosis, as this seemed to indicate more advanced disease and often carcinomatosis. Of patients with port site involvement, 77% also had peritoneal metastasis.[80]

Port sites other than the original extraction port can be involved, with tumor highlighting the potential for diffuse peritoneal dissemination in addition to direct tumoral seeding. Although extraction site, mode of gallbladder extraction, and occurrence of perforation may impact the decision to resect trocar sites at the time of subsequent operation, resection is unlikely to improve survival; port site involvement remains a marker of poor prognosis.

ADJUVANT THERAPY/PALLIATIVE THERAPY

Clearly, complete surgical resection offers the best chance of cure for patients with gallbladder cancer. There are currently no recommendations for neoadjuvant treatment in patients with locally advanced gallbladder malignancy. Adjuvant treatment, however, continues to be recommended regularly.[2,63,81,82] Per the NCCN's guidelines, there are no definite standard regimens supported by randomized controlled trials and no proven benefit to any adjuvant treatment. Multiple adjuvant therapy regimens are used, and observation continues to be an acceptable option after resection.[63]

The Mayo Clinic reviewed their outcomes in patients with R0 resectional therapy, comparing those with subsequent adjuvant therapy with those without.[83] There were 73 patients included in this retrospective review spanning 20 years, with 43 (59%) T1-2N0M0 and 30 (41%) T3N0M0 or T1-3N1M0. Adjuvant therapy usually consisted of combined chemotherapy and radiation. The overall survival was similar in the group receiving adjuvant therapy and the group that underwent surgery alone, although patients with more advanced disease tended to have adjuvant therapy.[83]

Although evidence to definitively support adjuvant treatment in gallbladder cancer is lacking, Sharma and colleagues[81] randomly assigned 81 unresectable patients to one of 3 arms: best supportive care, fluorouracil and folinic acid, and modified gemcitabine and oxaliplatin. The median overall survival was 4.5, 4.6, and 9.5 months, respectively.[81]

Given the overall poor prognosis of this disease, palliative strategies continue to evolve. Palliative percutaneous or endoscopic biliary drainage may improve symptoms related to malignant biliary obstruction. Combinations of chemotherapy and radiation may improve survival and quality of life, with gemcitabine used in most adjuvant and palliative regimens for gallbladder cancer.[82] Clearly improved systemic therapy is paramount to improving overall survival in patients with gallbladder cancer.

SUMMARY

A historical series in the natural history of gallbladder cancer published in *Cancer* in 1978 reported an overall median survival of 5.2 months.[4] Although this is similar to the 5-year survival seen in current stage III and IV patients, more gallbladder cancers are presently being diagnosed incidentally, at earlier stages, and with better prognoses. Gallbladder cancer remains a challenging disease in terms of prognosis, preoperative diagnosis, surgical management, and systemic treatment.

Surgical management, with R0 resection as the objective, offers the best prognosis with the only hope of cure. With T1a tumors, this usually occurs at the time of cholecystectomy accounting for the significantly better survival in this group despite the typical recommendation for no additional operation. Many T2 patients are not treated based on current recommendations, leaving room for improvement in the surgical treatment of gallbladder cancer.[74,84]

Studies suggest that if R0 resection is achieved with reoperation for incidental gallbladder cancer, survival is improved. No residual disease at the time of reoperation is also a marker for improved prognosis[3]; in the setting of R0 resection, more radical liver and bile duct resections do not seem, in some series, to improve survival.[1,70,76,78] The stage of disease, as a surrogate for tumor biology, is the most important predictor of complete resectability and, therefore, outcome in gallbladder carcinoma.[3,70,78] Improved systemic therapy will be critical in improving long-term outcomes for these patients.

REFERENCES

1. Shih SP, Schulick RD, Cameron JL, et al. Gallbladder cancer: the role of laparoscopy and radical resection. Ann Surg 2007;245:893–901.
2. Hueman MT, Vollmer CM, Pawlik TM. Evolving treatment strategies for gallbladder cancer. Ann Surg Oncol 2009;16:2101–15.
3. Pawlik TM, Gleisner AL, Vigano L, et al. Incidence of finding residual disease for incidental gallbladder carcinoma: implications for re-resection. J Gastrointest Surg 2007;11:1478–86.
4. Perpetuo MD, Valdivieso M, Heilbrun LK, et al. Natural history study of gallbladder cancer: a review of 36 years experience at M.D. Anderson Cancer Center. Cancer 1978;42:330–5.
5. Hawkins WG, DeMatteo RP, Jarnagin WR, et al. Jaundice predicts advanced disease and early mortality in patients with gallbladder cancer. Ann Surg Oncol 2004;11:310–5.
6. Siegel R, Naishadham D, Jemal A. Cancer statistics, 2013. CA Cancer J Clin 2013;63:11–30.
7. Randi G, Malvezzi M, Levi F, et al. Epidemiology of biliary tract cancers: an update. Ann Oncol 2009;20:146–59.
8. Castro FA, Koshiol J, Hsing AN, et al. Biliary tract cancer incidence in the United States – demographic and temporal variations by anatomic site. Int J Cancer 2013;133:1664–72.
9. Devor EJ, Buechley RW. Gallbladder cancer in Hispanic New Mexicans. Cancer 1980;45:1705–12.

10. Strom BL, Soloway RD, Rios-Dalenz JL, et al. Risk factors for gallbladder cancer and international collaborative case-control study. Cancer 1995;76:1747–56.
11. Ries LA, Young JL, Keel GE, et al, editors. SEER survival monograph: cancer survival among adults: U.S. SEER Program, 1988-2001, patient and tumor characteristics. National Cancer Institute, SEER Program. Bethesda (MD): NIH; 2007. Pub. No. 07–6215.
12. Zatonski WA, Lowenfels AB, Boyle P, et al. Epidemiologic aspects of gallbladder cancer: a case-control study of the SEARCH program of international agency for research on cancer. J Natl Cancer Inst 1997;89:1132–8.
13. Hamdani NH, Qadri SK, Aggarwalla R, et al. Clinicopathological study of gall-bladder carcinoma with special reference to gallstones: our 8 year experience from eastern India. Asian Pac J Cancer Prev 2012;13:5613–7.
14. Albores-Saaverdra J, Alcantra-Vazqauez A, Cruz-Ortiz H, et al. The precursor lesions of invasive gallbladder carcinoma. Hyperplasia, atypical hyperplasia and carcinoma in situ. Cancer 1980;45:919–27.
15. Everhart JE, Khare M, Hill M, et al. Prevalence and ethnic differences in gall-bladder disease in the United States. Gastroenterology 1999;117:632–9.
16. Venneman NG, VanErpecum KJ. Pathogenesis of gallstones. Gastroenterol Clin North Am 2010;39:171–83.
17. Miguel JF, Covarrubias C, Villaroel L, et al. Genetic epidemiology of cholesterol cholelithiasis among Chilean Hispanics, Amerindians, and Maoris. Gastroenterology 1998;115:937–46.
18. Andia ME, Hsing AW, Andreotti G, et al. Geographic variation of gallbladder cancer mortality and risk factors in Chile: a population-based ecologic study. Int J Cancer 2008;123:1411–6.
19. Hsing AW, Gao YT, Han TQ, et al. Gallstones and the risk of biliary tract cancer; a population-based study in China. Br J Cancer 2007;97:1577–82.
20. Gracie WA, Ransohoff DF. The natural history of silent gallstones-the innocent gallstone is not a myth. N Engl J Med 1982;307:798–800.
21. Pandey M. Risk factors for gallbladder cancer; a reappraisal. Eur J Cancer Prev 2003;12:15–24.
22. Pilgrim CH, Groeschl RT, Christians KK, et al. Modern perspectives on factors predisposing to the development of gallbladder cancer. HPB (Oxford) 2013; 15:839–44.
23. Piehler JM, Crichlow RW. Primary carcinoma of the gallbladder. Surg Gynecol Obstet 1978;147:929–42.
24. Diehl AK. Gallstone size and the risk of gallbladder cancer. JAMA 1983;250: 2323–6.
25. Roa I, Ibacache G, Roa J, et al. Gallstones and gallbladder cancer-volume and weight of gallstones are associated with gallbladder cancer: a case-control study. J Surg Oncol 2006;93:624–8.
26. Pilgrim CH, Groeschl RT, Pappas SG, et al. An often overlooked diagnosis: im-aging features of gallbladder cancer. J Am Coll Surg 2013;216:333–9.
27. Adsay NV. Neoplastic precursors of the gallbladder and extra-hepatic biliary system. Gastroenterol Clin North Am 2007;36:889–900.
28. Kubota K, Bandai Y, Noie T, et al. How should polypoid lesions of the gallbladder be treated in the era of laparoscopic cholecystectomy. Surgery 1995;117:481–7.
29. Shin SR, Lee JK, Lee KH, et al. Can the growth rate of a gallbladder polyp pre-dict a neoplastic polyp. J Clin Gastroenterol 2009;43:865–8.
30. Lee KF, Wong J, Li JC, et al. Polypoid lesions of the gallbladder. Am J Surg 2004;188:186–90.

31. Ito H, Hann LE, D'Angelica M, et al. Polypoid lesions of the gallbladder: diagnosis and follow-up. J Am Coll Surg 2009;208:570–5.

32. Yeh CN, Jan YY, Chao TC, et al. Laparoscopic cholecystectomy for polypoid lesions of the gallbladder. Surg Laparosc Endosc Percutan Tech 2001;11:176–81.

33. He ZM, Hu XQ, Zhou ZX. Considerations on indications for surgery in patients with polypoid lesions of the gallbladder. Di Yi Jun Yi Da Xue Xue Bao 2002; 22:951–2.

34. Terzi C, Sokmen S, Seckin S, et al. Polypoid lesions of the gallbladder: report of 100 cases with special reference to operative indications. Surgery 2000;127:622–7.

35. Caygill CP, Hill MJ, Braddick M, et al. Cancer mortality in chronic typhoid and paratyphoid carriers. Lancet 1994;343:83–4.

36. Kumar S, Kumar S, Kumar S. Infection as a risk for gallbladder cancer. J Surg Oncol 2006;93:633–9.

37. Sharma V, Chauhan VS, Nath G, et al. Role of bacteria in gallbladder carcinoma. Hepatogastroenterology 2007;54:1622–5.

38. Dutta U, Garg PK, Kumar R, et al. Typhoid carriers among patients with gallstones are at increased risk for carcinoma of the gallbladder. Am J Gastroenterol 2000;95:784–7.

39. Nagat E, Sakai K, Kinoshita K, et al. The relation between carcinoma of the gallbladder and an anomalous connection between the choledochus and the pancreatic duct. Ann Surg 1985;202:182–90.

40. Tanaka K, Ikoma A, Hamada N, et al. Biliary tract cancer accompanied by anomalous junction of the pancreaticobiliary ductal system in adults. Am J Surg 1998;175:218–20.

41. Kang CM, Kim KS, Choi JS, et al. Gallbladder carcinoma associated with anomalous pancreaticobiliary duct junction. Can J Gastroenterol 2007;21:383–7.

42. Etala E. Cancer de la vesicula bilia. Prensa Med Argent 1962;49:2283–99.

43. Stephen AE, Berger DL. Carcinoma in the porcelain gallbladder: a relationship revisited. Surgery 2001;129:699–703.

44. Schnelldorfer T. Porcelain gallbladder: a benign process or concern for malignancy. J Gastrointest Surg 2013;17:1161–8.

45. Towfigh S, McFadden DW, Cortina GR, et al. Porcelain gallbladder is not associated with gallbladder carcinoma. Am Surg 2001;67:7–10.

46. Fernanadez E, La Vecchia C, D'Avanzo B, et al. Family history and risk of liver, gallbladder, and pancreatic cancer. Cancer Epidemiol Biomarkers Prev 1994;3: 209–12.

47. Hemminki K, Li X. Familial liver and gallbladder cancer: a nationwide epidemiological study from Sweden. Gut 2003;52:592–6.

48. Goldgar DE, Easton DF, Cannon-Albright LA, et al. Systematic population-based assessment of cancer risk in first-degree relatives of cancer probands. J Natl Cancer Inst 1994;86:1600–8.

49. Carriaga MT, Henson DE. Liver, gallbladder, extrahepatic bile ducts, and pancreas. Cancer 1995;75:171–90.

50. Rai R, Sharma KL, Misra S, et al. PSCA gene variants (rs2294008 and rs2978974) confer increased susceptibility of gallbladder carcinoma in females. Gene 2013;530:172–7.

51. Malker HS, McLaughlin JK, Malker BK, et al. Biliary tract cancer and occupation in Sweden. Br J Ind Med 1986;43:257–62.

52. Kuzmickiene I, Didziapetris R, Stukonis M. Cancer incidence in the workers cohort of textile manufacturing factory in Alytus, Lithuania. J Occup Environ Med 2004;46:147–53.

53. Lazcano-Pance EC, Miqel JF, Munoz N, et al. Epidemiology and molecular pathology of gallbladder cancer. CA Cancer J Clin 2001;51:349–64.

54. Mancuso TF, Brennan MJ. Epidemiological considerations of cancer of the gallbladder, bile ducts and salivary glands in the rubber industry. J Occup Med 1970;12:333–41.

55. Varshney S, Buttirini G, Gupta R. Incidental carcinoma of the gallbladder. Eur J Surg Oncol 2002;28:4–10.

56. AJCC. Gallbladder (chapter 20). In: Edge S, Byrd DR, Compton CC, et al, editors. AJCC cancer staging manual. 7th edition. New York: Springer; 2010. p. 211–7.

57. Odze RD, Crawford JM, Glickman JN, et al. Gastrointestinal specimens (including hepatobiliary and pancreatic specimens): gallbladder. In: Lester SC, editor. Manual of surgical pathology. 2nd edition. Philadelphia: Elsevier; 2006. p. 354–8.

58. Paolucci V, Schaeff B, Schneider M, et al. Tumour seeding following laparoscopy: international survey. World J Surg 1999;23:989–97.

59. Nevin JE, Moran TJ, Kay S, et al. Carcinoma of the gallbladder: staging, treatment, and prognosis. Cancer 1976;37:141–8.

60. Oh TG, Chung MJ, Bang S, et al. Comparison of the sixth and seventh editions of the AJCC TNM classification for gallbladder cancer. J Gastrointest Surg 2013; 17:925–30.

61. Chan CP, Chang HC, Chen YL, et al. A 10 year experience of unsuspected gallbladder cancer after laparoscopic cholecystectomy. Int Surg 2003;88:175–9.

62. D'Hondt M, Lapointe R, Benamira Z, et al. Carcinoma of the gallbladder: patterns of presentation, prognostic factors and survival rate. An 11 year single center experience. Eur J Surg Oncol 2013;39:548–53.

63. NCCN-National Comprehensive Cancer Network. NCCN guidelines version 1. 2013. Gallbladder cancer. Available at: http://www.nccn.org/professionals/physician_gls/f_guidelines.asp#hepatobiliary. Accessed September, 2013.

64. Duffy A, Capanu M, Abou-Alfa GK, et al. Gallbladder cancer (GBC): 10-year experience at Memorial Sloan-Kettering Cancer Centre (MSKCC). J Surg Oncol 2008;98:485–9.

65. Corvera CU, Blumgart LH, Akhurst T, et al. 18F-fluorodeoxyglucose positron emission tomography influences management decision in patients with biliary cancer. J Am Coll Surg 2008;206:57–65.

66. Anderson CD, Rice MH, Pinson CW, et al. Fluorodeoxyglucose PET imaging in the evaluation of gallbladder carcinoma and cholangiocarcinoma. J Gastrointest Surg 2004;8:90–7.

67. Zhang WJ, Xu GF, Zou XP, et al. Incidental gallbladder carcinoma diagnosed during or after laparoscopic cholecystectomy. World J Surg 2009;33:2651–6.

68. Kwon AH, Imamura A, Kitade H, et al. Unsuspected gallbladder cancer diagnosed during or after laparoscopic cholecystectomy. J Surg Oncol 2008;97:241–5.

69. Panebianco A, Volpi A, Lozito C, et al. Incidental gallbladder carcinoma: our experience. G Chir 2013;34:167–9.

70. D'Angelica M, Dalal KM, DeMatteo RP, et al. Analysis of the extent of resection for adenocarcinoma of the gallbladder. Ann Surg Oncol 2009;16:806–16.

71. Fong Y, Jarnagin W, Blumgart LH. Gallbladder cancer: comparison of patients presenting initially for definitive operation with those presenting after prior non-curative intervention. Ann Surg 2000;232:557–69.

72. Weber SM, DeMatteo RP, Fong Y, et al. Staging laparoscopy in patients with extrahepatic biliary carcinoma. Analysis of 100 patients. Ann Surg 2002;235: 392–9.

73. Hari DM, Howard JH, Keung AM, et al. A 21-year analysis of stage I gallbladder carcinoma: is cholecystectomy alone adequate? HPB (Oxford) 2013;15:40–8.

74. Wright BE, Lee CC, Iddings DM, et al. Management of T2 gallbladder cancer: are practice patterns consistent with national recommendations? Am J Surg 2007;194:820–5 [discussion: 825–6].

75. Foster JM, Hoshi H, Gibbs JF, et al. Gallbladder cancer: defining the indications for primary radical resection and radical re-resection. Ann Surg Oncol 2007;14: 833–40.

76. Fuks D, Regimbeau JM, Le Treut YP, et al. Incidental gallbladder cancer by the AFC-GBC-2009 Study Group. World J Surg 2011;35(8):1887–97.

77. Dixon E, Vollmer CM, Sahajpal A, et al. An aggressive surgical approach leads to improved survival in patients with gallbladder cancer. Ann Surg 2005;241: 385–94.

78. Pawlik TM, Choti MA. Biology dictates prognosis following resection of gallbladder carcinoma: sometimes less is more. Ann Surg Oncol 2009;16:787–8.

79. Zhu AX, Hong TS, Hezel AR, et al. Current management of gallbladder carcinoma. Oncologist 2010;15:168–81.

80. Maker AV, Butte JM, Oxenberg J, et al. Is port site resection necessary in the surgical management of gallbladder cancer? Ann Surg Oncol 2012;19:409–17.

81. Sharma A, Dwary AD, Mohanti BK, et al. Best supportive care compared with chemotherapy for unresectable gall bladder cancer: a randomized controlled study. J Clin Oncol 2010;28:4581–6.

82. Daines WP, Rajagopalan V, Grossbard ML, et al. Gallbladder and biliary tract carcinoma: a comprehensive update, part 2. Oncology 2004;18:1049–68.

83. Gold DG, Miller RC, Haddock MG, et al. Adjuvant therapy for gallbladder carcinoma: the Mayo Clinic experience. Int J Radiat Oncol Biol Phys 2009;75:150–5.

84. Jensen EH, Abraham A, Habermann EB, et al. A critical analysis of the surgical management of early-stage gallbladder cancer in the United States. J Gastrointest Surg 2009;13:722–7.

Bile Metabolism and Lithogenesis

Kathleen O'Connell, MD[a], Karen Brasel, MD, MPH[b],*

KEYWORDS

- Gallstones • Gallbladder • Cholelithiasis • Bile • Bile acids

KEY POINTS

- Bile acids play a prominent role in expression of genes involved in their own uptake and secretion within the enterohepatic circulation.
- Bile acids serve as ligands for the nuclear receptor farnesoid X receptor and transmembrane protein TGR5, through which they exert their regulatory effects in hepatic and extrahepatic tissues.
- Cholelithiasis is a disease associated with the metabolic syndrome and is the result of both modifiable and nonmodifiable risk factors.
- Different types of gallstones (cholesterol, black pigment, brown pigment stones) are associated with separate risk factors and disease processes.
- Disease states and therapies can alter bile metabolism, leading to an increased risk of gallstone formation.

INTRODUCTION

Gallstone disease affects 20 to 25 million adults in the United States.[1,2] Although most patients remain asymptomatic, some patients do eventually progress to symptomatic or complicated disease, leading to more than 750,000 cholecystectomies in the United States every year.[3] Of all hospital admissions in 2009, cholelithiasis and cholecystitis were the second most common discharge diagnoses among patients admitted with gastrointestinal illnesses.[4] Cholelithiasis poses a significant economic burden in this country, with direct and indirect costs totaling $6.2 billion annually.[2,5] As our population continues to age and the obesity epidemic persists, the incidence of gallstone disease is increasing. A thorough understanding of the underlying physiology of bile metabolism and lithogenesis is necessary to provide optimal management of these patients and for developing new strategies to prevent gallstone formation.

BILE METABOLISM

The synthesis of bile acids, the formation of bile, the enterohepatic circulation, and the modifications of bile acids throughout their lifespan all contribute in the metabolism of

[a] Department of Surgery, Medical College of Wisconsin, 9200 West Wisconsin Avenue, Milwaukee, WI 53226, USA; [b] Surgery, Bioethics and Medical Humanities, Medical College of Wisconsin, 9200 West Wisconsin Avenue, Milwaukee, WI 53226, USA
* Corresponding author.
E-mail address: kbrasel@mcw.edu

Surg Clin N Am 94 (2014) 361–375
http://dx.doi.org/10.1016/j.suc.2014.01.004
0039-6109/14/$ – see front matter © 2014 Elsevier Inc. All rights reserved.
surgical.theclinics.com

bile. In recent years, many advances have been made in the understanding of the widespread activities of bile acids on a cellular and molecular level.

Function of Bile Acids

Bile acids function as the detergent component of bile, emulsifying dietary fats, fat-soluble vitamins, and drugs to allow intestinal absorption. Bile acids and phosphatidylcholine maintain the solubility of cholesterol in bile; the excretion of bile acids is the primary pathway for cholesterol catabolism, accounting for 50% of the daily turnover.[6] Recently, many studies have shown that bile acids have other important physiologic activities beyond fat digestion, including regulation of their own synthesis, endocrine and paracrine functions.[7–9] Bile acids serve as ligands for nuclear receptors, mainly farnesoid X receptor (FXR) and pregnane X receptor, which are involved in carbohydrate, triglyceride, and sterol metabolism.[10–13] Bile acids have also been shown to interact with cell surface receptors, namely TGR5, and be involved in energy expenditure, lipid metabolism, glucose homeostasis, and inflammatory/immune responses.[14] TGR5 receptors are located in brown adipose tissue, skeletal muscle, nervous system tissue, immune tissue, and colonic tissue, demonstrating the widespread effects of bile acids beyond the biliary system.[15,16] The molecular structure of TGR5 consists of a unique ligand-binding pocket for bile acids, making this receptor a potential drug target for new pharmaceuticals developed to treat metabolic syndrome.[17]

Bile Composition

The liver produces 600 to 750 mL of bile daily. The major lipid components of bile include bile acids (72%), phospholipids (24%), and cholesterol (4%).[18] The bile acid pool consists of primary bile acids (cholic acid and chenodeoxycholic acid) and secondary bile acids (deoxycholic acid and lithocholic acid). Primary bile acids are those that are produced de novo by the liver, and secondary bile acids are primary bile acids that have undergone deconjugation by intestinal bacteria. Phospholipids in healthy individuals consist mainly of phosphatidylcholine (>95%). These proportions are altered in chronic cholestatic conditions, such as primary sclerosis cholangitis or primary biliary cirrhosis.

Bile Acid Synthesis

Bile acids, the main lipid component of bile, are formed in the perivenous hepatocytes. Formation of all bile acids begins with a steroid nucleus, to which subsequent modifications are made. The amphipathic nature of bile salts is caused by the combination of hydrophilic hydroxyl groups and hydrophobic methyl groups, which are oriented opposite each other around the steroid nucleus.[16]

There are 2 pathways by which bile acid biosynthesis occurs: the classic or neutral pathway and the alternative or acidic pathway. The classic pathway begins with hydroxylation of the steroid nucleus, which is the rate-limiting step controlled by cholesterol 7α-hydroxylase (CYP7A1).[19] This enzyme is only found in hepatocytes; thus, the classic pathway only takes place in the liver. This pathway is regulated by a negative feedback loop with bile acids inhibiting CYP7A1 activity and expression.[7]

The alternative pathway is controlled by oxysterol 7α-hydroxylases (CYP7B1), which are constitutively expressed in extrahepatic tissue, such as macrophages, kidney, and vascular endothelium. These enzymes oxidize cholesterol to oxysterols in the peripheral tissues, which are then transported to the liver for final modification to form primary bile acids.[20] Normally, the alternative pathway contributes approximately 10% to overall daily bile acid synthesis; however, this pathway may become more prominent in patients with liver disease.[16]

Bile acid intermediates from both the classic and alternative pathways are then hydroxylated by sterol 12-α-hydroxylase (CYP8B1), which determines the ratio of primary bile acids, cholic acid versus chenodeoxycholic acid.[19] The primary bile acids are then conjugated with glycine (75%) or taurine (25%), increasing the hydrophilicity of the molecules.[21,22] At this point, the conjugated bile acids are then ready for transport into the bile canalicular lumen.

ENTEROHEPATIC CIRCULATION

Bile acids follow a circular pathway passing through the liver, biliary tree, intestine, and portal blood. The purpose of this enterohepatic circulation (EHC) is to recover and recycle bile acids. Ninety-five percent of the bile acid pool is recovered by the EHC, and 5% is excreted in stool. The rate-limiting step of EHC is bile acid secretion from hepatocytes, an ATP-dependent process governed by the bile salt export pump (BSEP).[23]

Interorgan Transport

When stimulated by a meal, the gallbladder contracts, releasing the stored bile containing conjugated bile acids, into the duodenum. Here they form mixed micelles with other biliary lipids and dietary lipids. Once in the ileum, a small amount of bile acids are deconjugated and subsequently passively reabsorbed in the terminal ileum. Most of the bile acids remain conjugated in the small intestine and are reabsorbed by an active transporter in the ileal enterocytes, the apical sodium-dependent bile acid transporter (ASBT).[21] The bile acids that escape reabsorption in the terminal ileum enter the colon where they are subjected to modifications introduced by the gut microflora. After reabsorption by either the ileum or colon, the bile acids enter the portal blood and are transported back to the liver. Conjugated and unconjugated bile acids are extracted from portal blood at the sinusoidal membrane of hepatocytes via the sodium/taurocholate cotransporting polypeptide and via the organic anion–transporting polypeptides (OATP1B1, OATP1B3), respectively.[21] Recycled unconjugated bile acids are then reconjugated to glycine or taurine, and re-secreted into the bile canaliculi along with newly synthesized bile acids by the BSEP. The cycle then repeats itself, with the bile acids completing multiple cycles before they undergo excretion in the stool. A small amount of bile acids spill into the systemic circulation and are transported in the blood via serum albumin.[24] In the peripheral tissues, bile acids interact with TGR5 receptors to regulate gene expression outside of the biliary system as discussed previously. Bile acids have been detected in brain, heart, kidney, thyroid, and ovarian tissues.[25–27] Details of the molecular modifications that take place throughout various points in the EHC are found later.

Intracellular Transport

As depicted in **Fig. 1**, bile acids enter the apical pole of the ileal enterocytes through the ASBT, an energy-dependent process. Once inside the cell, transport to the opposite pole is mediated by proteins including fatty acid–binding protein (FABP1) and ileal lipid–binding protein (ILBP).[28,29] FABP1 is abundant in the liver and small bowel and preferentially binds fatty acids as opposed to bile acids. ILBP is predominantly located in enterocytes in the distal ileum and has greater affinity for conjugated bile acids. Once the bile acids are transported to the basal membrane, they exit the enterocyte via the basolateral heterodimeric organic solute transporter (OSTα/OSTβ) into the portal blood.[30]

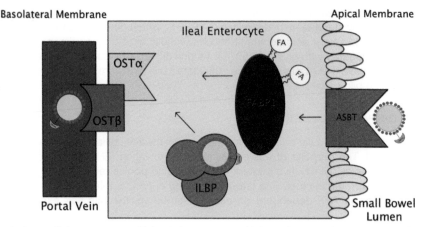

Fig. 1. Intracellular transport of bile acids. Conjugated bile acids enter the apical pole of the ileal enterocytes through ASBT. Inside the cell, bile acid transport is mediated by the ileal lipid–binding protein (ILBP), while the fatty acid–binding protein (FABP1) transports fatty acids. Exit at the basolateral membrane into the portal system is mediated by the organic solute transporter (OSTα/OSTβ).

Modifications by Gut Bacteria

Bile acids have multiple mechanisms by which they exert bactericidal activity. First, antibacterial effects are inherent in the detergent molecular structure of bile acids. Second, conjugated bile acids bind to FXR receptors in the ileum, inducing gene expression of angiogenin, nitric oxide synthase, and interleukin 18, all enzymes known to have antimicrobial effects.[31] Through this mechanism, it is thought that conjugated bile acids assist in controlling bacterial overgrowth in the gut. Colonic bacteria metabolize bile acids and, thus, decrease the bactericidal activity.

As stated previously, the small amount of conjugated bile acids that escape to the colon are deconjugated by bile acid hydrolases, enzymes produced by colonic bacteria (**Fig. 2**). The process of deconjugation includes enzymatic hydrolysis of the C-24 N-acyl amide bond linking bile acids to their amino acid conjugates (glycine and taurine).[16] Deconjugation and subsequent oxidation converts the primary bile acids, cholic acid and chenodeoxycholic acid, to secondary bile acids, deoxycholic and lithocholic acids, respectively. This biotransformation decreases the toxicity of the bile acids to the bacteria while increasing the toxicity to enterocytes and hepatocytes. The carcinogenic effects of secondary bile acids on the cells of the colon and liver are mediated by various cell signaling pathways resulting in the inhibition of DNA repair enzymes, interference of tumor suppressor genes, and stimulation of growth promoters.[32] Bile acids have been well established in the carcinogenesis of colorectal cancer.[33,34]

FXR

FXR is a nuclear receptor that is highly expressed in the liver, intestine, and kidney. In hepatocytes, bile acids activate FXR to suppress their own de novo synthesis, producing a negative feedback loop.[20,35] There are 2 known bile acid/FXR–dependent pathways that inhibit CYP7A1 (rate-limiting enzyme in bile acid synthesis in the neutral pathway) and CYP8B1 (enzyme responsible for production of cholic acid). First, bile acids activate FXR, leading to upregulation of small heterodimer partner (SHP). SHP interacts with multiple transcription factors that, in turn, bind to bile acid response elements located in the promoter region of CYP7A1 and CYP8B1, leading to the

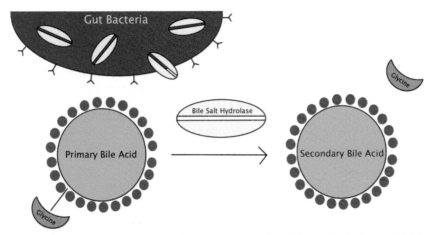

Fig. 2. Deconjugation of bile acids. Colonic bacteria produce bile acid hydrolyses, which lyse the bond to glycine or taurine in primary bile acids, resulting in the formation of secondary bile acids.

inhibition of bile acid synthesis.[36–38] Second, binding of bile acids to FXR causes increased expression of fibroblast growth factor 19, which binds to fibroblast growth factor receptor 4 (FGFR4) receptors on hepatocytes. This activity initiates a cascade of events leading to the activation of the JNK (c-Jun N-terminal Kinase) pathway, ultimately repressing CYP7A1 transcription.[39]

The activation of FXR in hepatocytes also enhances the conjugation and detoxification of bile acids in addition to increasing bile acid efflux to prevent hepatic accumulation. FXR is involved in the conjugation of bile acids via the regulation of bile acid coenzyme A synthetase and bile acid coenzyme A amino acid N-acetyltransferase.[40] Bile acids promote their own excretion from hepatocytes into the canalicular lumen through FXR-activated expression of the BSEP in the hepatocyte membrane, thus, preventing hepatocyte toxicity.

GALLBLADDER DISEASE

Gallstone disease affects 10% to 20% of American adults within their lifetime and is one of the leading indications for surgery in the United States.[41] Eighty percent of people with gallstones remain asymptomatic, with the diagnosis usually made by ultrasound or computed tomography for an unrelated cause. However, 2% to 3% of patients progress to symptomatic disease per year, with 10% of patients considered symptomatic at 5 years.[42] A total of 1% to 2% of patients with gallstones develop complicated disease (ie, cholecystitis, pancreatitis, cholangitis) annually.[43]

Lithogenesis

Gallstones form in the gallbladder and in the bile ducts. The gallbladder is the site of the formation of most gallstones and its functions are essential to the process of lithogenesis. Filling of the gallbladder occurs with tonic contraction of the ampullary sphincter at 10 to 15 mm Hg. Bile flow is increased during periods of partial emptying (in between meals) and involves the activity of the migrating motor complex and motilin. After a meal, cholecystokinin (CCK) is released from the duodenum, stimulating contraction of the gallbladder. The contraction empties 50% to 70% of the volume into the duodenum and refills within 60 to 90 minutes.[44]

The mucosa of the gallbladder functions in absorption of electrolytes and water, concentration of bile, and secretion of proteins. The volume of the gallbladder is 40 to 50 mL; however, it is capable of storing up to 750 mL of bile because it has the greatest absorptive capacity per unit of any bodily tissue. Concentration of bile occurs by active sodium chloride transport, resulting in passive water absorption and concentration of the bile to 5 to 10 times its native form. Hydrogen ions are secreted by the gallbladder to decrease the pH of the bile from approximately 7.5 to 7.8 to 7.1 to 7.3, leading to increased calcium solubility.[44] The secretion of mucous glycoproteins provides a resistant barrier to the concentrated bile salts as well as a nidus for cholesterol nucleation.

Cholesterol stones

Eighty percent of all gallstones are classified as cholesterol stones. The formation of cholesterol gallstones is multifactorial and involves cholesterol supersaturation in bile, crystal nucleation, gallbladder dysmotility, and gallbladder absorption and secretion. First, as bile is concentrated in the gallbladder, there is a transfer of cholesterol and phospholipids from vesicles to micelles. The phospholipids preferentially transfer to the micelles, leaving behind cholesterol-rich vesicles, which then precipitate into crystals. Second, crystallization is accelerated by pronucleating factors in the gallbladder, including mucin glycoproteins, immunoglobulins, and transferrin. Third, incomplete emptying or dysmotility of the gallbladder allows concentrated bile to stagnate, increasing the residence time within the gallbladder. Dismotility of the gallbladder also permits an increase in the size of existing gallstones, thus, increasing the probability of transforming into symptomatic disease. Lastly, alteration in the concentrations of sodium, chloride, and bicarbonate changes the saturation of cholesterol leading to precipitation of calcium and crystal formation (**Fig. 3**).[44]

Risk factors There are various well-established risk factors leading to the development of cholesterol gallstones. Modifiable risk factors include diet, sedentary lifestyle, rapid weight loss, and obesity. Nonmodifiable risk factors include ethnicity, genetics, advancing age, and female sex (**Table 1**).[45]

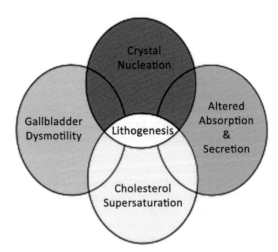

Fig. 3. Lithogenesis. Gallstone formation consists of 4 components: cholesterol supersaturation, crystal nucleation, gallbladder dysmotility, and abnormal gallbladder absorption/secretion.

Table 1 Modifiable and nonmodifiable risk factors for cholesterol gallstone formation	
Cholesterol Gallstone Risk Factors	
Modifiable	**Nonmodifiable**
Diet	Genetics
Physical activity	Ethnicity
Rapid weight loss	Advancing age
Obesity	Female sex
Dyslipidemia	Chronic disease states

Ethnicity/geography Cholesterol gallstones are most prevalent in developed countries, and this is attributed to the popularization of the Western diet. The Third National Health and Nutrition Examination Survey, a large cross-sectional ultrasonographic study, established the prevalence of gallstone disease in the United States.[46] This study demonstrated that North American Indians have the highest rates of cholelithiasis, with women at 64.1% and men at 29.5% prevalence rates. Mexican Americans have a higher prevalence of gallstones compared with non-Hispanic groups in the United States, with rates equal to 8.9% in men and 26.7% in women. Caucasian woman have a prevalence of 16.6% and men at 8.6%, which is higher than African American women at 13.9% and men at 5.0%. On a global scale, Asians have an overall prevalence of 3% to 15%, with multiple recent studies reporting a significant increase in cholesterol gallstone disease over the past few decades, largely attributed to adoption of a Westernized diet.[45] The lowest rates of gallstones are in sub-Saharan Africans at less than 5%.[41]

Genetics The contribution of hereditary versus environmental factors to the development of gallstones has yet to be determined. Familial studies have demonstrated that people with first-degree relatives with gallstones are 2 to 4 times more likely to develop gallstones compared with controls.[47,48] The Swedish twin study, published in 2005, included 43,141 pairs of monozygotic and dizygotic twins. This study revealed significantly higher rates of gallstone disease in monozygotic twins compared with dizygotic twins, especially in the younger cohort. The researchers concluded that heritability accounts for 25%, shared environmental influences for 13%, and unique environmental influences for 62% of gallstone disease variance among the twins.[49] Another study of 358 Midwestern families found the heritability of symptomatic gallstones to be at least 30%, similar to what was found in the Swedish study.[50] These studies demonstrated that, although family members share common environmental exposures, including dietary habits, genetic predisposition is a major risk factor to the development of stones.

Sex Women are twice as likely as men to form gallstones, a process related to female sex hormones, birth control medications, parity, and hormone replacement therapies. Estrogens increase cholesterol secretion and decrease bile salt secretion, and progesterone also reduces bile salt secretion and impairs gallbladder emptying. The combination of these 2 hormones creates a high cholesterol-cholestatic environment, optimal for lithogenesis.

Additionally, women who are pregnant are more likely to suffer from symptomatic gallstones. The increased levels of estrogen and progesterone lead to cholesterol hypersecretion and gallbladder stasis. During pregnancy, it is estimated that 30% of women develop biliary sludge and 2% develop gallstones. In the postpartum period when gallbladder motility and bile composition return to normal, there is complete resolution of sludge in 61% of women and in 28% of women with gallstones.[51]

Age The risk of developing gallstones increases markedly with advancing age. After 40 years of age, the incidence of gallstones increases by 1% to 3% per year.[52] With increasing age, hepatic cholesterol secretion is increased, cholesterol saturation increases, and bile acid synthesis is decreased. These alterations are attributed to decreased activity of the rate-limiting enzyme for bile acid synthesis CYP7A1.[53] There is also a higher prevalence of black pigment stones compared with cholesterol stones in people of increasing age.

Dietary factors Multiple large global epidemiologic studies have identified that diets high in refined carbohydrates, high in triglycerides, and low in fiber are associated with the development of gallstones. Diets high in protein and fiber have been shown to have the opposite effect, actually protecting against gallstone development.[54,55] Fiber, by increasing bulk, accelerates intestinal transit time, leading to decreased formation of secondary bile acids. Because secondary bile acids are associated with an increased cholesterol saturation index in bile, increased consumption of dietary fiber hinders the development of gallstones.[45] Other dietary factors with an inverse association to gallstone development include alcohol and caffeine.[56,57] Moderate amounts of alcohol, 1 to 2 drinks daily, is protective in that the conversion of cholesterol to bile acids is increased. Caffeine, on the other hand, stimulates CCK release from the duodenum, effectively increasing gallbladder motility.

Total parenteral nutrition (TPN) is a well-known risk factor for the development of sludge and gallstones. A possible explanation for this strong correlation is that the loss of enteric stimulation of gallbladder contraction leads to gallbladder stasis. One study demonstrated that after 4 weeks of TPN, 50% of patients developed gallbladder sludge, which progressed to 100% with sludge at 6 weeks.[58] Most of these patients are asymptomatic, and there is resolution with discontinuation of TPN.

Obesity Obesity is an epidemic in developed nations and is a strong risk factor for gallstone disease. This factor may be, in part, caused by the increased activity of 3-hydroxy-3-methylglutaryl–coenzyme A (HMG-CoA) reductase, the rate-limiting enzyme in cholesterol synthesis, leading to increased cholesterol synthesis in the liver and secretion into the bile.[59] Although obese individuals hypersecrete bile salts and phospholipids in addition to cholesterol, the rate of cholesterol hypersecretion exceeds that of the other factors, leading to supersaturation of the bile with increased lithogenicity.

Abdominal adiposity, especially in women, has been identified as a major risk factor for gallstone development. Waist circumference and waist-to-hip ratio have been shown to be better predictors of gallstone development compared with body mass index or overall total body fat.[60] Individuals with obesity in their late teenage years carry the greatest risk of developing gallstone disease throughout their lifetime. The prevalence of gallstone disease among obese children and adolescents may be as high as 2%, whereas the prevalence among unselected pediatric groups is between 0.1% and 1.0%.[61,62]

Rapid weight loss Bariatric surgery patients with rapid postoperative weight loss develop gallstones in 30% to 71% of cases. The incidence of gallstones is highest within the first 2 years after surgery. Most of these stones are asymptomatic, but weight loss exceeding 25% of total body weight is predictive of symptomatic disease.[63] The mechanism for increased lithogenesis in bariatric patients is unclear; however, one hypothesis implicates increased secretion of mucin and calcium from the gallbladder as contributing factors to the formation of gallstones.[64]

Patients with a history of low-caloric dieting and extreme fluctuations in weight are also at risk for stone formation. Weight reduction leads to mobilization of hepatic stores of cholesterol. In combination with decreased gallbladder emptying and reduced bile acid synthesis, supersaturation of bile and rapid stone formation takes place.

Dyslipidemia Cholesterol gallstone formation is a metabolic issue that is correlated with lipid abnormalities. Hypertriglyceridemia and low high-density lipoprotein concentration are associated with increased cholesterol saturation of bile and increased risk for cholesterol stone formation.[64–66] Both of these dyslipidemias have been shown to be independent risk factors for cholelithiasis. Hypercholesterolemia is not strongly associated with cholesterol stone disease.

Drugs Certain drugs interfere with cholesterol and bile acid synthesis. Clofibrate, used to treat hypertriglyceridemia, is an inhibitor of hepatic acyl coenzyme A: cholesterol acyltransferase (ACAT). The inhibition of ACAT increases the concentration of free cholesterol in bile, thus, lowering the threshold for gallstone formation. Statins, also used in patients with dyslipidemia, inhibit HMG-CoA reductase, decreasing cholesterol synthesis in the liver. Statins seemingly protect against gallstone formation by decreasing the amount of cholesterol in the bile.[67] Ceftriaxone, a third-generation cephalosporin, is secreted unmetabolized into bile. Especially in children, ceftriaxone leads to sludge and pseudolithiasis, which spontaneously resolves on discontinuation of the antibiotic. Octreotide, used clinically for its global gastrointestinal inhibitory properties, also inhibits contraction of the gallbladder resulting in stasis. The inhibition of CCK by octreotide leads to decreased small bowel motility and enhancement of secondary bile acid formation. An increased ratio of secondary bile acids results in enhanced cholesterol secretion and gallbladder mucin production. Lastly, octreotide stimulates calcium release into bile, creating a more lithogenic environment.

Diabetes mellitus Diabetes mellitus (DM) has frequently been associated with cholelithiasis, although the relationship has not been fully delineated. There is evidence that bile acid composition and size of the pool are altered in humans with type 1 and type 2 DM.[68,69] In large series of patients with diabetes, gallstone disease is significantly higher than observed in the general population. Independent risk factors for gallstone formation in patients with diabetes include advancing age, higher body mass index, and positive family history.

On a molecular level, bile acids regulate gluconeogenesis, glycogen synthesis, and insulin sensitivity via FXR gene expression. CYP7A1 is negatively regulated by FXR. With the dysregulation of FXR expression as is seen in patients with diabetes, CYP7A1 activity is increased and the size of the bile acid pool increases. Additionally, evidence suggests glucose and insulin are involved in the modulation of bile acid synthesis. Glucose has been shown to enhance FXR gene expression, whereas insulin represses FXR gene expression.[70]

Pigment stones
Pigment stones account for 20% of all gallstones. This group consists of brown and black pigment stones.

Brown stones Brown pigment gallstones are associated with biliary dysmotility and bacterial infection of the bile. They are composed of calcium bilirubinate, fatty acid soaps (calcium palmitate and calcium stearate), cholesterol, and mucinous glycoproteins (products of bacterial biofilms). The most common risk factor is bile duct stasis, which is encountered in the following disease states: sclerosing cholangitis, congenital cysts, strictures, chronic pancreatitis, and duodenal diverticula. Unlike cholesterol stones, brown pigment stones are mostly identified as primary ductal stones, with patients suffering from choledocholithiasis and hepatolithiasis.[41]

Brown pigment stones also result from bacterial infections and biliary parasites. East Asians traditionally have higher rates of brown pigment stones secondary to recurrent pyogenic cholangitis, also known as *Oriental cholangiohepatitis*, characterized by biliary obstruction with recurrent cholangitis. The bacteria produce a film containing glucuronidase, which hydrolyses conjugated bilirubin to free bilirubin. Free bilirubin then precipitates when mixed with calcium. Recently there has been an increase in cholesterol stones in East Asia, likely attributable to improved hygiene with reduced biliary infections and consumption of a westernized diet.

Black stones Black pigment stones account for 2% of all gallstones and are associated with chronic liver disease and hemolytic conditions.[71] These stones develop exclusively in the gallbladder and consist of calcium bilirubinate with mucin glycoproteins. The prevalence of gallstones in patients with chronic liver disease is near 30%.[72] Cholelithiasis associated with liver disease is secondary to altered pigment secretion, abnormal gallbladder motility, and increased estrogen levels.[2] Sickle cell disease results in excessive unconjugated bilirubin excretion, which precipitates with calcium. Prophylactic cholecystectomy may be considered in this patient population because differentiating the cause of abdominal pain in this group can be difficult. Although infrequent, black pigment stones are also identified in children born prematurely and those that require TPN.[41]

Complications of Cholelithiasis

Most gallstones remain clinically silent, with a risk of progression of 2% to 3% per year, including 1% to 2% of patients who develop major complications.[42,73] Within 5 years of diagnosis, 10% of patients with gallstones will become symptomatic, which increases to 20% at 20 years.[43] The longer gallstones remain silent, the less likely patients are to develop symptoms. At one end of the disease spectrum is biliary colic, of which 10% to 20% of patients will go on to develop cholecystitis. At the other end of the spectrum is cholangitis, which occurs with biliary obstruction and bactibilia. Bile is normally sterile, but bacteria can reflux from the duodenum into the biliary system, enter the hepatic veins and perihepatic lymphatics causing systemic bacteremia. Other disease processes secondary to gallstone complications include choledocholithiasis, gallstone pancreatitis, and gallstone ileus.

Gallstone disease is a known risk factor for gallbladder carcinoma, with a relative risk of 4.9.[74] Most people with gallbladder cancer have gallstones, suggesting stones may function as a cofactor in the development of cancer. One hypothesis is that the presence of gallstones creates chronic inflammation of the mucosa, which over time leads to dysplasia. Increased risk of gallbladder carcinoma is associated with stones larger than 3 cm, and increased number, volume, and weight of the stones.[75] Patients with stones greater than 3 cm should be considered for a prophylactic cholecystectomy because the risk of cancer is 4% over 20 years.

Disease States Causing Altered Bile Acid Metabolism

Crohn's disease with ileocecal involvement or surgical resection of the terminal ileum leads to diminished ileal reabsorption of bile acids. This diminished reabsorption allows more bile acids to escape to the colon, where they solubilize unconjugated bilirubin, facilitating passive absorption and transport back to the liver. The liver then secretes excess pigment (bilirubin) into the bile, leading to a higher proportion of black pigment stones in patients with Crohn's disease. Reduced hepatic secretion of bile acids, supersaturation with cholesterol, and increased enterohepatic cycling of bile pigment results in gallstone formation in 13% to 34% of all patients with Crohn's disease. The prevalence of gallstones is lower in patients with colonic Crohn's disease and is highest in patients with terminal ileal disease.[76–78]

Patients with cystic fibrosis (CF) are known to have excessive loss of bile acids through fecal excretion. The mechanism by which mutations in CF transmembrane conductase regulator (CFTR) affect EHC have not been fully delineated. Dysfunction of CFTR in the apical plasma membranes of cholangiocytes impairs chloride/bicarbonate exchange, thus, altering the composition of bile. Studies in CF mice have demonstrated significantly decreased pH in the ileum, leading to increased loss of bile salts in the feces. This increased loss, in turn, results in hyperbilirubinbilia (elevated secretion of conjugated bilirubin into bile) and increased proportion of hydrophobic bile acids. Additionally these mice had higher concentrations of biliary cholesterol, although the gallstones that form are considered more of a black pigment stone. The overall prevalence of gallstones in patients with CF is between 10% and 30%.[79]

Individuals with spinal cord injury (SCI) have an increased risk of developing gallstone disease, with a prevalence of 30%.[80,81] The gallbladder receives sympathetic innervation via the splanchnic nerves originating from T7-T10, which allow relaxation of the gallbladder smooth muscle. Interruption of this pathway, especially in high SCI, is thought to cause gallbladder dysfunction. In addition, patients with SCI also frequently have neurogenic bowel resulting in slow intestinal transit times, which results in an increase in the formation of secondary bile acids, thus, promoting the formation of gallstones.

SUMMARY

Cholelithiasis is a disease process affecting a significant number of American adults, accounting for a considerable burden on the health care system. The development of gallstones is largely multifactorial, consisting of both modifiable and nonmodifiable risk factors. There have been major advances in uncovering the molecular basis of bile metabolism and lithogenesis in recent years; however, because of the complexity of the pathways involved, investigations are ongoing. Understanding the pathogenesis of gallstone formation will direct the development of targeted therapies for the prevention and treatment of this disease.

REFERENCES

1. Tazuma S. Gallstone disease: epidemiology, pathogenesis, and classification of biliary stones (common bile duct and intrahepatic). Best Pract Res Clin Gastroenterol 2006;20:1075–83.
2. Shaffer EA. Epidemiology and risk factors for gallstone disease: has the paradigm changed in the 21st century? Curr Gastroenterol Rep 2005;7:132–40.
3. Graves EJ, Owings MF. 1995 summary: National Hospital Discharge Survey. Adv Data 1997;(291):1–10.
4. Peery E, Dellon S, Lund J, et al. Burden of gastrointestinal disease in the United States: 2012 update. Gastroenterology 2012;143:1179–87.
5. Everhart JE, Ruhl CE. Burden of digestive diseases in the United States part I: overall and upper gastrointestinal diseases. Gastroenterology 2009;136: 376–86.

6. Insull W Jr. Clinical utility of bile acid sequestrants in the treatment of dyslipidemia: a scientific review. South Med J 2006;99:257–73.
7. Keitel V, Kubitz R, Häussinger D. Endocrine and paracrine role of bile acids. World J Gastroenterol 2008;14:5620–9.
8. Nguyen A, Bouscarel B. Bile acids and signal transduction: role in glucose homeostasis. Cell Signal 2008;20:2180–97.
9. Trauner M, Claudel T, Fickert P, et al. Bile acids as regulators of hepatic lipid and glucose metabolism. Dig Dis 2010;28:220–4.
10. Wang H, Chen J, Hollister K, et al. Endogenous bile acids are ligands for the nuclear receptor FXR/BAR. Mol Cell 1999;3:543–53.
11. Makishima M, Okamoto AY, Repa JJ, et al. Identification of a nuclear receptor for bile acids. Science 1999;284:1362–5.
12. Staudinger JL, Goodwin B, Jones SA, et al. The nuclear receptor PXR is a lithocholic acid sensor that protects against liver toxicity. Proc Natl Acad Sci U S A 2001;98:3369–74.
13. Halilbasic E, Claudel T, Trauner M. Bile acid transporters and regulatory nuclear receptors in the liver and beyond. J Hepatol 2013;58:155–68.
14. Pols TW, Noriega LG, Nomura M, et al. The bile acid membrane receptor TGR%: a valuable metabolic target. Dig Dis 2011;29:37–44.
15. Kawamata Y, Fujii R, Hosoya M, et al. A G protein-coupled receptor responsive to bile acids. J Biol Chem 2003;278:9435–40.
16. Monte MJ, Marin JJ, Antelo A, et al. Bile acids: chemistry physiology, and pathophysiology. World J Gastroenterol 2009;15:804–16.
17. Macchiarulo A, Gioiello A, Thomas C, et al. Molecular field analysis and 3D-quantitative structure-activity relationship study (MFA3D-QSAR) unveil novel features of bile acid recognition at TGR5. J Chem Inf Model 2008;48:1792–801.
18. Hay DW, Carey MC. Chemical species of lipids in bile. Hepatology 1990;12:6S–14S.
19. Staels B, Fonseca VA. Bile acids and metabolic regulation: mechanisms and clinical responses to bile acid sequestration. Diabetes Care 2009;32:S237–45.
20. Russell DW. The enzymes, regulation, and genetics of bile acid synthesis. Annu Rev Biochem 2003;72:137–74.
21. Zwicker BL, Agellon LB. Transport and biological activities of bile acids. Int J Biochem Cell Biol 2013;45:1389–98.
22. Warren DB, Chalmers DK, Hutchison K, et al. Molecular dynamics simulations of spontaneous bile salt aggregation. Colloids Surf A Physicochem Eng Asp 2006;280:182–93.
23. Gerloff T, Stieger B, Hagenbuch B, et al. The sister of P-glycoprotein represents the canalicular bile salt export pump of mammalian liver. J Biol Chem 1998;273:10046–50.
24. Rudman D, Kendall FE. Bile acid content of human serum. The binding of cholanic acids by human plasma proteins. J Clin Invest 1957;36:538–42.
25. Smith LP, Nierstenhoefer M, Yoo SW, et al. The bile acid synthesis pathway is present and functional in the human ovary. PLoS One 2009;4:e7333.
26. Khurana S, Raufman JP, Pallone TL. Bile acids regulate cardiovascular function. Clin Transl Sci 2011;4:210–8.
27. Mukaisho K, Araki Y, Sugihara H, et al. High serum bile acids cause hyperthyroidism and goiter. Dig Dis Sci 2008;53:1411–6.
28. Sacchettini JC, Hauft SM, Van Camp SL, et al. Developmental and structural studies of an intracellular lipid binding protein expressed in the ileal epithelium. J Biol Chem 1990;265:19199–207.

29. Levy E, Menard D, Delvin E, et al. Localization, function and regulation of the two intestinal fatty acid-binding protein types. Histochem Cell Biol 2009;132:351–67.
30. Dawson PA, Hubbert M, Haywood J, et al. The heteromeric organic solute transporter alpha-beta, Ostalpha-Ostbeta, is an ileal basolateral bile acid transporter. J Biol Chem 2005;280:6960–8.
31. Inagaki T, Maschetta A, Lee YK, et al. Regulation of antibacterial defense in the small intestine by the nuclear bile acid receptor. Proc Natl Acad Sci U S A 2006; 103:3920–5.
32. McGarr SE, Ridlong JM, Hylemon PB. Diet, anaerobic bacterial metabolism, and colon cancer: a review of the literature. J Clin Gastroenterol 2005;39:98–109.
33. Roberton A. Roles of endogenous substances and bacteria in colorectal cancer. Mutat Res 1993;290:71–8.
34. Bernstein C, Bernstein H, Garewal H, et al. A bile acid-induced apoptosis assay for colon cancer risk and associated quality control studies. Cancer Res 1999; 59:2353–7.
35. Heuman DM, Hylemon PB, Vlahcevic ZR. Regulation of bile acid synthesis. III. Correlation between biliary bile salt hydrophobicity index and the activities of enzymes regulating cholesterol and bile acid synthesis in the rat. J Lipid Res 1989;30:1161–71.
36. Stroup D, Crestani M, Chiang JY. Identification of a bile acid response element in the cholesterol 7 alpha-hydroxylase gene CYP7A. Am J Physiol 1997;273: G508–17.
37. Yang Y, Zhang M, Eggertsen G, et al. On the mechanism of bile acid inhibition of rat sterol 12alpha-hydroxylase gene (CYP8B1) transcription: role of alpha-fetoprotein transcription factor and hepatocyte nuclear factor 4alpha. Biochim Biophys Acta 2002;1583:63–73.
38. Goodwin B, Jones SA, Price RR, et al. A regulatory cascade of the nuclear receptors FXR, SHP-1, and LRH-1 represses bile acid biosynthesis. Mol Cell 2000; 6:517–26.
39. Holt JA, Luo G, Billin AN, et al. Definition of a novel growth factor-dependent signal cascade for the suppression of bile acid biosynthesis. Genes Dev 2003;17:1581–91.
40. Pircher PC, Kitto JL, Petrowski ML, et al. Farnesoid X receptor regulates bile acid-amino acid conjugation. J Biol Chem 2003;278:27703–11.
41. Stinton LM, Shaffer EA. Epidemiology of gallbladder disease: cholelithiasis and cancer. Gut Liver 2012;6:172–87.
42. Ransohoff DF, Gracie WA, Wolfenson LB, et al. Prophylactic cholecystectomy or expectant management for silent gallstones. A decision analysis to assess survival. Ann Intern Med 1983;99:199–204.
43. Thistle JL, Cleary PA, Lachin JM, et al. The natural history of cholelithiasis: the National Cooperative Gallstone Study. Ann Intern Med 1984;101:171–5.
44. Pitt HA, Ahrendt SA, Nakeeb A. Calculous biliary disease. In: Mulholland MW, editor. Greenfield's surgery: scientific principles and practice. Philadelphia: Lippincott Williams & Wilkins; 2011. Chapter 60.
45. Yoo EH, Lee SY. The prevalence and risk factors for gallstone disease. Clin Chem Lab Med 2009;47:795–807.
46. National Center for Health Statistics, Plan and operation of the Third National Health and Nutrition Examination Survey 1988-94. Vital Health Stat 1 1994;(32): 1–407.
47. Gilat T, Feldman C, Halpem Z, et al. An increased familial frequency of gallstones. Gastroenterology 1983;84:242–6.

48. Sarin SK, Negi VS, Dewan R. High familial prevalence of gallstones in the first-degree relatives of gallstone patients. Hepatology 1995;22:138–41.

49. Katsika D, Grijibovski A, Einarsson C, et al. Genetic and environmental influences on symptomatic gallstone disease: a Swedish study of 43,141 twin pairs. Hepatology 2005;41:1138–43.

50. Nakeeb A, Comuzzie AG, Martin L, et al. Gallstones: genetics versus environment. Ann Surg 2002;235:842–9.

51. Maringhini A, Ciambra M, Baccelliere P, et al. Biliary sludge and gallstones in pregnancy: incidence, risk factors, and natural history. Ann Intern Med 1993; 119:116–20.

52. Einarsson K, Nilsell K, Leijd B, et al. Influence of age on secretion of cholesterol and synthesis of bile acids by the liver. N Engl J Med 1985;313:277–82.

53. Bertolotti M, Gabbi C, Anzivino C, et al. Age-related changes in bile acid synthesis and hepatic nuclear receptor expression. Eur J Clin Invest 2007;37: 501–8.

54. Kritchevsky D, Dlurfeld DM. Gallstone formation in hamsters: effect of varying animal and vegetable protein levels. Am J Clin Nutr 1983;37:802–4.

55. Attili AF, Scafato E, Marchioli R, et al. Diet and gallstones in Italy: the cross-sectional MICOL results. Hepatology 1998;27:1492–8.

56. Nestel PJ, Simons LA, Homma Y. Effects of ethanol on bile acid and cholesterol metabolism. Am J Clin Nutr 1976;29:1007–15.

57. Leitzmann MF, Willett WC, Rimm EB. A prospective study of coffee consumption and the risk of symptomatic gallstone disease in men. JAMA 1999;22:2106–12.

58. Messing B, Bories C, Kunstlinger F, et al. Does total parenteral nutrition induce gallbladder sludge formation and lithiasis? Gastroenterology 1983; 84:1012–9.

59. Erlinger S. Gallstones in obesity and weight loss. Eur J Gastroenterol Hepatol 2000;12:1347–52.

60. Tsai CJ, Leitzmann MF, Willett WC, et al. Central adiposity, regional fat distribution, and the risk of cholecystectomy in women. Gut 2006;55:708–14.

61. Kaechele V, Wabitsch M, Thiere D, et al. Prevalence of gallbladder stone disease in obese children and adolescents: influence of the degree of obesity, sex, and pubertal development. J Pediatr Gastroenterol Nutr 2006;42:66–70.

62. Kratzer W, Walcher T, Arnold F, et al. Gallstone prevalence and risk factors for gallstone disease in an urban population of children and adolescents. Z Gastroenterol 2010;48:683–7.

63. Li VK, Pulido N, Fajnwaks P, et al. Predictors of gallstone formation after bariatric surgery: a multivariate analysis of risk factors comparing gastric bypass, gastric banding, and sleeve gastrectomy. Surg Endosc 2009;23:1640–4.

64. Shiffman ML, Shamburek RD, Schwartz CC, et al. Gallbladder mucin, arachidonic acid, and bile lipids in patients who develop gallstones during weight reduction. Gastroenterology 1993;105:1200–8.

65. Petitti DB, Friedman GD, Klatsky AL. Association of a history of gallbladder disease with a reduced concentration of high-density-lipoprotein cholesterol. N Engl J Med 1981;304:1396–8.

66. Thijs C, Knipschild P, Brombacher P. Serum lipids and gallstones: a case-control study. Gastroenterology 1990;99:843–9.

67. Tsai CJ, Leitzmann MF, Willet WC, et al. Statin use and the risk of cholecystectomy in women. Gastroenterology 2009;136:1593–600.

68. Andersen E, Karlaganis G, Sjovalll J. Altered bile acid profiles in duodenal bile and urine in diabetic subjects. Eur J Clin Invest 1988;18:166–72.

69. Brufau G, Stellaard F, Prado K, et al. Improved glycemic control with colesevelam treatment in patients with type 2 diabetes is not directly associated with changes in bile acid metabolism. Hepatology 2010;52:1455–64.

70. Duran-Sandoval D, Mautino G, Martin G, et al. Glucose regulates the expression of the farnesoid X receptor in liver. Diabetes 2004;53:890–8.

71. Lammert F, Miquel JF. Gallstone disease: from genes to evidence-based therapy. J Hepatol 2008;48:S124–35.

72. Acalovschi M, Badea R, Dumitraçcu D, et al. Prevalence of gallstones in liver cirrhosis: a sonographic survey. Am J Gastroenterol 1988;83:954–6.

73. Friedman GD. Natural history of asymptomatic and symptomatic gallstones. Am J Surg 1993;165:399–404.

74. Randi G, Franceschi S, La Vecchia C. Gallbladder cancer worldwide: geographical distribution and risk factors. Int J Cancer 2006;118:1591–602.

75. Shrikhande SV, Barreto SG, Singh S, et al. Cholelithiasis in gallbladder cancer: coincidence, cofactor, or cause! Eur J Surg Oncol 2010;36:514–9.

76. Cohen S, Kaplan M, Gottlieb L, et al. Liver disease and gallstones in regional enteritis. Gastroenterology 1971;60:237–45.

77. Whorwell PJ, Hawkins R, Dewbury K, et al. Ultrasound survey of gallstones and other hepatobiliary disorders in patients with Crohn's disease. Dig Dis Sci 1984; 29:930–3.

78. Hutchinson R, Tyrrell PN, Kumar D, et al. Pathogenesis of gallstones in Crohn's disease: an alternative explanation. Gut 1994;35:94–7.

79. Angelico M, Gandin C, Canuzzi P, et al. Gallstones in cystic fibrosis: a critical reappraisal. Hepatology 1991;14:768–75.

80. Moonka R, Stiens SA, Resnick WJ, et al. The prevalence and natural history of gallstones in spinal cord injured patients. J Am Coll Surg 1999;189:274–81.

81. Apstein MD, Dalecki-Chipperfield K. Spinal cord injury is a risk factor for gallstone disease. Gastroenterology 1987;92:966–8.

Unusual Complications of Gallstones

Minh B. Luu, MD*, Daniel J. Deziel, MD

KEYWORDS

- Gallstones • Complications • Lost stones • Fistula • Obstruction

KEY POINTS

- Extrinsic compression of the bile duct from gallstone disease is associated with bilio-biliary fistulization requiring biliary-enteric reconstruction.
- Biliary-enteric fistulas are associated with intestinal obstruction at various levels. The primary goal of therapy is relief of intestinal obstruction; definitive repair is performed for selected patients.
- Hemobilia from gallstone-related pseudoaneurysms is preferentially controlled by selective arterial embolization.
- Rapidly increasing jaundice with relatively normal liver enzymes is a diagnostic hallmark of bilhemia.
- Acquired thoraco-biliary fistulas are primarily treated by percutaneous and endoscopic interventions.

INTRODUCTION

Gallstones are a routine commodity for general surgeons. Symptomatic disease presentations in their common forms of biliary colic, acute cholecystitis, choledocholithiasis, and gallstone pancreatitis are well known. This does not imply that these daily conditions are without difficult challenges, even for the most experienced biliary surgeons. However, when stones migrate to involve adjacent viscera or vascular structures, the clinical challenge is far less familiar. Biliary eruption into the gut, into the chest, or into the pelvis is a confounding situation; and, in circumstances that violate major blood vessels, a rapidly catastrophic one. Most surgeons will encounter few, if any, of these baffling patients during the course of their career. Yet, such occurrences have been recognized for centuries and will continue. This article is a simple primer to aid in the recognition and management of some of these gallstone oddities.

Department of General Surgery, Rush University Medical Center, Rush Medical College, 1633 West Congress Parkway, Chicago, IL 60612, USA
* Corresponding author.
E-mail address: minh_luu@rush.edu

Surg Clin N Am 94 (2014) 377–394
http://dx.doi.org/10.1016/j.suc.2014.01.002
0039-6109/14/$ – see front matter © 2014 Elsevier Inc. All rights reserved.

BILIARY FISTULA

Biliary fistulas are abnormal communications of the biliary system to an internal or external location. These conditions share a common pathophysiology of biliary obstruction, infection, necrosis, and fistulization. Internal fistulas can form to the gastrointestinal (GI) tract, thoracic cavity, genitourinary (GU) structures, or the vascular system. External fistulas are communications of the biliary system to the skin either spontaneously or by way of operatively lost stones. Bowel obstruction can result on passage of large stones through bilioenteric fistulas with enlodgement in the small intestine or colon (gallstone ileus) or the pyloric region (Bouveret syndrome). Fistulization between the gallbladder and extrahepatic bile ducts can also occur (Mirizzi syndrome). Although rare, these conditions may cause significant morbidity and mortality that warrant attention.

Internal Fistula

Bilio-biliary fistula
Mirizzi syndrome
Background Although Hans Kehr[1] in 1905 first reported on patients with partial bile duct obstruction due to an impacted stone in the gallbladder, it was Pablo Luis Mirizzi's article in 1948 entitled "Sindrome del conducto hepatico"[2] that called attention to this condition.

Pathophysiology The eponym Mirizzi syndrome (MS) is used to describe mechanical obstruction of the common hepatic duct due to extrinsic compression (with or without an associated fistula) from stones in the gallbladder or cystic duct. The actual obstruction is usually from a large impacted stone in the gallbladder neck or infundibulum adjacent to the extrahepatic ducts (**Fig. 1**). Sometimes the extrinsic obstruction is caused by a small stone impacted in the cystic duct that has a long parallel course to the common hepatic duct or even by a tensely distended gallbladder itself. In his famous article, Mirizzi[2] incorrectly postulated a functional spasm of the common hepatic duct as the cause of the bile duct obstruction. MS occurs in approximately 0.2% to 1.5% of patients with gallstones. Beltran[3] theorized that the external compression of the bile duct and the later development of cholecystobiliary and cholcystoenteric fistulas are different stages of the same disease process.

Classification Classification schemes are founded on the presence or absence of fistulous erosion between the gallbladder and common bile duct and the extent of

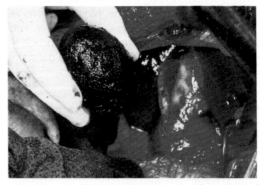

Fig. 1. An intraoperative picture of a large stone removed from the infundibulum of a patient with Mirizzi syndrome.

common duct destruction. MS was classified by Mc Sherry and colleagues[4] in 1982 into 2 types and reclassified by Csendes and colleagues[5] in 1989 into 4 types. A more recent modification added a fifth type that includes the presence of a bilioenteric fistula with or without gallstone ileus (**Fig. 2**).[6]

Clinical presentation Patients with MS present in the fifth to seventh decade and are usually women. A long-standing history of gallstone disease is usually elicited and the presenting symptoms are those of obstructive jaundice. Additionally, patients with MS also can present in the setting of acute cholecystitis, cholangitis, or pancreatitis.

Diagnosis Preoperative diagnosis of MS can be difficult, but careful surgical planning and intraoperative recognition may avoid the high incidence of bile duct injuries.[7] Ultrasound and abdominal computed tomography (CT) are nonspecific but may be suggestive when there is dilation of the proximal common hepatic or intrahepatic ducts only. The accuracy of endoscopic retrograde cholangiopancreatography (ERCP) to diagnose MS ranges from 55% to 90%. Because of the difficulty of preoperative diagnosis, more than one-half of MS cases are not diagnosed until operation.[8] Characteristic findings of MS at surgery are fibrosis and obliteration of the Calot triangle due to impacted stones in the infundibulum or cystic duct. The gallbladder may be contracted or dilated with a thickened wall. Intraoperative cholangiography and ultrasonography are useful tools to delineate the abnormal anatomy in the midst of fibrosis and inflammation (**Fig. 3**).

Treatment The goals of treatment for patients with MS are to decompress the biliary tree and prevent recurrence. Temporary stenting of the bile duct during ERCP has

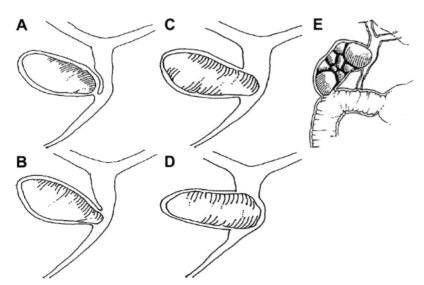

Fig. 2. Mirizzi syndrome type I to V. (*A*) Type I is the extrinsic compression of the common bile duct by an impacted gallstone. (*B*) Type II involves one-third the circumference of the bile duct. (*C*) Type III involves two-thirds the circumference of the bile duct. (*D*) Type IV involves the whole circumference of the bile duct. (*E*) Type V involves types I to IV with the addition of a bilioenteric fistula. (*From* Beltran MA, Csendes A, Cruces KS. The relationship of Mirizzi syndrome and cholecystoenteric fistula: validation of a modified classification. World J Surg 2008;32:2237–43; with permission.)

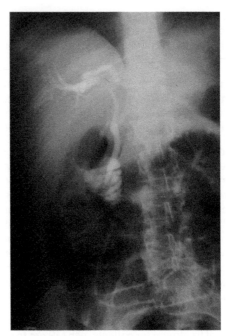

Fig. 3. A percutaneous transhepatic cholangiography showing a smooth external compression of the common hepatic duct due to a large stone in a patient with Mirizzi syndrome.

been used to allow time for surgical planning and medical optimization. Surgical treatment is required and the extent based on the type of MS. Type I can be managed with cholecystectomy or subtotal cholecystectomy alone, whereas types II, III, and IV often require biliary reconstruction. Suggested surgical treatment based on Beltran's classification of MS is outlined in **Table 1**.[9] Although the laparoscopic management of MS has been described,[10] surgeons should be wary because of the high risk of bile duct injury. When diagnosed preoperatively, serious consideration should be given to transferring the patient to a facility capable of major biliary reconstruction. Because gallbladder cancer can be found in up to 25% of MS cases, an intraoperative frozen section of the gallbladder wall should be performed and capability for an appropriate oncologic resection available.[11]

Biliary-enteric fistula
Spontaneous internal biliary fistula: Most internal biliary fistulas are due to chronic or neglected gallstone disease. Cholecystoduodenal fistulas are the most frequent, followed by cholecystocolonic fistulas. Less common fistula sites are cholecystogastric, cholecystocholedochal, choledochoduodenal, cholecystojejunal, and hepaticobronchial fistulas.[12–16] Choledochoduodenal fistulas are most commonly due to dorsal erosion of a duodenal ulcer. A systematic review by Petrowsky and Clavien[17] summarized the distribution of biliary-enteric fistulas shown in **Table 2**.

Cholecystoduodenal fistulas account for 75% to 80% of cholecystoenteric fistulas. Most are clinically silent or have vague digestive symptoms. Passage of large stones can result in gallstone ileus. Cholecystocolic fistulas are the second most common type.[18] Costi and colleagues[19] reviewed literature between 1950 and 2006 and found 231 cases. Only 7.9% of these cases were diagnosed preoperatively. In contrast to the

Table 1
New classification and suggested surgical treatment of Mirizzi syndrome

Type of Mirizzi	Description	Treatment
I	External compression of the bile duct	Open cholecystectomy Open subtotal cholecystectomy Laparoscopic cholecystectomy Laparoscopic subtotal cholecystectomy
IIa	Cholecystobiliary fistula <50% the diameter of the bile duct	Open cholecystectomy Open subtotal cholecystectomy
IIb	Cholecystobiliary fistula >50% the diameter of the bile duct	Open subtotal cholecystectomy Biliary-enteric derivation: Side-to-side to the duodenum En-Y-de-Roux to the jejunum
IIIa	Cholecystobiliary fistula and cholecystoenteric fistula without gallstone ileus	Simple closure of the fistula and treatment of the gallbladder according to the presence of Mirizzi I, IIa, or IIb
IIIb	Cholecystobiliary fistula and cholecystoenteric fistula with gallstone ileus	Treatment of the gallstone ileus and deferred treatment of the gallbladder according to the presence of Mirizzi I, IIa or IIb

From Beltrán MA. Mirizzi syndrome: history, current knowledge and proposal of a simplified classification. World J Gastroenterol 2012;18(34):4639–50.

benign presentations of most cholecystoduodenal fistulas, patients with fistulas to the colon often report a sudden change from mild biliary symptoms to acute attacks. The influx of bacteria from the colon into the biliary system is thought to be the cause of the change in clinical condition. During the acute episode, most patients will have fever, chills, and abdominal pain. Nausea, weight loss, and diarrhea may be present due to bile acid loss. In some circumstances, choleretic diarrhea caused by the irritant effect of bile acids on the colonic mucosa may be the primary symptom and indication for surgery. Surgical treatment consisting of cholecystectomy with resection of the fistula tract should be performed. Laparoscopic management has been described but not widely used.[20]

Gallstone ileus

Background Gallstone ileus is classically described as the impaction of gallstone(s) in the distal ileum and accounts for 1% to 3% of all mechanical bowel obstruction.[21] The anatomist Thomas Bartholin first described gallstone ileus in 1654.[22] In a series of 131 cases, Courvoisier,[23] in 1890, reported a surgical mortality rate of 44%. More contemporary mortality rates of 15% to 18% are still considerable and reflect the associated afflictions of many patients with this condition.[17,24,25]

Clinical presentation Most cholecystoenteric fistulas are clinically silent, but if larger (≥2 cm) stones enter the intestine, a mechanical obstruction results. Half of the patients with gallstone ileus will have a history of prior biliary symptoms and 20% to 30% of the patients have associated acute cholecystitis. Approximately 85% of affected people are women and the median age is 70 years. Obstructive symptoms may be partial and intermittent as the gallstone progresses aborally. This has been referred to as a "tumbling" obstruction and may be responsible for the diagnostic delay for several days that is characteristic in these patients. The Rigler triad, consisting of small bowel obstruction (SBO), pneumobilia, and an aberrant stone in the GI

Table 2
Incidence and frequency of biliary-enteric fistulas

Author,[Ref.] year	Incidence (%)	Total	Biliary-enteric Fistulas (%)				
			Cholecystoduodenal	Cholecystocolic	Cholecystogastric	Choledochoduodenal	Others
Glenn, 1957	0.9	40	30 (76)	3 (7.5)	1 (2.5)	2 (5)	4 (10)
Half, 1971	0.4	24	13 (54)	4 (17)	1 (4)	4 (17)	2 (8)
Safaie, 1973	—	92	70 (76)	10 (11)	5 (5)	4 (4)	3 (3)
Patrassi, 1975	1.6	58	32 (55)	7 (12)	2 (3)	3 (5)	14 (24)
Yamashita, 1997	1.7	33	6 (18)	3 (9)	—	20 (61)	4 (12)
Total	1.0	247	151 (61)	27 (11)	9 (4)	33 (13)	27 (11)

From Petrowsky H, Clavien P. Biliary fistula, gallstone ileus, and Mirizzi's syndrome. In: Clavien P, Baillie J, editors. Diseases of the gallbladder and bile ducts: diagnosis and treatment. 2nd edition. Malden (MA): Blackwell Publishing; 2006. p. 239–51.

tract, is present in only 20% to 35% of reported cases.[26–28] Radiographic evidence of pneumobilia should be carefully looked for, as it is present (sometimes only in retrospect) in most patients with gallstone ileus (**Fig. 4**). Its presence should tip off the preoperative diagnosis particularly when a mature woman presents with SBO without a history of prior abdominal surgery or biliary tract intervention. Colonic obstruction, usually the sigmoid, is often associated with a colonic stricture. CT (**Fig. 5**) has a sensitivity of 93% to diagnose gallstone ileus, but the diagnosis is often delayed 3 to 8 days after the onset of symptoms.[29]

Treatment Following adequate fluid and electrolyte resuscitation, surgery is indicated. Relief of intestinal obstruction is the primary objective. The stone can usually be gently manipulated proximal to the site of obstruction and removed by enterotomy (**Fig. 6**). Concomitant definitive cholecystectomy and closure of the biliary-enteric fistula is controversial. In most instances, operative treatment has been limited to relief of obstruction; however, the potential for recurrent symptoms should prompt consideration of definitive resection and repair for fit patients with residual stones. Reisner and Cohen[24] reported a higher mortality rate in a 1 stage (16.9%) compared with enterolithotomy alone (11.7%). Follow-up of those who underwent enterolithotomy alone showed a 5% to 9% recurrence rate but only 10% of those who recurred required reoperation. Spontaneous closure of the fistula may explain the low need for operative intervention but is open to question. Marko Doko and colleagues[29] also compared the 2 surgical management pathways and found that although mortality rates were similar, patients who underwent index cholecystectomy had a higher rate of complications. They concluded that cholecystectomy in the setting of gallstone ileus should be reserved only for those with acute or gangrenous cholecystitis and residual stones. If a cholecystectomy is done, the common bile duct must be evaluated for an obstruction that may have contributed to fistula formation. The surgeon can anticipate that cholecystectomy in the setting of gallstone ileus will always be a more difficult operation. Interval cholecystectomy and fistula repair is considered for patients with residual stones or symptoms after enterolithotomy alone. In reality, this is practiced infrequently because of the general medical status of many of these patients.

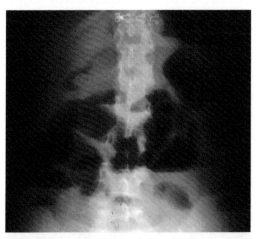

Fig. 4. Plain abdominal film demonstrating central pneumobilia and dilated small intestine in gallstone ileus.

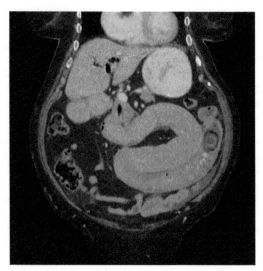

Fig. 5. Coronal CT of an obstructing gallstone in the small intestine.

Bouveret syndrome Bouveret syndrome is a variant of gallstone ileus that was described by Leon Bouveret in 1896[30] in 2 patients with gastric outlet obstruction due to gallstones.[31] The mechanism of obstruction is similar to gallstone ileus except the site of obstruction is the duodenal bulb, postbulbar duodenum, pylorus, or pre-pyloric area. Typical symptoms include nausea/emesis (86%) and abdominal pain (71%). Other nonspecific signs and symptoms include anorexia, weight loss, abdominal distension, and hematemesis. Endoscopic examination will often confirm gastric outlet or duodenal obstruction (**Fig. 7**). Visualization of an impacted stone, however, occurs in only 69% of cases because some stones can become deeply embedded within the mucosa. CT is often used to confirm endoscopic findings and delineate the anatomy of the biliary-enteric fistula. Despite the low success rate, endoscopic retrieval of the obstructing stone should be attempted to minimize morbidity in a high-risk patient population. Advances in endoscopic technology and instrumentation should improve the success rate.[32] Laser lithotripsy, mechanical lithotripsy, or extracorporal shock wave lithotripsy have been tried. Operation by laparoscopic or open lithotomy (**Fig. 8**) with or without cholecystectomy and fistula closure is usually

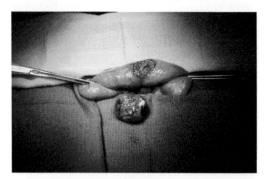

Fig. 6. Intraoperative picture of an enterolithotomy in a patient with gallstone ileus.

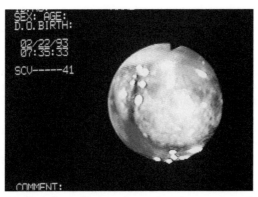

Fig. 7. An endoscopic view of a gallstone obstructing the gastric outlet in a patient with Bouveret syndrome.

necessary. Roux-en-Y duodenojejunostomy has been described to manage large fistulas.[33]

Biliary-vascular fistula
Hemobilia Hemorrhage into the biliary system was recognized by Francis Glisson in 1654 as a potential consequence of blunt or penetrating injury to the liver.[34] Antoine Portal, Professor of Anatomy and Surgery at College Royale de France, is credited with the first ante mortem diagnosis of the condition in 1777 while he was treating a servant of the Marquise de Cambis who suffered from hepatic abscesses.[35] In the modern era, Swedish surgeon Philip Sandblom made comprehensive study of this problem in his 1972 monograph.[36] It was he who coined the term "hemobilia" to denote bleeding into or through the biliary tract.

Hemobilia may originate from the liver, the gallbladder, the intrahepatic or extrahepatic bile ducts, or from the pancreas (hemosuccus pancreaticus). Bleeding may range from occult to massive and has a tendency to occur periodically. Clinically significant hemobilia is usually from an arterial source, although venous bleeding can be significant in cases of portal hypertension. Trauma is the most frequent antecedent of hemobilia; either accidental trauma or, more commonly, iatrogenic trauma from any of a litany of transhepatic or endoscopic interventions, including cholangiography,

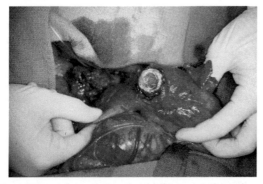

Fig. 8. Intraoperative picture of an obstructing gallstone at the pylorus in a patient with Bouveret syndrome.

biopsy, drainage, stent placement, balloon dilatation, and lithotripsy. Other causes include hepatobiliary malignancy, inflammatory conditions, vascular disorders, and, of course, gallstones.

The symptoms of hemobilia depend on the rate of bleeding and the presence of bile duct obstruction from clots. Flowing bile has natural fibrinolytic activity that dissolves clots unless the bleeding is too rapid. Conversely, minor hemobilia may persist with fibrinolysis and remain asymptomatic except for chronic anemia. The classic clinical triad of biliary tract hemorrhage was highlighted by Quincke[37] in 1871: gastrointestinal hemorrhage, biliary colic, and jaundice. Gastrointestinal hemorrhage is most commonly manifested as melena (90%), sometimes as hemetemesis (60%), with biliary colic present in 70% of patients and jaundice in 60% of patients with clinically apparent symptoms.[36] Rarely, clot obstruction has caused acute cholecystitis or pancreatitis.[38–44] There is a tendency to overlook the biliary tract as a source of significant gastrointestinal hemorrhage. Indeed, Professor Sandblom lamented that "Blind resection of a healthy stomach has been performed many times because of misinterpreted hemorrhage into the biliary tract."[36]

Hemobilia from gallstones is usually microscopic and not uncommon. Fecal occult blood has been demonstrated in one-quarter of patients with cholelithiasis.[45] The mechanism is direct trauma to the biliary mucosa from the stones. Gallstone disease accounts for up to 10% of cases of major hemobilia.[36,46] This occurs when gallstones erode through the gallbladder wall or bile duct into an adjacent portion of the gut with fistula formation and/or into an adjacent blood vessel with creation of a pseudoaneurysm. Rupture of a pseudoaneurysm results in massive hemobilia, gastrointestinal bleeding, and occasionally intraperitoneal bleeding as well.[47] Not surprisingly, this complication has frequently proven fatal.

Spontaneous gallstone erosion can involve various arteries, including the cystic artery, hepatic artery, replaced right hepatic artery (originating from the superior mesenteric artery), gastroduodenal artery, or even the aorta.[36,47–53] Pseudoaneurysms resulting from operative trauma may cause life-threatening hemobilia as a late or early complication following either open or laparoscopic cholecystectomy.[54–63] Post cholecystectomy pseudoaneurysms have been associated with bile leaks and formation of late bile duct strictures.[64] Three gallstones were discovered in the portal vein of Ignatius of Loyola at the time of his autopsy.[65] Gallstones have been found in portal venous collaterals along the common bile duct in a patient with portal vein thrombosis.[36]

When hemobilia is suspected, upper gastrointestinal endoscopy is the initial examination to exclude other sources and to directly visualize blood issuing from the ampulla of Vater. Imaging by transabdominal ultrasonography, CT, magnetic resonance imaging, or direct cholangiography via various routes can demonstrate blood in the gallbladder or bile ducts and identify vascular anomalies. Selective hepatic arterial angiography is the most specific method for identifying the source of an active bleed and affords the opportunity for therapeutic embolization.

Treatment of gallstone-related hemobilia is by cholecystectomy and removal of bile duct stones. When major arterial hemorrhage is identified, selective arterial embolization is the mainstay of therapy today. Arterial injury discovered intraoperatively is managed by vessel ligation or aneurysm repair. Bile duct obstruction caused by hemobilia is successfully treated with endoscopic biliary drainage in most cases.[66]

Bilhemia Bilhemia is direct flow of bile into the blood through a biliary-vascular fistula. This occurs when there is an abnormal communication between the higher-pressure, typically obstructed, biliary system and the lower-pressure portal vein, hepatic veins, or inferior vena cava. Clinically significant bilhemia is rare but has often resulted in fatal pulmonary embolization of bile or sepsis.[67] The cause is most often blunt trauma with central liver rupture or iatrogenic penetrating injury associated with percutaneous transhepatic interventions, such as biopsy, drainage, and placement of biliary stents or transjugular intrahepatic porto-systemic shunts.[68–70] In exceptionally rare instances, bilhemia may be caused by venous erosion of gallstones.[36,65]

The cardinal diagnostic feature of bilhemia is rapidly increasing jaundice and pronounced direct hyperbilirubinemia without a substantial elevation of liver enzymes.[68] Cholangiography by endoscopic retrograde or transhepatic approaches is the best method for imaging the fistula. Unlike hemobilia, arteriography is not diagnostic. Hepatobiliary scintigraphy may also indicate the diagnosis.[71]

Treatment of bilhemia is founded on relief of bile duct obstruction by endoscopic, transhepatic, or surgical means, which may result in spontaneous closure of the fistula. Interruption of the fistula by placement of covered stents or by balloon tamponade or angiographic coil occlusion has been successful.[72,73] Although not applicable to gallstone bilhemia, operative solutions have included liver resection, liver transplantation, and external drainage of the bile duct or disrupted liver.[68]

Biliary-thoracic fistula

Biliary-thoracic fistulas are abnormal communications between the biliary tract and the thoracic cavity. The end point within the thoracic cavity can be either the pleural space or the bronchial tree. The causes of biliary-thoracic fistulas are many and can be categorized into thoracoabdominal trauma, parasitic liver disease, suppurative biliary tract obstruction, or iatrogenic due to external drainage procedures. In Western countries, gallbladder perforation, leading to subhepatic abscesses or postoperative bile duct stenosis, is the primary cause of biliary-thoracic fistulas, whereas in developing countries, liver abscesses due to echinococcal or amebic infections are more common.[17] Patients often present with right upper quadrant and pleuritic pain, but sometimes only vague symptoms, such as shortness of breath, are present.[74] In patients with bronchobiliary fistulas, bitter taste and productive yellow sputum may be present, suggesting bile pigments in sputum, known as biliptysis.[75] Signs of systemic infection, such as fever, chills, or leukocytosis, may be present in only half of the patients. Imaging will often show a right pleural effusion.[76] Percutaneous and endoscopic interventions should first be attempted to treat acquired fistulas and surgery should be reserved as second-line treatment.[77] Singh and colleagues[78] suggested a treatment algorithm for thoracobiliary fistulas, as shown in **Fig. 9**.

Biliary-genitourinary fistula

Fistulous connections between the biliary tract and GU organs may occur spontaneously or consequent to accidental or operative trauma but are extremely unusual. Connections have been described between the gallbladder or common bile duct and the right renal pelvis, the urinary bladder, and the embryonic remnant urachus.[79–82] Rabinowitz and colleagues[82] reported on an elderly man with multiple episodes of urinary tract infections who was found to have gallstones in his urinary bladder. Retrograde injection of a sinus at the dome of the bladder confirmed a connection between the urachal remnant and the gallbladder. Definitive repair involved resection of the gallbladder, bladder dome, and the urachal remnant. Fistulization between the common bile duct and a neobladder ileal conduit has been successfully managed endoscopically.[83] Gallstone migration into GU structures has been observed as a complication of gallstones lost at the time of cholecystectomy.[84–86] Symptoms include recurrent urinary tract infections and passage of gallstones through the urethra. Gallstones in the urinary bladder may be amenable to cystoscopic

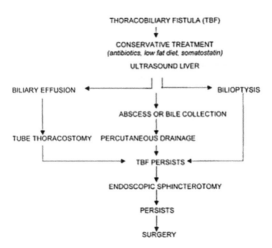

THORACOBILIARY FISTULA (TBF)

CONSERVATIVE TREATMENT
(antibiotics, low fat diet, somatostatin)

ULTRASOUND LIVER

BILIARY EFFUSION ← ——— | |——— → BILIOPTYSIS

ABSCESS OR BILE COLLECTION

TUBE THORACOSTOMY   PERCUTANEOUS DRAINAGE

TBF PERSISTS ←

ENDOSCOPIC SPHINCTEROTOMY

PERSISTS

SURGERY

Fig. 9. Suggested approach to the management of thoracobiliary fistulas. (*From* Singh B, Moodley J, Sheik-Gafoor MH, et al. Conservative management of thoracobiliary fistula. Ann Thorac Surg 2002;73(4):1088–91.)

extraction with spontaneous closure of the fistula tract. If the stones are multiple or embedded in the bladder wall, operative removal may be necessary.

Although not specifically due to gallstone disease, a host of other rare urinary fistulas have been described involving upper abdominal organs, including nephrohepatic fistulas,[87] pyelo-duodenal fistulas from pyonephrosis,[88,89] and unusual fistulas from migration of biliary stents.[90] Posttraumatic nephro-bilary fistula has been treated by percutaneous embolization.[91]

External

Spontaneous cholecystocutaneous fistula was once a common complication of gallstone disease but now is a rare condition because of early diagnosis and treatment. A total of 226 cases have been reported since the early twentieth century and fewer than 25 cases have been reported in the past 50 years.[92,93] Most patients are women older than 50 years and most fistulas drain externally to the right upper quadrant. Other locations, such as chest wall, umbilicus, right groin, or gluteus, have been reported.[92,94,95]

LOST GALLSTONES

Spillage of bile and gallstones during a laparoscopic cholecystectomy is not infrequent. The presence of cholecystitis, patient age, pigmented stones, number of stones more than 15, and resident participation are risk factors for stone spillage.[96–98] Control of bile and stone spillage is not a major issue in open cholecystectomy, but can be challenging laparoscopically. It is estimated that lost stones occur in 2% of laparoscopic cholecystectomy cases with 8.5% of those cases resulting in subsequent complications.[99] Although most lost stones are silent, they can cause wound infection, abscess, or cutaneous sinus formation. Fistulization of lost stones can occur internally to the GI tract or thoracic cavity or externally to the skin. Stones lost in the Morrison pouch tend to migrate posteriorly and those lost in the gastrocolic omentum may result in painful fibrotic masses. **Fig. 10** is a list of complications reportedly due to lost gallstones.[99]

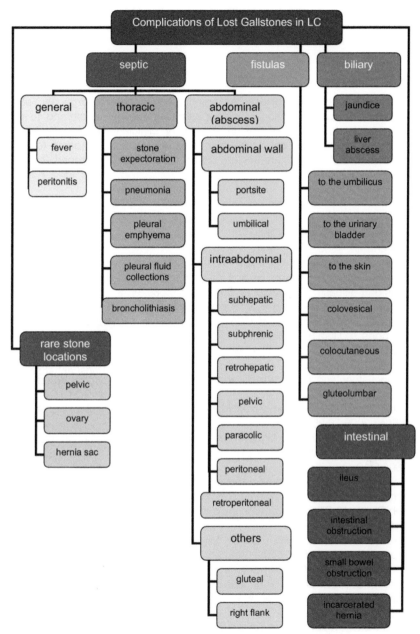

Fig. 10. Diagram of possible complications of lost gallstones. (*From* Zehetner J, Shamiyeh A, Wayand W. Lost gallstones in laparoscopic cholecystectomy: all possible complications. Am J Surg 2007;193(1):73–8.)

Suggestions to minimize the spillage of stones and the resulting complications are early controlled decompression of dilated gallbladders, early recognition and control of the operation by the attending physician during a difficult case or with an inexperienced trainee, and meticulous survey of the abdomen for spilled stones.

The treatment of lost gallstone complications usually involves drainage of infection and stone removal. Spontaneous closure of the fistula tract can be expected after removal of gallstones.

SUMMARY

The management of gallstone disease is commonplace for general surgeons. Yet, rarities exist and, although not unique, their appearances may be seldom and so separated in time as to elude recognition. The wary clinician who is cognizant of anomalous biliary passages and stone migrations will be better prepared to handle these unusual conditions that are benign, but potentially fatal and properly curable.

REFERENCES

1. Kehr H. Die in neiner klinik geubte technik de gallenstein operationen, mit einen hinweis auf die indikationen und die dauerersolge. Munchen (Germany): JF Lehman; 1905.
2. Mirizzi P. Sindrome del conducto hepatico. J Int Chir 1948;8:731–7.
3. Beltran MA. Mirizzi syndrome and gallstone ileus: an unusual presentation of gallstone disease. J Gastrointest Surg 2005;9:686–9.
4. Mc Sherry C, Ferstenberg H, Virhup M. The Mirizzi syndrome: suggested classification and surgical therapy. Surg Gastroenterol 1982;1:219–25.
5. Csendes A, Diaz JC, Burdiles P, et al. Mirizzi syndrome and cholecystobiliary fistula: a unifying classification. Br J Surg 1989;76:1139–43.
6. Beltran MA, Csendes A, Cruces KS. The relationship of Mirizzi syndrome and cholecystoenteric fistula: validation of a modified classification. World J Surg 2008;32:2237–43.
7. Lai EC, Lau WY. Mirizzi syndrome: history, present and future development. ANZ J Surg 2006;76:251–7.
8. Safioleas M, Stamatakos M, Safioleas P, et al. Mirizzi syndrome: an unexpected problem of cholelithiasis: our experience with 27 cases. Int Semin Surg Oncol 2008;5:12–5.
9. Beltran MA. Mirizzi syndrome: history, current knowledge and proposal of a simplified classification. World J Gastroenterol 2012;18:4639–50.
10. Yeh C, Jan Y, Chen M. Laparoscopic treatment for Mirizzi syndrome. Surg Endosc 2003;17:1573–8.
11. Redaelli CA, Buchler MW, Schilling MK, et al. High coincidence of Mirizzi syndrome and gallbladder carcinoma. Surgery 1997;121:58–63.
12. Judd ES, Burden VG. Internal biliary fistula. Ann Surg 1925;81:305–12.
13. Borman C, Rigler LG. Spontaneous internal biliary fistula and gallstone obstruction, with particular reference to roentgenologic diagnosis. Surgery 1937;1: 349–78.
14. Puestow CB. Spontaneous internal biliary fistulae. Ann Surg 1942;115:1043–54.
15. Levowitz BS. Spontaneous internal biliary fistulas. Ann Surg 1961;154:241–51.
16. Piedad OH, Wells PB. Spontaneous internal biliary fistula, obstructive and nonobstructive types. Ann Surg 1971;175:75–80.
17. Petrowsky H, Clavien P. Biliary fistula, gallstone ileus, and Mirizzi's syndrome. In: Clavien PA, Baillie J, editors. Diseases of the gallbladder and bile ducts: diagnosis and treatment. 2nd edition. Malden (MA): Blackwell Publishing; 2008. p. 239–51.
18. Antonacci N, Taffurelli G, Casadei R, et al. Asymptomatic cholecystocolonic fistula: a diagnostic and therapeutic dilemma. Case Rep Surg 2013;2013:1–3.

19. Costi R, Randone B, Violi V, et al. Cholecystocolonic fistula: facts and myths. A review of the 231 published cases. J Hepatobiliary Pancreat Surg 2009;16:8–18.
20. Gentileschi P, Forlini A, Rossi P, et al. Laparoscopic approach to cholecystocolic fistula: report of a case. J Laparoendosc Surg 1995;5:413–7.
21. Cooperman AM, Dickson ER, ReMine WH. Changing concepts in the surgical treatment of gallstone ileus: a review of 15 cases with emphasis on diagnosis and treatment. Ann Surg 1968;167:377–83.
22. Deckoff SL. Gallstone ileus: a report of 12 cases. Ann Surg 1955;142:52–65.
23. Courvoisier L. The pathology and surgery of the biliary tract. Leipzig (Germany): FCW Vogel; 1890. p. 58.
24. Reisner RM, Cohen JR. Gallstone ileus: a review of 1001 reported cases. Am Surg 1994;60:441–6.
25. Moss JF, Bloom AD, Mesleh GF, et al. Gallstone ileus. Am Surg 1987;53:424–8.
26. Balthazar EJ, Schechter LS. Air in gallbladder: a frequent finding in gallstone ileus. AJR Am J Roentgenol 1978;131:219–22.
27. Ripolles T, Miguel-Dasit A, Errando J, et al. Gallstone ileus: increased diagnostic sensitivity by combining plain film and ultrasound. Abdom Imaging 2001;26: 401–5.
28. Yu C, Lin C, Shyu R, et al. Value of CT in the diagnosis and management of gallstone ileus. World J Gastroenterol 2005;11:2142–7.
29. Marko Doko M, Zovak M, Kopljar M, et al. Comparison of surgical treatments of gallstone ileus: preliminary report. World J Surg 2003;27:400–4.
30. Bouveret L. Stenose du pylore adherent a la vesicule. Rev Med 1986;16:1–16.
31. Cappell MS, Davis M. Characterization of Bouveret's syndrome: a comprehensive review of 128 cases. Am J Gastroenterol 2006;101:2139–46.
32. Zhao J, Barrera E, Salabat M, et al. Endoscopic treatment for Bouveret syndrome. Surg Endosc 2013;27(2):655.
33. Erlandson MD, Kim AW, Richter HM III, et al. Roux-en-Y duodenojejunostomy in the treatment of Bouveret syndrome. South Med J 2009;102:963–5.
34. Glisson F. Anatomia hepatis. Amsterdam: J.J. Waesberge & E Weyerstraten; 1654.
35. Portal A. Observations sur la nature et le traitement des maladies du foie. Charleston (SC): Caille et Ravier; 1813.
36. Sandblom P. Hemobilia (biliary tract hemorrhage). Springfield (MA): Charles C Thomas; 1972.
37. Quincke H. Ein fall von aneurysma der leberarterie. Berl Klin Wochenschr 1871; 8:349–51.
38. Counihan TC, Islam S, Swanson RS. Acute cholecystitis resulting from hemobilia after tru-cut biopsy: a case report and brief review of the literature. Am Surg 1996;62:757–8.
39. Lee SL, Caruso DM. Acute cholecystitis secondary to hemobilia. J Laparoendosc Adv Surg Tech A 1999;9:347–9.
40. Parekh J, Corvera CU. Hemorrhagic cholecystitis. Arch Surg 2010;145:202–4.
41. Van Os EC, Petersen BT. Pancreatitis secondary to percutaneous liver biopsy-associated hemobilia. Am J Gastroenterol 1996;91:577–80.
42. Wolf DS, Wasan SM, Merhav H, et al. Hemobilia in a patient with protein S deficiency after laparoscopic cholecystectomy that caused acute pancreatitis: successful endoscopic management. Gastrointest Endosc 2005;62:163–6.
43. Kim JD, Lee KM, Chung WC, et al. Acute pancreatitis and cholangitis caused by hemobilia from biliary papillomatosis. Gastrointest Endosc 2007;65:177–80.
44. de Ribot X, Casellas F, Papo M, et al. Hemobilia causing acute pancreatitis after percutaneous liver biopsy. J Clin Gastroenterol 1995;21:171–2.

45. Gad P. Okkult blodning ved galdesten. Nord Med 1962;68:1069.
46. Blumgart LH. Hemobilia and bilhemia. In: Surgery of the liver, biliary tract and pancreas. 4th edition. Philadelphia: Saunders Elsevier; 2007. p. 1067–84.
47. Martinis A, Kalaitzis I, Basioukas P, et al. Vascular complications of large gallstones: proposal of a first classification. Hellenic J Surg 2012;84:318–9.
48. England RE, Marsh PJ, Ashleigh R, et al. Case report: pseudoaneurysm of the cystic artery: a rare cause of haemobilia. Clin Radiol 1998;53:72–5.
49. Bibyan M, Khandelwal RG, Reddy PK, et al. Gallstone causing pseudoaneurysm of accessory right hepatic artery. Indian J Gastroenterol 2012;31:213–4.
50. Broadbent NR, Taylor DE. Gallstone erosion of the aorta. ANZ J Surg 1975;45:207–8.
51. Siddiqui NA, Chawla T, Nadeem M. Cystic artery pseudoaneurysm secondary to acute cholecystitis as cause of haemobilia. BMJ Case Rep 2011;2011. pii: bcr0720114480.
52. Wang S, Wang X. Hemobilia secondary to acute gangrenous cholecystitis. Am Surg 2012;78:149–51.
53. Priya H, Anshul G, Alok T, et al. Emergency cholecystectomy and hepatic arterial repair in a patient presenting with haemobilia and massive gastrointestinal haemorrhage due to a spontaneous cystic artery gallbladder fistula masquerading as a pseudoaneurysm. BMC Gastroenterol 2013;13:43.
54. Larmi TK. Hemobilia associated with cholecystitis, postcholecystectomy conditions and trauma: review of 12 cases. Ann Surg 1966;163:373–81.
55. Zilberstein B, Cecconello I, Ramos AC, et al. Hemobilia as a complication of laparoscopic cholecystectomy. Surg Laparosc Endosc 1994;4:301–3.
56. Stewart BT, Abraham RJ, Thomson KR, et al. Post-cholecystectomy haemobilia: enjoying a renaissance in the laparoscopic era? Aust N Z J Surg 1995;65:185–8.
57. Saldinger PF, Wang JY, Boyd C, et al. Cystic artery stump pseudoaneurysm following laproscopic cholecystectomy. Surgery 2002;131:585–6.
58. Dogru O, Cetinkaya Z, Bulbuller N, et al. Hemobilia: a rare complication of laparoscopic cholecystectomy. Surg Endosc 2003;17:1495–6.
59. Stewart L, Robinson TN, Lee CM, et al. Right hepatic artery injury associated with laparoscopic bile duct injury: incidence, mechanism, and consequences. J Gastrointest Surg 2004;8:523–30.
60. Srinivasaiah N, Bhojak M, Jackson R, et al. Vascular emergencies in cholelithiasis and cholecystectomy: our experience with two cases and literature review. Hepatobiliary Pancreat Dis Int 2008;7:217–20.
61. Yao CA, Arnell TD. Hepatic artery pseudoaneurysm following laparoscopic cholecystectomy. Am J Surg 2010;199:10–1.
62. Hadj AK, Goodwin M, Schwalb H, et al. Pseudoaneurysm of the hepatic artery. J Gastrointest Surg 2011;15:1899–901.
63. Petrou A, Brenna N, Soonawalla Z, et al. Hemobilia due to cystic artery stump pseudoaneurysm following laparoscopic cholecystectomy: case presentation and literature review. Int Surg 2012;97:140–4.
64. Madanur MA, Battula N, Sethi H, et al. Pseudoaneurysm following laparoscopic cholecystectomy. Hepatobiliary Pancreat Dis Int 2007;6:294–8.
65. Ullman WH. Autopsy of Ignatius of Loyola. Monogr Soc Res Child Dev 1963;35:1758–63.
66. Kim KH, Kim TN. Etiology, clinical features, and endoscopic management of hemobilia: a retrospective analysis of 37 cases. Korean J Gastroenterol 2012;59:296–302.

67. Sandblom P, Jakobsson B, Lindgren H, et al. Fatal bilhemia. Surgery 2000;127: 354–7.
68. Glaser K, Wetscher G, Pointner R, et al. Traumatic bilhemia. Surgery 1994;116: 24–7.
69. Brown CY, Walsh GC. Fatal bile embolism following liver biopsy. Ann Intern Med 1952;36:1529–33.
70. Mallery S, Freeman ML, Peine CJ, et al. Biliary-shunt fistula following transjugular intrahepatic portosystemic shunt placement. Gastroenterology 1996;111:1353–7.
71. Francois D, Walrand S, Van Nieuwenhuyse JP, et al. Hepatobiliary scintigraphy in a patient with bilhemia. Eur J Nucl Med 1994;21:1020–3.
72. Struyven J, Cremer M, Pirson P, et al. Posttraumatic bilhemia: diagnosis and catheter therapy. AJR Am J Roentgenol 1982;138:746–7.
73. Rankin RN, Vellet DA. Portobiliary fistula: occurrence and treatment. Can Assoc Radiol J 1991;42:55–9.
74. Cunningham L, Grobman M, Paz H, et al. Cholecystopleural fistula with cholelithiasis presenting as a right pleural effusion. Chest 1990;97:751–2.
75. Gugenheim J, Ciardullo M, Traynor O, et al. Bronchobiliary fistulas in adults. Ann Surg 1988;207:90–4.
76. Delco F, Domenighetti G, Kauzlaric D, et al. Spontaneous biliothorax (thoracobilia) following cholecystopleural fistula presenting as an acute respiratory insufficiency: successful removal of gallstones from the pleural space. Chest 1994; 106:961–3.
77. Poullis M, Poullis A. Biliptysis caused by a bronchobiliary fistula. J Thorac Cardiovasc Surg 1999;118:971–2.
78. Singh B, Moodley J, Sheik-Gafoor MH, et al. Conservative management of thoracobiliary fistula. Ann Thorac Surg 2002;73:1088–91.
79. Op den Orth JO. A radiologically demonstrated fistula between the common bile duct and the right renal pelvis. Radiol Clin Biol 1969;38:402–5.
80. Holst S, Peterson NE, McCroskey BL. Pyelo-choledochal fistula accompanying operative-cholangiography. J Urol 1988;139:823–4.
81. Shah A, Salamut W, Rull G, et al. Spontaneous pelvi-cholecystic fistula. BJU Int 2002;89:322–3.
82. Rabinowitz CB, Song JH, Movson JS, et al. Cholecysto-urachal fistula. Abdom Imaging 2007;32:108–10.
83. Narayan S, Roslyn J, Raz S, et al. Successful endoscopic treatment of a fistula between the common bile duct and neobladder. Gastrointest Endosc 1993;39: 94–8.
84. Castro MG, Alves AS, Oliveira CA, et al. Elimination of biliary stones through the urinary tract: a complication of laparoscopic cholecystectomy. Rev Hosp Clin Fac Med Sao Paulo 1999;54:209–12.
85. Lutken W, Berggren P, Maltbak J. Passing of gallstones via the urethra: a complication of laparoscopic cholecystectomy. Surg Laparosc Endosc 1997;7:495–7.
86. Famulari C, Pirrone G, Macri A, et al. The vesical granuloma: rare and late complication of laparoscopic cholecystectomy. Surg Laparosc Endosc Percutan Tech 2001;11:368–71.
87. Abraham JI, Martin JL, Smith EH. Nephrohepatic fistula. N Y State J Med 1971; 71:2881–3.
88. Boardman KP. Duodenal and common bile duct obstruction with a pyeloduodenal fistula caused by renal calculus pyonephrosis. Br J Urol 1976;48:6.
89. Desmond JM, Evans SE, Couch A, et al. Pyeloduodenal fistulae: a report of two cases and review of literature. Clin Radiol 1989;40:267–70.

90. Basile A, Macri A, Lamberto S, et al. Duodenoscrotal fistula secondary to retroperitoneal migration of an endoscopically placed plastic biliary stent. Gastrointest Endosc 2003;57:136–8.

91. Ryu R, Novak Z, Coldwell D. Percutaneous embolization of a posttraumatic nephrobiliary fistula. J Trauma 1998;44:389–91.

92. Yuceyar S, Erturk S, Karabicak I, et al. Spontaneous cholecystocutaneous fistula presenting with an abscess containing multiple gallstones: a case report. Mt Sinai J Med 2005;72:402–4.

93. Sayed L, Sangal S, Finch G. Spontaneous cholecystocutaneous fistula: a rare presentation of gallstones. J Surg Case Rep 2010;2010:5.

94. Malik AH, Nadeem M, Ockrim J. Complete laparoscopic management of cholecystocutaneous fistula. Ulster Med J 2007;76:166–7.

95. Nicholson T, Born MW, Garber E. Spontaneous cholecystocutaneous fistula presenting in the gluteal region. J Clin Gastroenterol 1999;28:276–7.

96. Woodfield J, Rodgers M, Windsor J. Peritoneal gallstones following laparoscopic cholecystectomy. Surg Endosc 2004;18:1200–7.

97. Barrat C, Champault A, Matthyssens L, et al. Iatrogenic perforation of the gallbladder during laparoscopic cholecystectomy does not influence the prognosis: prospective study. Ann Chir 2004;129:25–9.

98. Brockmann J, Kocher T, Senninger N, et al. Complications due to gallstones lost during laparoscopic cholecystectomy. Surg Endosc 2002;16:1226–32.

99. Zehetner J, Shamiyeh A, Wayand W. Lost gallstones in laparoscopic cholecystectomy: all possible complications. Am J Surg 2007;193:73–8.

Endoscopic Management of Biliary Disorders

Diagnostic and Therapeutic

Todd H. Baron, MD

KEYWORDS

- Biliary disorders • Endoscopy • Endoscopic ultrasound
- Endoscopic retrograde cholangiopancreatography

KEY POINTS

- Endoscopy allows for diagnostic and therapeutic applications through endoscopic retrograde cholangiopancreatography (ERCP) and endoscopic ultrasound (EUS).
- Because of advancements in abdominal imaging ERCP is now almost an exclusive therapeutic procedure.
- EUS allows diagnosis by imaging and by tissue acquisition.
- EUS-guided therapeutics is becoming a viable alternative to percutaneous procedures.

INTRODUCTION

Hirschowitz's landmark article on fiberoptics[1] and subsequent application to flexible endoscopy changed the world of endoscopy. Decades later, the introduction of endoscopic retrograde cholangiopancreatography (ERCP) changed the management of biliary tract disorders.[2] ERCP slowly evolved from a purely diagnostic procedure and has matured to become a highly effective therapeutic procedure. Although the indications for diagnostic ERCP are now uncommon, technologic advances have extended its' diagnostic capabilities beyond simple cholangiography (**Box 1**). Similarly, endoscopic ultrasound (EUS), a less-invasive diagnostic tool than ERCP, has therapeutic capabilities that have only recently become realized (**Box 2**). Although ERCP has matured and its' growth plateaued, there continues to be enormous growth potential for therapeutic EUS. In this article the diagnostic and therapeutic applications of endoscopic techniques for patients with biliary disorders are discussed.

Funding Source: None.
Division of Gastroenterology and Hepatology, University of North Carolina, 41041 Bioinformatics Boulevard, CB 7080, Chapel Hill, NC 27599-0001, USA
E-mail address: todd_baron@med.unc.edu

Surg Clin N Am 94 (2014) 395–411
http://dx.doi.org/10.1016/j.suc.2013.12.005 **surgical.theclinics.com**

> **Box 1**
> **Applications of ERCP for biliary disease**
>
> Diagnostic
>   Primary sclerosing cholangitis
>   Indeterminate biliary strictures
>   Sphincter of Oddi manometry
> Therapeutic
>   Common bile duct stones
>   Bile duct leaks
>   Benign biliary strictures
>   Malignant biliary strictures
>   Transpapillary gallbladder drainage
>   Ampullary adenoma

DIAGNOSTIC ERCP

Diagnostic ERCP has been replaced by noninvasive imaging modalities, such as magnetic resonance imaging (MRI) and magnetic resonance cholangiopancreatography (MRCP), and less-invasive EUS. However, there are several indications for diagnostic ERCP (see **Box 1**).

> **Box 2**
> **Applications of EUS for biliary disease**
>
> Diagnostic
>   Gallbladder
>   Stones
>   Sludge
>   Microlithiasis
>   Bile duct stones
>   Indeterminate biliary strictures
>   Ampullary lesions
> Therapeutic
>   Transmural gallbladder drainage
>   Transgastric drainage of bilomas
>   Transgastric drainage of hepatic abscesses
>   Biliary drainage
>   Rendezvous
>   Hepaticogastrostomy
>   Choledochoduodenostomy

Primary Sclerosing Cholangitis

Primary sclerosing cholangitis (PSC) is a fibrosing disease of the biliary tree. The diagnosis rests on clinical features, liver biopsy, and cholangiography. ERCP remains the gold standard for cholangiography, although it has largely been replaced by MRCP.[3] ERCP is warranted when MRCP is nondiagnostic or normal when the diagnosis is highly suspected and when cytologic sampling and therapeutic intervention are needed. However, it is important that proper techniques are used to obtain optimal cholangiographic images.[4] Complete filling of the intrahepatics is essential to establish the diagnosis in early stages and best obtained when an occlusion balloon catheter (stone retrieval balloon) is positioned above the cystic duct takeoff when the gallbladder is intact (**Fig. 1**).

Patients with PSC are at increased risk for cholangiocarcinoma (CCA). Thus, ERCP is useful for obtaining cytologic and biopsy samples in patients with PSC undergoing ERCP in the presence of dominant strictures and/or a worsening in clinical course. Cytologic evaluation using fluorescent in situ hybridization analysis has proved to be useful in identifying underlying CCA,[5] which in turn may allow transplantation[6] and improvement in survival.

Indeterminate Biliary Strictures

An indeterminate biliary stricture is defined as one that has defied diagnosis despite serum laboratory examination, imaging studies, and histologic sampling. Repeat ERCP with cholangioscopy can be useful in visualizing the stricture and allowing directed biopsies to allow a diagnosis to be established.[7] It must be emphasized that cholangioscopy in the setting of PSC is less reliable than in those patients with de novo strictures, because the endoscopic appearance of benign strictures and malignant strictures can be similar.[8] There are two methods of cholangioscopy: passage of a cholangioscope through the working channel of the ERCP scope (**Fig. 2**); and

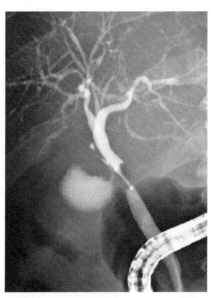

Fig. 1. Diagnostic cholangiogram for primary sclerosing cholangitis. Note occlusion balloon is inflated below cystic duct take off to maximize contrast filling of the intrahepatic ducts.

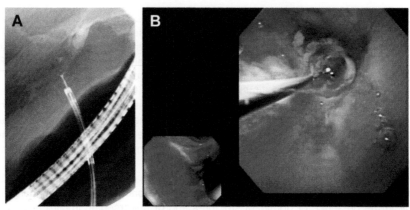

Fig. 2. Cholangioscopy using a prototype video cholangioscope. (*A*) Radiographic image showing the cholangioscope passed to the bifurcation. A biopsy forceps is seen extending from the cholangioscope. (*B*) Cholangioscopic image (*right*) of stricture. Note inset from of the endoscopic image from the ERCP scope shows the cholangioscope in the duodenum entering the papilla.

passage of a small-caliber forward-viewing endoscope (4.9 mm) directly into the bile duct.[9,10] The latter is referred to as direct peroral cholangioscopy[11,12] and can be technically challenging because the mechanics and angulation do not easily permit a forward-viewing endoscope to be passed directly into the bile duct. However, the optics achieved with these forward-viewing endoscopes are superior (video rather than fiberoptic) and the endoscope has a larger working channel than do cholangio-scopes passed through the ERCP channel.

Another, recently introduced technologic advancement is the use of probe-based confocal laser endomicroscopy. The probe is passed into the bile duct through the endoscope and allows real-time histologic images of the biliary epithelium. It has shown promise for determining malignancy in patients with and without PSC.[13,14]

Sphincter of Oddi Manometry

Postcholecystectomy biliary-type pain may be a manifestation of sphincter of Oddi dysfunction (SOD).[15] SOD is classified clinically as type I, II, or III. Type I SOD patients have elevated liver tests during an attack that normalize between attacks and a dilated bile duct by imaging. Type II SOD patients have either abnormal liver tests during an attack or a dilated bile duct, but not both. Type III SOD patients have pain only and no objective pancreaticobiliary laboratory or imaging abnormalities. Type I SOD patients respond uniformly to endoscopic sphincterotomy (ES) and manometry is not needed for diagnosis or therapy. Elevated biliary pressures found during SOD manometry at the time of ERCP can predict response to ES in patients with type II SOD.[15] The data to support the use of SOD manometry in patients with type III SOD are lacking,[15,16] but is offered for those patients who have disabling pain and who understand the risks of potentially fatal and/or disabling adverse effects.

THERAPEUTIC ERCP

The most common therapeutic uses of ERCP are the management of common bile duct (CBD) stones and relief of malignant obstruction. However, the range of therapeutic options for biliary disease has exploded (see **Box 1**).

CBD Stones

The success rate of ERCP for removal and clearance of CBD stones less than 1.5 cm in the absence of underlying strictures, using ES, balloons, and/or baskets, is nearly 100% when performed by experienced endoscopists. The need for mechanical lithotripsy or intraductal therapy (laser and electrohydraulic lithotripsy) for extraction of large bile duct stones has become less common with the use of combined ES and large-diameter balloon dilation[17,18] ($\geq$12 mm and up to 20 mm) (**Fig. 3**). This combination enlarges the lumen of the distal bile duct and sphincterotomy opening, the major limitations to successful extraction of large stones. The use of endoscopic balloon dilation alone to extract stones as an alternative to ES has fallen out of favor in the United States because of the higher risk of post-ERCP pancreatitis.[19] However, it is useful for selected patients with smaller stones who are at high risk of bleeding (coagulopathy, thrombocytopenia, antithrombotic agents), and perforation (Billroth II anatomy).

Benign Biliary Strictures

There are a variety of causes of benign biliary strictures (BBS). Endoscopic therapy for most BBS consists of balloon dilation and placement of plastic biliary stents.[20,21] It has

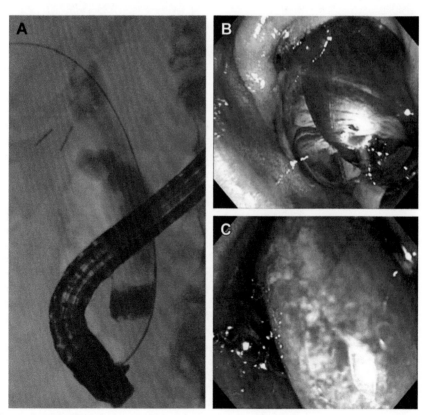

Fig. 3. Combined endoscopic sphincterotomy and large diameter balloon dilation for removal of large bile duct stone. (*A*) Cholangiogram shows large filling defect. (*B*) Endoscopic view of 15-mm balloon inflated across sphincterotomy site. (*C*) Large stone extracted and in the duodenum.

been shown that placement of multiple side-by-side plastic stents (**Fig. 4**) that remain in place for 6 to 12 months provides the best results and avoids surgery in more than 90% of patients. Recurrences can be retreated with more aggressive and longer-duration stent placement. The use of fully covered self-expandable metal stents (SEMS), which reach diameters up to three times that of rigid plastic stents, has shown

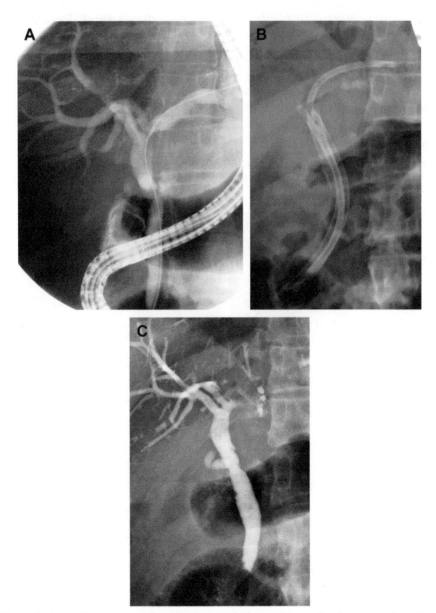

Fig. 4. Endoscopic treatment of an anastomotic biliary stricture after liver transplantation. (*A*) Initial cholangiogram demonstrates anastomotic stricture. (*B*) After balloon dilation placement of multiple plastic stents are seen across the stricture. (*C*) Final cholangiogram at the time of stent removal shows resolution of stricture.

promise in the treatment of BBS not involving the bifurcation,[20] although they are expensive and not approved in the United States for use in benign disease.

Bile Duct Leaks

Nearly all bile leaks are postsurgical and occur after biliary surgery, usually cholecystectomy. Leaks are maintained by the high-pressure biliary sphincter. Ablation of the pressure gradient is achieved by endoscopic biliary sphincterotomy, placement of short length biliary stents,[22] or a combination of the two (**Fig. 5**). Placement of a biliary stent across the leak site is generally only necessary when the leak site involves the main duct or biliary anastomosis. As in the treatment of BBS fully covered metal stents can be effective, but are not approved for such treatment and if used should be reserved for cases refractory to standard endoscopic therapy.[22,23]

Transpapillary Gallbladder Drainage

Transpapillary gallbladder drainage is achieved by ERCP after cannulation and passage of a guidewire across the cystic duct into the gallbladder. A plastic stent is placed with one end in the gallbladder lumen and the other in the duodenum (**Fig. 6**).[24] In some cases of severe cholecystitis a nasocholecystic tube is initially placed and later exchanged to an internal transpapillary stent. The success rate for placement is high in centers with experience in advanced endoscopy. The procedure can be completed without performing an ES in patients with high risk of bleeding and is especially useful when percutaneous drainage fails or is not feasible.[25]

Ampullary Adenoma

Ampullary adenomas are being increasingly discovered incidentally during endoscopy performed for other reasons. Although the term endoscopic ampullectomy is typically used, the anatomically correct term is endoscopic papillectomy.[26] Complete endoscopic resection is feasible even for large lesions (**Fig. 7**). The main

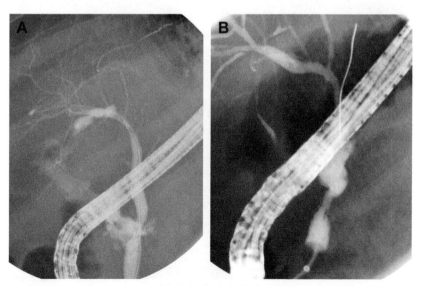

Fig. 5. Treatment of a postsurgical bile leak. (*A*) Cholangiogram shows extravasation of contrast. A 10F catheter transpapillary biliary stent was placed across the leak site. (*B*) Follow-up cholangiogram after stent removal shows absence of leak, but with mild stricture.

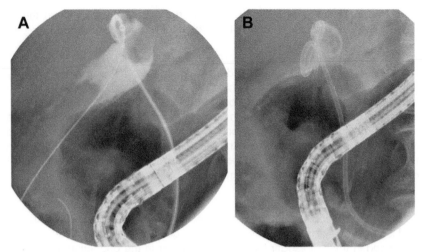

Fig. 6. Endoscopic transpapillary drainage of nonoperative drainage of cholecystitis in a 91-year-old nonoperative patient. (*A*) Cholangiogram showing guidewire passed into gallbladder passed across obstructing stone in the neck of the gallbladder and cystic duct. (*B*) Radiographic image with stent placed into gallbladder neck beyond the stone.

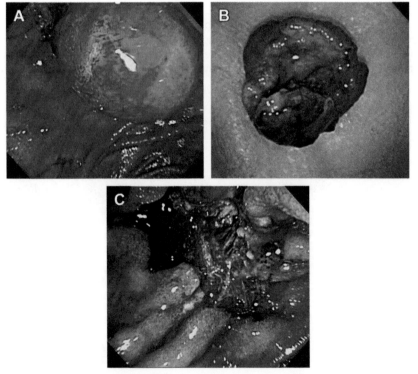

Fig. 7. Endoscopic papillectomy. (*A*) Endoscopic appearance of large periampullary lesion. (*B*) Gross picture of lesion after endoscopic resection. (*C*) Endoscopic appearance of resection site.

limitation to eradication is intraductal extension greater than 1 cm. The presence of cancer can be anticipated if ulceration, firmness, or spontaneous bleeding is identified at the time of endoscopy and is suspected preprocedurally with a presentation of obstructive jaundice in the absence of underlying choledocholithiasis. Resection techniques are similar to polypectomy in other areas except for the use of a side-viewing endoscope. Prophylactic pancreatic duct stents are placed to prevent post-ERCP pancreatitis. For large polyps, especially those with lateral extensions along the duodenal wall, more than one endoscopic procedure is often necessary for complete eradication. Surveillance endoscopy is necessary with the intervals based on histopathology and presence of residual disease on initial follow-up endoscopy.[27]

Malignant Biliary Obstruction

Distal (nonhilar) malignant obstruction

Malignant distal biliary obstruction is effectively treated using a single stent. Obstruction is relieved as effectively as surgical biliary bypass with lower morbidity and mortality, although with an increased rate of reobstruction when 10F catheter plastic stents are used.[28] These 10F catheter stents are fixed and are the largest that are passed through a standard therapeutic channel endoscope. Because of the three-fold increase in final diameter biliary SEMS have significantly longer patency durations than 10F catheter plastic stents and decrease the need for reintervention when used for palliation of malignant distal obstructive jaundice (**Fig. 8**). They are also cost-effective when used for patients who survive more than 3 to 4 months.[28] The first available biliary SEMS were bare metal; later covered SEMS were introduced to reduce tumor ingrowth through the stent spaces (interstices) and potentially prolong patency. The superior patency of covered SEMS remains unproven with contrasting results seen between two meta-analyses.[29,30] Advantages of covered SEMS are removability and ease of revision compared with uncovered SEMS, which become imbedded into the surrounding bile duct. Removability may become of upmost importance in patients in whom a tissue diagnosis was not confirmed at the time of placement and who are later found to have benign disease (eg, autoimmune pancreatitis) or curable malignancy (eg, lymphoma[31]).

In patients undergoing biliary stent placement for preoperative decompression, plastic stents are generally used.[32,33] SEMS are useful for those patients who will have delay in surgery, such as those patients with pancreatic cancer undergoing neoadjuvant therapy.[33,34] Short-length uncovered (nonremovable) SEMS do not preclude subsequent pancreaticoduodenectomy.[34]

Hilar malignant obstruction

The approach to hilar biliary obstruction is much less straightforward than for distal obstruction[28,35] and may be more likely to require percutaneous drainage, depending on endoscopist expertise. Factors that determine unilateral versus bilateral stent placement for palliation of hilar obstruction include potential resectability, Bismuth classification, presence and location of liver atrophy, intrahepatic tumor burden (**Fig. 9**), and presence of PSC.[36] Hilar cases are technically challenging for a variety of reasons. Avoidance of widespread contrast injection is essential to minimize contamination of intrahepatic ducts, and thereby minimize cholangitis resulting from a contaminated, undrained system. Thus, to avoid contrast injection guidewires are passed into intrahepatic ducts without contrast injection using an image-guided approach (computed tomography, MRI). The advantages of SEMS placement are not as clear-cut as for nonhilar obstruction, and reintervention for management of

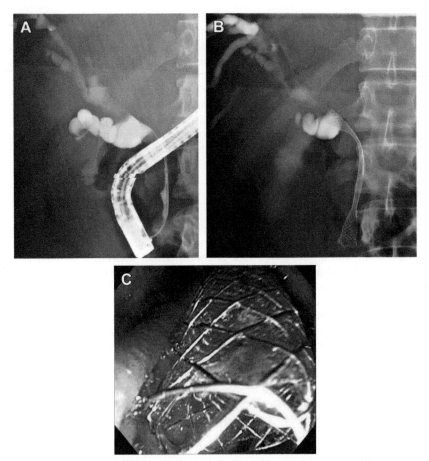

Fig. 8. Endoscopic palliation of a distal malignant biliary stricture caused by metastatic breast cancer. (*A*) Cholangiogram shows long distal bile duct stricture involving the cystic duct take off. Note dilated cystic duct. (*B*) Radiograph immediately after covered self-expandable metal stent placement. (*C*) Endoscopic photo of stent exiting the papilla.

stent occlusion when bilateral stents are placed is often difficult.[28] In patients who have SEMS placed for palliation of more advanced hilar CCA there is a greater need for reintervention because of stent occlusion.[37]

Therapies that can be delivered endoscopically for hilar CCA to prolong palliation include photodynamic therapy[38] and, more recently, radiofrequency ablation.[39] The use of endoscopically delivered brachytherapy, either low- or high-dose, is now reserved predominately for protocols that allow subsequent liver transplantation.[6,40]

Therapeutic ERCP in Patients with Surgically Altered Anatomy

ERCP was once considered impossible in patients with altered surgically anatomy. Initially, patients with Billroth II anatomy and biliary disease were successfully approached. With increasing experience, initially using colonoscopes,[41] followed by advances in endoscopic technology, particularly balloon enteroscopy, endoscopic biliary therapy can be achieved in patients with post-Whipple anatomy and patients

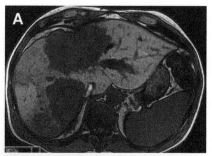

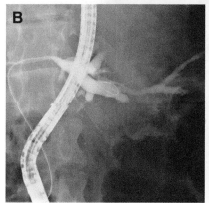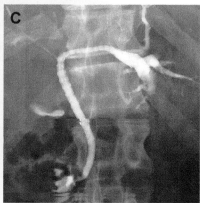

Fig. 9. Palliation of malignant hilar obstruction with unilateral metal stent. (*A*) MRI shows extensive tumor into right system. A dilated left duct can be seen. (*B*) Access into left system with avoidance of extensive contrast into right system. (*C*) Placement of uncovered expandable metal stent across stricture into left system proximally and bile duct distally.

with Roux-en-Y anastomoses with high success rates in centers with experience (**Fig. 10**).[42] Unfortunately, biliary cannulation is technically difficult in patients with native papillae because colonoscopes and balloon enteroscopes are forward-viewing rather than side-viewing. ERCP can be performed in patients with Roux-en-Y gastric bypass using a laparoscopic-assisted approach that allows access to the excluded stomach and antegrade passage of a standard side-viewing duodenoscope into the duodenum.[43]

Novel Percutaneous-Endoscopic Access Approaches

Novel percutaneous-endoscopic access approaches have recently been described to treat biliary diseases.[44] Recently termed "percutaneous assisted translumenal endoscopic therapy"[45] has been used to treat gallbladder disease and to access the excluded stomach to pass antegrade duodenoscopes in patients with Roux-en-Y gastric bypass anatomy such that management of CBD stones can be achieved entirely endoscopically.[46]

ENDOSCOPIC ULTRASOUND
Diagnostic EUS

EUS has now become a standard part of biliary diagnostics because it is less-invasive than ERCP. EUS is extremely sensitive for the diagnosis of gallbladder sludge, cholelithiasis, and microlithiasis and can establish these diagnoses in patients with

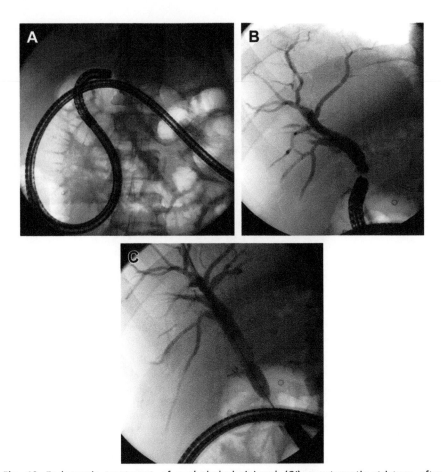

Fig. 10. Endoscopic treatment of a choledochojejunal (CJ) anastomotic stricture after pylorus-sparing Whipple. (*A*) Radiographic image on reaching the CJ using a single balloon enteroscope. (*B*) Cholangiogram showing focal narrowing of CJ. (*C*) Balloon dilation of CJ stricture yielded excellent result.

suspected biliary pancreatitis who have negative transabdominal ultrasound studies.[47] EUS is also sensitive for the diagnosis of CBD stones and is especially useful for patients with suspected CBD stones in whom other imaging studies (transabdominal ultrasound, MRCP) are nondiagnostic.

Linear-array EUS allows directed tissue acquisition using fine-needle aspiration techniques and is helpful in establishing a tissue diagnosis of malignant biliary strictures when other modalities are negative,[48] for staging of CCA[49] and other biliary malignancies, and to evaluate for the presence of lymph node involvement in patients with malignant biliary strictures.

Therapeutic EUS

Biliary drainage

Applications of therapeutic EUS for biliary disease are now becoming realized. Although EUS to provide biliary access for ERCP using a rendezvous approach is well-established, direct biliary drainage is now becoming an increasingly used approach.[50] This is because newer accessories specifically designed to access and drain the biliary tree through fine-needle aspiration wire-guided entry are emerging. This allows reliable and safe drainage accessing intrahepatics ducts through the stomach into the left lobe (hepaticogastrostomy), through the duodenum into the bile duct (choledochoduodenostomy), and by accessing these sites and internalizing drainage through the papilla without a rendezvous approach.[51,52] EUS-guided biliary drainage is especially helpful where access to the papilla is not possible because of duodenal obstruction.[53]

Gallbladder drainage

Transgastric and transduodenal drainage of the gallbladder using EUS guidance is an alternative to percutaneous cholecystostomy in patients with acute cholecystitis[54] who are poor operative candidates for cholecystectomy. The main advantage of an EUS approach is avoidance of percutaneous drains, which may be life-long if patients are not operative and/or have underlying malignancies.[55] Indeed, gallbladder stone clearance can be achieved endoscopically across such internally created tracts.[56]

Drainage of liver abscesses

Historically liver abscesses have been performed nonsurgically using percutaneous approaches. Recently, transgastric drainage using EUS-guided transgastric approaches have been described and can be performed when percutaneous therapy fails.[57]

Drainage of bilomas

Similar to liver abscesses, bilomas are usually drained percutaneously. EUS-guided drainage of bilomas through the stomach is an alternative approach.[58]

ADVERSE EVENTS

Adverse events (AEs) of ERCP and EUS are well-known and include sedation, bleeding, perforation, pancreatitis, infection, bile leakage, and death.[59–61] Risk factors for AEs include operator characteristics, patient risk factors, and degree of invasiveness of the procedure. In patients at high risk for post-ERCP pancreatitis the use of rectally administered indomethacin immediately after the ERCP significantly reduces the risk, as does placement of a temporary pancreatic duct stent.[62] Fortunately, most AEs can be managed medically, with repeat endoscopy, and/or by percutaneous means. Several types of perforations may occur after ERCP and most can be managed nonsurgically.[63] Improved recognition and closure devices allow nonoperative treatment of lateral wall perforations. However, it is important to have all disciplines available (hospitalists, critical care intensivists, interventional radiologists, and surgeons) to manage patients with AEs. Other ERCP-related AEs include stent migration (proximally or distally). EUS-transmural therapies can result in leakage between the puncture site and the biliary tree, perforation, and bleeding.

SUMMARY

Endoscopic therapy for biliary diseases has progressed markedly over the last 30 years and has become a mature field. A wide array of biliary diseases can be treated endoscopically using ERCP, with high success rates and low AE rates in experienced centers. EUS is now established as a diagnostic tool for biliary diseases and is also emerging as a therapeutic tool for biliary diseases. Future advancements in ERCP and EUS are expected.

REFERENCES

1. Hirschowitz BI, Peters CW, Curtiss LE. Preliminary report on a long fiberscope for examination of stomach and duodenum. Med Bull (Ann Arbor) 1957;23(5):178–80.
2. McCune WS. ERCP–the first twenty years. Gastrointest Endosc 1988;34(3): 277–8.
3. Eaton JE, Talwalkar JA, Lazaridis KN, et al. Pathogenesis of primary sclerosing cholangitis and advances in diagnosis and management. Gastroenterology 2013;145(3):521–36. http://dx.doi.org/10.1053/j.gastro.2013.06.052. pii: S0016-5085(13)00996-7.
4. Gardner TB, Baron TH. Optimizing cholangiography when performing endoscopic retrograde cholangiopancreatography. Clin Gastroenterol Hepatol 2008;6(7):734–40.
5. Barr Fritcher EG, Voss JS, Jenkins SM, et al. Primary sclerosing cholangitis with equivocal cytology: fluorescence in situ hybridization and serum CA 19–9 predict risk of malignancy. Cancer Cytopathol 2013;121(12):708–17. http://dx.doi.org/10.1002/cncy.21331.
6. Gores GJ, Darwish Murad S, Heimbach JK, et al. Liver transplantation for perihilar cholangiocarcinoma. Dig Dis 2013;31(1):126–9.
7. Draganov PV, Chauhan S, Wagh MS, et al. Diagnostic accuracy of conventional and cholangioscopy-guided sampling of indeterminate biliary lesions at the time of ERCP: a prospective, long-term follow-up study. Gastrointest Endosc 2012; 75(2):347–53.
8. Petersen BT. Cholangioscopy for special applications: primary sclerosing cholangitis, liver transplant, and selective duct access. Gastrointest Endosc Clin N Am 2009;19(4):579–86.
9. Osanai M, Itoi T, Igarashi Y, et al. Peroral video cholangioscopy to evaluate indeterminate bile duct lesions and preoperative mucosal cancerous extension: a prospective multicenter study. Endoscopy 2013;45(8):635–42.
10. Moon JH, Terheggen G, Choi HJ, et al. Peroral cholangioscopy: diagnostic and therapeutic applications. Gastroenterology 2013;144(2):276–82.
11. Itoi T, Moon JH, Waxman I. Current status of direct peroral cholangioscopy. Dig Endosc 2011;23(Suppl 1):154–7.
12. Nishikawa T, Tsuyuguchi T, Sakai Y, et al. Comparison of the diagnostic accuracy of peroral video-cholangioscopic visual findings and cholangioscopy-guided forceps biopsy findings for indeterminate biliary lesions: a prospective study. Gastrointest Endosc 2013;77(2):219–26.
13. Heif M, Yen RD, Shah RJ. ERCP with probe-based confocal laser endomicroscopy for the evaluation of dominant biliary stenoses in primary sclerosing cholangitis patients. Dig Dis Sci 2013;58(7):2068–74.
14. Wani S, Shah RJ. Probe-based confocal laser endomicroscopy for the diagnosis of indeterminate biliary strictures. Curr Opin Gastroenterol 2013;29(3):319–23.
15. Hall TC, Dennison AR, Garcea G. The diagnosis and management of sphincter of Oddi dysfunction: a systematic review. Langenbecks Arch Surg 2012;397(6): 889–98.
16. Cotton PB, Durkalski V, Orrell KB, et al. Challenges in planning and initiating a randomized clinical study of sphincter of Oddi dysfunction. Gastrointest Endosc 2010;72(5):986–91.
17. Meine GC, Baron TH. Endoscopic papillary large-balloon dilation combined with endoscopic biliary sphincterotomy for the removal of bile duct stones (with video). Gastrointest Endosc 2011;74(5):1119–26 [quiz: 1115.e1–5].

18. Teoh AY, Cheung FK, Hu B, et al. Randomized trial of endoscopic sphincterotomy with balloon dilation versus endoscopic sphincterotomy alone for removal of bile duct stones. Gastroenterology 2013;144(2):341–5.e1.
19. Liu Y, Su P, Lin Y, et al. Endoscopic sphincterotomy plus balloon dilation versus endoscopic sphincterotomy for choledocholithiasis: a meta-analysis. J Gastroenterol Hepatol 2013;28(6):937–45.
20. Baron TH Sr, Davee T. Endoscopic management of benign bile duct strictures. Gastrointest Endosc Clin N Am 2013;23(2):295–311.
21. Zepeda-Gómez S, Baron TH. Benign biliary strictures: current endoscopic management. Nat Rev Gastroenterol Hepatol 2011;8(10):573–81.
22. Dumonceau JM, Tringali A, Blero D, et al, European Society of Gastrointestinal Endoscopy. Biliary stenting: indications, choice of stents and results: European Society of Gastrointestinal Endoscopy (ESGE) clinical guideline. Endoscopy 2012;44(3):277–98.
23. Akbar A, Irani S, Baron TH, et al. Use of covered self-expandable metal stents for endoscopic management of benign biliary disease not related to stricture (with video). Gastrointest Endosc 2012;76(1):196–201.
24. Pannala R, Petersen BT, Gostout CJ, et al. Endoscopic transpapillary gallbladder drainage: 10-year single center experience. Minerva Gastroenterol Dietol 2008;54(2):107–13.
25. Itoi T, Sofuni A, Itokawa F, et al. Endoscopic transpapillary gallbladder drainage in patients with acute cholecystitis in whom percutaneous transhepatic approach is contraindicated or anatomically impossible (with video). Gastrointest Endosc 2008;68(3):455–60.
26. Will U, Müller AK, Fueldner F, et al. Endoscopic papillectomy: data of a prospective observational study. World J Gastroenterol 2013;19(27):4316–24.
27. Ahn DW, Ryu JK, Kim J, et al. Endoscopic papillectomy for benign ampullary neoplasms: how can treatment outcome be predicted? Gut Liver 2013;7(2):239–45. http://dx.doi.org/10.5009/gnl.2013.7.2.239.
28. Ferreira LE, Baron TH. Endoscopic stenting for palliation of malignant biliary obstruction. Expert Rev Med Devices 2010;7(5):681–91.
29. Saleem A, Leggett CL, Murad MH, et al. Meta-analysis of randomized trials comparing the patency of covered and uncovered self-expandable metal stents for palliation of distal malignant bile duct obstruction. Gastrointest Endosc 2011;74(2):321–7.e1–3.
30. Almadi MA, Barkun AN, Martel M. No benefit of covered vs uncovered self-expandable metal stents in patients with malignant distal biliary obstruction: a meta-analysis. Clin Gastroenterol Hepatol 2013;11(1):27–37.e1.
31. Bakken JC, Baron TH. Metal stents and biliary obstruction secondary to lymphoma: a tale of caution. Dig Dis Sci 2010;55(12):3636.
32. van der Gaag NA, Rauws EA, van Eijck CH, et al. Preoperative biliary drainage for cancer of the head of the pancreas. N Engl J Med 2010;362(2):129–37.
33. Bonin EA, Baron TH. Preoperative biliary stents in pancreatic cancer. J Hepatobiliary Pancreat Sci 2011;18(5):621–9.
34. Baron TH, Kozarek RA. Preoperative biliary stents in pancreatic cancer–proceed with caution. N Engl J Med 2010;362(2):170–2.
35. Rerknimitr R, Angsuwatcharakon P, Ratanachu-ek T, et al. Asia-Pacific consensus recommendations for endoscopic and interventional management of hilar cholangiocarcinoma. J Gastroenterol Hepatol 2013;28(4):593–607.
36. Kozarek RA. Malignant hilar strictures: one stent or two? Plastic versus self-expanding metal stents? The role of liver atrophy and volume assessment as

a predictor of survival in patients undergoing endoscopic stent placement. Gastrointest Endosc 2010;72(4):736–8.

37. Siddiqui A, Shahid H, Sarkar A, et al. Stage of hilar cholangiocarcinoma predicts recurrence of biliary obstruction in patients with metal stents. Clin Gastroenterol Hepatol 2013;11(9):1169–73. http://dx.doi.org/10.1016/j.cgh.2013.05.035. pii: S1542–3565(13)00873-2.

38. Leggett CL, Gorospe EC, Murad MH, et al. Photodynamic therapy for unresectable cholangiocarcinoma: a comparative effectiveness systematic review and meta-analyses. Photodiagnosis Photodyn Ther 2012;9(3):189–95.

39. Figueroa-Barojas P, Bakhru MR, Habib NA, et al. Safety and efficacy of radiofrequency ablation in the management of unresectable bile duct and pancreatic cancer: a novel palliation technique. J Oncol 2013;2013:910897.

40. Simmons DT, Baron TH, Petersen BT, et al. A novel endoscopic approach to brachytherapy in the management of hilar cholangiocarcinoma. Am J Gastroenterol 2006;101(8):1792–6.

41. Chahal P, Baron TH, Poterucha JJ, et al. Endoscopic retrograde cholangiography in post-orthotopic liver transplant population with Roux-en-Y biliary reconstruction. Liver Transpl 2007;13(8):1168–73.

42. Azeem N, Tabibian JH, Baron TH, et al. Use of a single-balloon enteroscope compared with variable-stiffness colonoscopes for endoscopic retrograde cholangiography in liver transplant patients with Roux-en-Y biliary anastomosis. Gastrointest Endosc 2013;77(4):568–77.

43. Saleem A, Levy MJ, Petersen BT, et al. Laparoscopic assisted ERCP in Roux-en-Y gastric bypass (RYGB) surgery patients. J Gastrointest Surg 2012;16(1):203–8.

44. Abu Dayyeh BK, Baron TH. Development of a hybrid percutaneous-endoscopic approach for the complete clearance of gallstones. Clin Gastroenterol Hepatol 2012;10(8):947–9.

45. Baron TH, Song LM. Percutaneous assisted transprosthetic endoscopic therapy (PATENT): expanding gut access to infinity and beyond! (with video). Gastrointest Endosc 2012;76(3):641–4.

46. Law R, Wong Kee Song LM, Petersen BT, et al. Single-session ERCP in patients with previous Roux-en-Y gastric bypass using percutaneous-assisted transprosthetic endoscopic therapy: a case series. Endoscopy 2013;45(8):671–5.

47. Chan HH, Wang EM, Sun MS, et al. Linear echoendoscope-guided ERCP for the diagnosis of occult common bile duct stones. BMC Gastroenterol 2013; 13:44.

48. Ohshima Y, Yasuda I, Kawakami H, et al. EUS-FNA for suspected malignant biliary strictures after negative endoscopic transpapillary brush cytology and forceps biopsy. J Gastroenterol 2011;46(7):921–8.

49. Levy MJ, Heimbach JK, Gores GJ. Endoscopic ultrasound staging of cholangiocarcinoma. Curr Opin Gastroenterol 2012;28(3):244–52.

50. Sarkaria S, Lee HS, Gaidhane M, et al. Advances in endoscopic ultrasound-guided biliary drainage: a comprehensive review. Gut Liver 2013;7(2):129–36. http://dx.doi.org/10.5009/gnl.2013.7.2.129.

51. Gupta K, Perez-Miranda M, Kahaleh M, et al, InEBD Study Group. Endoscopic ultrasound-assisted bile duct access and drainage: multicenter, long-term analysis of approach, outcomes, and complications of a technique in evolution. J Clin Gastroenterol 2013;48(1):80–7.

52. Kahaleh M, Artifon EL, Perez-Miranda M, et al. Endoscopic ultrasonography guided biliary drainage: summary of consortium meeting, May 7th, 2011, Chicago. World J Gastroenterol 2013;19(9):1372–9.

53. Khashab MA, Fujii LL, Baron TH, et al. EUS-guided biliary drainage for patients with malignant biliary obstruction with an indwelling duodenal stent (with videos). Gastrointest Endosc 2012;76(1):209–13.

54. Jang JW, Lee SS, Song TJ, et al. Endoscopic ultrasound-guided transmural and percutaneous transhepatic gallbladder drainage are comparable for acute cholecystitis. Gastroenterology 2012;142(4):805–11.

55. Baron TH, Topazian MD. Endoscopic transduodenal drainage of the gallbladder: implications for endoluminal treatment of gallbladder disease. Gastrointest Endosc 2007;65(4):735–7.

56. Kamata K, Kitano M, Kudo M, et al. Endoscopic ultrasound (EUS)-guided transluminal endoscopic removal of gallstones. Endoscopy 2010;42(Suppl 2):E331–2.

57. Noh SH, Park do H, Kim YR, et al. EUS-guided drainage of hepatic abscesses not accessible to percutaneous drainage (with videos). Gastrointest Endosc 2010;71(7):1314–9.

58. Shami VM, Talreja JP, Mahajan A, et al. EUS-guided drainage of bilomas: a new alternative? Gastrointest Endosc 2008;67(1):136–40.

59. Balmadrid B, Kozarek R. Prevention and management of adverse events of endoscopic retrograde cholangiopancreatography. Gastrointest Endosc Clin N Am 2013;23(2):385–403.

60. Glomsaker T, Hoff G, Kvaløy JT, et al, Norwegian Gastronet ERCP Group. Patterns and predictive factors of complications after endoscopic retrograde cholangiopancreatography. Br J Surg 2013;100(3):373–80.

61. ASGE Standards of Practice Committee, Early DS, Acosta RD, Chandrasekhara V, et al. Adverse events associated with EUS and EUS with FNA. Gastrointest Endosc 2013;77(6):839–43.

62. Akbar A, Abu Dayyeh BK, Baron TH, et al. Rectal nonsteroidal anti-inflammatory drugs are superior to pancreatic duct stents in preventing pancreatitis after endoscopic retrograde cholangiopancreatography: a network meta-analysis. Clin Gastroenterol Hepatol 2013;11(7):778–83.

63. Baron TH, Wong Kee Song LM, Zielinski MD, et al. A comprehensive approach to the management of acute endoscopic perforations (with videos). Gastrointest Endosc 2012;76(4):838–59.

Biliary Issues in the Bariatric Population

Brandon T. Grover, DO, Shanu N. Kothari, MD*

KEYWORDS

- Bariatric surgery • Obesity • Cholelithiasis • Biliary tract • Ursodeoxycholic acid
- Cholangiography • Endoscopy • Laparoscopic-assisted percutaneous transgastric endoscopic retrograde cholangiopancreatography

KEY POINTS

- Biliary disease is common in the obese population and increases after bariatric surgery.
- Management of the gallbladder at the time of bariatric surgery remains controversial. It is reasonable to remove the gallbladder in conjunction with bariatric surgery only if patients have symptoms and a documented disorder on imaging.
- Transabdominal imaging for biliary disease has limitations in the morbidly obese patient, and may underestimate gallbladder disease.
- The use of ursodeoxycholic acid has been shown to be effective in decreasing the risk of formation of gallstones and gallbladder sludge if used during the rapid weight loss phase after bariatric surgery.
- After Roux-en-Y gastric bypass, access to the biliopancreatic ducts by standard endoscopic retrograde cholangiopancreatography (ERCP) is compromised. The use of laparoscopic-assisted percutaneous transgastric ERCP is highly successful in providing access to the duodenum, to the bile, and to the pancreatic ducts.

INTRODUCTION

Bariatric surgery has recently become the most common elective operation in the United States.[1] Cholecystectomy is one of the most common operations performed by general surgeons.[2] Some bariatric operations, including Roux-en-Y gastric bypass (RYGBP), alter the normal foregut and midgut anatomy, making subsequent management of biliary tract disease more challenging. In addition, morbidly obese patients and patients who have had bariatric surgery have a higher incidence of biliary disease. All general surgeons should be familiar with the post-RYGBP anatomy and the potential for subsequent biliary tract disorder. As in the general population, many

There are no conflicts of interest to disclose.
Department of General and Vascular Surgery, Gundersen Health System, 1900 South Avenue, C05-001, La Crosse, WI 54601, USA
* Corresponding author.
E-mail address: snkothar@gundersenhealth.org

Surg Clin N Am 94 (2014) 413–425
http://dx.doi.org/10.1016/j.suc.2014.01.003
0039-6109/14/$ – see front matter © 2014 Elsevier Inc. All rights reserved.

stone-related complications can occur, including biliary colic (symptomatic cholelithiasis), acute and chronic cholecystitis, biliary pancreatitis, and choledocholithiasis.

CHOLELITHIASIS

The incidence of cholelithiasis in the general population found by ultrasonography ranges from 2% to 15%.[3-7] Obesity, female gender, age more than 40 years, white ethnicity, and premenopausal state have been shown to increase the incidence of cholelithiasis.[5] Other risk factors include rapid weight gain or weight loss (as seen after bariatric surgery), pregnancy, use of oral contraceptives, estrogen replacement, diabetes, and family history.[8-10]

Among the various types of gallstones, cholesterol stones are the most common. Cholesterol stone formation is multifactorial. Regardless of the associated causes, lithogenesis is related to supersaturation of bile with cholesterol. Other contributing factors that can occur within the gallbladder include bile stasis, decreased concentration of bile salts, infection, and increased glycoprotein secretion.[11]

Many patients considering bariatric surgery have multiple preoperative risk factors. Following cholecystectomy, the prevalence of any gallbladder disorder in the morbidly obese population has been reported to be as high as 87% to 97%.[12-16] Patients with a body mass index (BMI) more than 40 kg/m^2 have been shown to have a risk of having gallstones 8 times higher than those with lower BMI.[17] Rapid weight loss after surgery increases the chance of developing cholelithiasis if not already present. The reported incidence of cholelithiasis after RYGBP ranges from 6.7% to 52.8%,[17,18] with most studies showing rates around 30%.[12,19-22] Multiple physiologic changes occur after bariatric surgery that contribute to gallstone formation, including hypersaturation of bile with cholesterol, increased mucin production acting to decrease nucleation time,[23] and gallbladder hypomotility.[24] Significant decrease in gallbladder emptying after RYGBP contributes to biliary sludge and/or gallstone formation.[22]

In the early days of open bariatric surgery, it was common practice to perform a cholecystectomy at the time of weight loss surgery.[15,25-27] Because of the high incidence of gallbladder disease after biliopancreatic diversion, cholecystectomy is routinely performed as a component of this operation.[28] In the current era of laparoscopic bariatric surgery, most surgeons do not routinely perform a cholecystectomy at the time of weight loss surgery.[29]

To date, there is no consensus on the management of the gallbladder at the time of bariatric surgery, leaving the decision for concomitant cholecystectomy to the discretion of the surgeon. Many factors must be considered.

Some surgeons advocate routine prophylactic cholecystectomy at the time of bariatric surgery. This approach may be reasonable given the high incidence of gallbladder disorders seen in this patient population; the challenging management of stone-related complications in the anatomically altered patient; and the potential for avoiding a second operation, which is a benefit from the perspectives of both patient recovery and cost.

Some bariatric surgeons perform a cholecystectomy if a disorder is identified on preoperative imaging or intraoperatively via imaging or palpation. This strategy assumes that, if a disorder is present before surgery, the likelihood of developing symptoms or of the worsening of disease in the postoperative period is high.[30-32] It also precludes the difficulty in addressing the common bile duct with Roux-en-Y anatomy, should a subsequent stone disorder arise.

Other surgeons perform a cholecystectomy at the time of bariatric surgery only for patients with both pathology and symptoms consistent with biliary disease. Reasons for this approach include shorter operative times, avoiding complications related to cholecystectomy, avoiding prolonged hospital stay,[16] low incidence of future cholecystectomy, and increased ease of cholecystectomy after substantial weight loss.[16,33–35]

It is our practice to perform a cholecystectomy at the time of bariatric surgery only if the patient has a documented pathology and has symptoms that seem to correlate with the disease process. In our institution, the incidence of patients requiring cholecystectomy after bariatric surgery is 4%.[34] Many of these patients have lost significant weight, which makes performing an elective operation easier because the abdominal wall compliance becomes favorable and a large dome of pneumoperitoneum can be achieved. We routinely perform an intraoperative cholangiogram on patients undergoing RYGBP because this is the last easy look at the biliary tree.

BILIARY IMAGING IN THE BARIATRIC POPULATION

For advocates of concomitant cholecystectomy in patients with documented biliary disease, evaluation of the gallbladder is an important consideration. Ultrasonography has been shown to be the most reliable method of detecting cholelithiasis in nonobese patients.[36,37] Ultrasonography can be performed transabdominally in the preoperative setting or by direct interrogation intraoperatively. Other modalities used to evaluate for cholelithiasis preoperatively are computed tomography (CT) cholecystography and endoscopic ultrasonography.

Studies have shown decreased sensitivity of finding cholelithiasis by transabdominal ultrasonography in the morbidly obese patient.[12,38] Increased amounts of fat within the abdominal wall and around the intra-abdominal organs can obscure the view of the gallbladder. Furthermore, image quality is diminished because of the increased thickness of the abdominal wall. These factors may lead to underestimating or misdiagnosing biliary disorders. The use of transabdominal ultrasonography can have a false-negative rate as high as 20%.[39] Alternatively, a recent study by Kothari and colleagues[34] found that intraoperative laparoscopic ultrasonography and transabdominal ultrasonography were equally sensitive in identifying cholelithiasis, but intraoperative laparoscopic ultrasonography found significantly more gallbladder polyps.

Transabdominal ultrasonography is readily available, well tolerated, causes no exposure to radiation, and has a negligible complication profile. For these reasons, it is the most common imaging modality used to evaluate the gallbladder, despite its potential limitations in the obese patient. Obtaining imaging preoperatively facilitates counseling the patients with biliary disorders regarding risks and benefits of cholecystectomy planned concomitantly with bariatric surgery. An acceptable alternative is the use of intraoperative ultrasonography, if resources are available and the surgeon is experienced. However, if this approach is used, all patients who still have a gallbladder need an appropriate informed consent discussion and documentation for possible cholecystectomy.

Because of the potential false-negative rate in detecting stones by transabdominal ultrasonography, Neitlich and Neitlich[40] sought to find a better imaging modality to evaluate the gallbladder in the preoperative bariatric patient. In their small series of 16 patients, CT cholecystography had 100% sensitivity and 91% specificity for identifying cholelithiasis compared with a 50% sensitivity for ultrasonography. Although accuracy in detecting stones was favorable, this modality has the potential for increased complications related to contrast and radiation exposure and higher costs.

PREVENTION OF CHOLELITHIASIS

Given the high rate of cholelithiasis in patients having bariatric surgery, attempts have been made to decrease the incidence of gallstone formation. Ursodeoxycholic acid, commonly known as ursodiol, is a bile acid that works by inhibiting biliary cholesterol crystallization. It has been used in varying doses and durations after bariatric surgery in attempts to prevent subsequent stone formation. The risk of developing gallstones is highest during the rapid weight loss phase after surgery and generally decreases as weight loss stabilizes.[17,41,42]

Sugerman and colleagues[21] designed a multicenter, double-blinded, randomized, placebo-controlled, prospective trial that evaluated the efficacy of ursodiol in the prevention of gallstones in patients after RYGBP. They randomized patients with a negative intraoperative gallbladder ultrasonography into 4 different treatment groups. Postoperative ultrasonography was then performed at 2, 4, and 6 months, or until cholelithiasis was found. Group 1, consisting of 56 patients randomized to placebo, experienced a 43% rate of gallstone or gallbladder sludge formation by 6 months after surgery. Group 2 included 53 patients who were treated with 300 mg of ursodiol daily and, by 6 months after surgery, 21% had developed cholelithiasis or sludge. Group 3, consisting of 61 patients, was given 600 mg of ursodiol, divided twice daily, and only 8% of patients developed gallstones or sludge by 6 months. Group 4 contained 63 patients who were given 1200 mg of ursodiol, divided twice daily, and by 6 months 17% developed gallstones or sludge. Statistical significance was found at all treatment levels versus placebo, with the lowest rate of gallstone and sludge formation found with 600-mg divided dosing. They reported a similar compliance rate, approximately 85%, among each of the 4 groups.

A subset of 54 patients who had not formed stones or sludge by 6 months was followed with subsequent ultrasonography at 12 months. With good representation of all 4 treatment groups, patients who had received any dose of ursodiol had a 12% chance of forming stones or sludge compared with 46% of those who had not.

Although their study was not directly designed to determine the duration of prophylactic treatment, the recommendation from this trial was to treat patients undergoing bariatric surgery with 600 mg of ursodiol, divided twice daily, for 6 months, to decrease the incidence of cholelithiasis and gallbladder sludge formation.[21]

A meta-analysis by Uy and colleagues[43] sought to assess the effectiveness of ursodiol in the prevention of gallstones in the postbariatric patient. They identified 5 randomized controlled trials that compared the use of ursodiol with placebo in patients after bariatric surgery.[21,44-47] Of the 521 patients, 322 were randomized to ursodiol and 199 to placebo. The meta-analysis found that 8.8% of patients in the ursodiol group developed cholelithiasis compared with 27.7% in the placebo group. The dose and duration of treatment were different in each study, ranging from 300 mg/d to 1200 mg/d and 3 months to 24 months, respectively. All of the studies performed routine postoperative transabdominal ultrasonography at regular intervals to assess for the development of gallstones. Most of the studies showed a similar compliance rate and adverse reaction rate between treatment and placebo groups. Common adverse events included diarrhea, constipation, headache, skin rash, dizziness, and upper respiratory tract infections. For patients who still have their gallbladder, it is our practice to prescribe 300 mg of ursodiol twice daily for 6 months after surgery.

POST–GASTRIC BYPASS MANAGEMENT OF GALLSTONE DISEASE
Cholelithiasis

Cholelithiasis is common in bariatric patients. Rates of subsequent cholecystectomy in the literature vary widely, between 4% and 52.8%.[17,34] Iglézias Brandão de Oliveira and colleagues[17] reported a 52.8% cholecystectomy rate performed for findings of gallstones on scheduled postoperative imaging, regardless of patient symptoms.

Surgeons who perform a cholecystectomy only when patients have symptoms that seem to correlate with imaging findings have a lower surgical rate of 4% to 8%.[34,48,49]

Proper management of biliary disease in patients after bariatric surgery is critical. Gallstone-related complications are the most commonly encountered biliary issues in these patients. In most patients, routine laparoscopic cholecystectomy can be performed safely and in the same fashion as in patients who have not undergone bariatric surgery. For those who have undergone RYGBP, the investigators advocate the routine use of intraoperative cholangiogram because this is the last easy look at the biliary tree. It is also appropriate to evaluate the mesocolic, jejunojejunostomy, and Petersen defects, because an occult internal hernia can masquerade as biliary colic. If an internal hernia is identified, it can be repaired at the time of diagnosis.

Choledocholithiasis

One of the biggest challenges with regard to biliary stone disease in patients after RYGBP is acquiring access to the biliary tree when choledocholithiasis is known or suspected. Diagnosis can be made during surgery via cholangiography, choledochoscopy, or ultrasonography performed at the time of cholecystectomy, or before surgery by ultrasonography, CT, or magnetic resonance cholangiopancreatography (MRCP). Endoscopic access to the ampulla of Vater can be difficult after RYGBP because the stomach is divided and the duodenum is excluded (**Fig. 1**).[50] If choledocholithiasis is discovered at the time of laparoscopic cholecystectomy, multiple

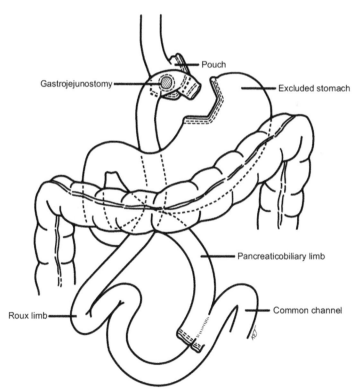

Fig. 1. Roux-en-Y gastric bypass anatomy. (*Reprinted from* Kothari SN. Bariatric surgery and postoperative imaging. Surg Clin North Am 2011;91:156; with permission.)

intraoperative steps can be taken to clear the common bile duct. First, the ductal system can be flushed with saline. Intravenous administration of glucagon may allow relaxation of the sphincter of Oddi. If this is unsuccessful, minimally invasive exploration of the biliary ductal system can be accomplished via fluoroscopic methods, endoscopic methods, or a combination of both, depending on operator experience. Most commonly, a transcystic duct approach is undertaken, but the exploration can alternatively be performed directly through a ductotomy on the common bile duct. For the transcystic approach, a guide wire is initially placed through the cystic duct under fluoroscopy with attempts to advance it into the duodenum. A small balloon catheter is then used to dilate the cystic duct to facilitate access to the common bile duct and aid in stone extraction. A combination of wires, balloon catheters, and baskets can then be used in attempts to extract the stone from the duct. If a choledochoscope is available, this can be placed through the dilated cystic duct and advanced into the common bile duct. This technique allows direct visualization of any stones or debris within the ductal system. Through the working channel of the scope, balloon catheters or baskets can be used to pull or grasp the stone(s) for extraction. If the stone appears to be impacted at the ampulla of Vater, the choledochoscope can be used to apply gentle pressure to the stone in an effort to push it into the duodenum. If laparoscopic methods are unsuccessful, open common bile duct exploration or transgastric endoscopic retrograde cholangiopancreatography (ERCP) should be considered. This decision depends on available resources and surgeon experience.

BILIARY TRACT ACCESS AFTER RYGBP

In many patients with biliary tract disease having RYGBP, the diagnosis is not made during surgery. If choledocholithiasis or other bile duct disorder is found or suspected outside the operating room, the altered anatomy can create a challenge to obtaining access to the common bile duct. Access options include, but are not limited to, percutaneous transhepatic cholangiography, balloon-assisted endoscopy, and percutaneous transgastric ERCP.

Percutaneous Transhepatic Cholangiography

Although not widely published for patients who have had RYGBP, percutaneous transhepatic cholangiography can be considered in patients with suspected biliary disorders who are found to have dilated intrahepatic ducts on ultrasonography or other imaging modalities such as MRCP. The procedure is most commonly performed by an interventional radiologist. Percutaneous access is obtained and the needle is advanced under ultrasonography or fluoroscopic guidance through the liver capsule and into a peripherally dilated duct. Contrast medium can be injected to verify position. A wire can subsequently be fed into the more central ductal system. A plastic cannula is then fed over the wire, which may require serial dilations of the tract. A catheter can then be fed through the cannula and various interventions can be performed through the catheter under radiologic imaging to assess and clear the hepatic and common bile ducts. If access to the ducts is successfully achieved there is a high sensitivity in diagnosing the cause of obstruction.[51] Complications such as infection or bleeding secondary to injury to a major hepatic artery can occur.[52,53]

Balloon-assisted Endoscopy

Attempts to access the duct in the standard transoral fashion have been reported. This technique involves passing the endoscope through the mouth, down the esophagus, across the gastrojejunal anastomosis, down the Roux limb, across the jejunojejunal anastomosis, and up the biliopancreatic limb to the ampulla of Vater. Depending on the length of the Roux limb, this may not be possible. Single or double balloons and specialized overtubes (**Fig. 2**) have been used to facilitate this procedure with varying success. The challenge of long Roux limbs (>100 cm) and angulation of the intestine at the jejunojejunal anastomosis contribute to the difficulty of standard ERCP. These adjunct devices aid in overcoming the anatomic changes seen after RYGBP surgery. Lennon and colleagues[54] reported their experience comparing single-balloon ERCP with a spiral-overtube ERCP. They found similar success rates in cannulation of the ampulla of Vater between the two methods, with an overall success rate in patients after RYGBP of 38.9%. Others have shown success rates as high as 66%, but these patients had Roux-en-Y anatomy for nonbariatric reasons, such as total gastrectomy with esophagojejunostomy for gastric cancer.[55] This reconstruction typically has a shorter Roux limb, allowing an increased likelihood of reaching the ampulla.

The major disadvantage of this method is the low success rate in cannulation of the biliary ductal system. Furthermore, the use of balloons and overtubes requires specialized equipment that is not available in many institutions, and complication rates increase with more aggressive endoscopic procedures. Complications of bleeding, pancreatitis, and perforation have been reported.[54,56] The technology and experience required may limit availability of this approach even in centers that offer standard ERCP.

Percutaneous Transgastric ERCP

Access to the biliary tree can be achieved through the remnant stomach in patients who have had RYGBP, and can be performed either through a gastrostomy tube or by laparoscopic-assisted access. Some surgeons routinely place a radiopaque ring

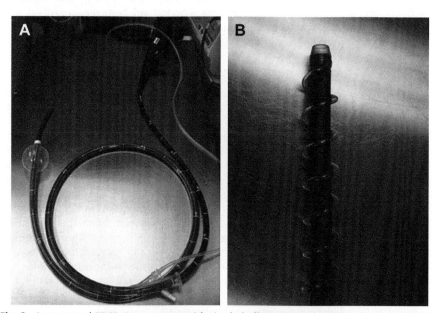

Fig. 2. Augmented ERCP. Enteroscope with single balloon overtube (*A*) and spiral overtube (*B*). (*Reprinted from* Lennon AM, Kapoor S, Khashab M, et al. Spiral assisted ERCP is equivalent to single balloon assisted ERCP in patients with Roux-en-Y anatomy. Dig Dis Sci 2012;57:1393; with permission.)

or perform a gastropexy at the time of RYGBP to facilitate future interventional radiologic access.[17,57] As an alternative, laparoscopic-assisted percutaneous transgastric ERCP is a well-documented, feasible, and safe option to gain access to the remnant stomach, duodenum, and pancreaticobiliary ductal system (**Fig. 3**). This approach is performed under general anesthesia and involves intraoperative coordination with the surgeon and an ERCP-trained specialist. Once the patient is under general anesthesia, positioned supine, and appropriately prepped and sterilely draped, the procedure is performed as follows:

- Laparoscopic access to the peritoneal cavity is achieved and a pneumoperitoneum is created by insufflation with CO_2. Typically, 3 ports are used initially: 1 for the laparoscope, and 2 working ports.
- Laparoscopic exploration of the abdomen is conducted to look for internal hernias or other obvious disorders.
- The remnant stomach is identified and positioned with graspers under the left lateral abdominal wall below the costal margin.
- Stay sutures are placed in the body of the stomach to provide countertraction.
- A 15-mm trocar is placed percutaneously through the left lateral abdominal wall and then directly into the remnant stomach. The gastrotomy is positioned along the greater curvature, allowing the endoscopist a straight path to the pylorus.
- A clamp is placed across the small bowel, just distal to the ligament of Treitz to prevent excessive bowel dilatation, and the pneumoperitoneum is evacuated.
- The endoscopist can use a standard side-viewing ERCP scope through the 15-mm trocar and perform any necessary procedures.
- Once the endoscopist has finished, the pneumoperitoneum is reestablished and the trocar is removed from the stomach.
- The gastrotomy is closed with a linear stapling device or intracorporeal suturing.
- Suctioning of any spilled gastric contents is performed, hemostasis verified, and the pneumoperitoneum is evacuated.
- The 15-mm trocar site fascia and all skin incisions are then closed.

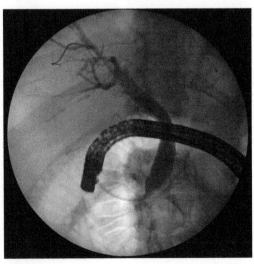

Fig. 3. Laparoscopic-assisted transgastric ERCP showing a dilated common bile duct. (*Reprinted from* Kothari SN. Bariatric surgery and postoperative imaging. Surg Clin North Am 2011;91:158; with permission.)

Table 1
Review of case reports of transgastric endoscopy

Author, Publication Year	Transgastric Endoscopy N	CBD Success	Complications
Pimentel et al,[59] 2004	1	1	None
Ceppa et al,[60] 2007	10	4	None
Nakao et al,[61] 2007	1	1	None
Patel et al,[62] 2008	8	8	None
Roberts et al,[63] 2008	6	6	None
Dapri et al,[64] 2009	1	1	None
Gutierrez et al,[65] 2009	32	28	Gastrostomy leak (n = 2), pancreatitis (n = 1), wound infection (n = 1)
Peeters & Himpens,[66] 2009	1	1	Pancreatitis (n = 1)
Sebastian et al,[67] 2009	1	1	None
Badaoui et al,[68] 2010	1	1	None
Bertin et al,[69] 2011	22	20	Abdominal wall hematoma (n = 1), retroperitoneal perforation (n = 1)
Saleem et al,[70] 2012	15	15	None
Richardson et al,[58] 2012	13	11	None

Abbreviation: CBD, common bile duct.
Adapted from Richardson JF, Lee JG, Smith BR, et al. Laparoscopic transgastric endoscopy after Roux-en-Y gastric bypass: case series and review of the literature. Am Surg 2012;78:1184.

Outcomes from this approach have been highly successful in accessing the biliary tree with low overall complication rates. Richardson and colleagues[58] published a review of the literature and their experience with this procedure in patients after RYGBP. Their review, from 13 different published studies and including patients from their institution, consisted of 112 patients who underwent laparoscopic or open transgastric ERCP (**Table 1**).[58–70] All but 1 patient had successful cannulation of the common bile duct. Reported complications included 2 gastrostomy leaks, 2 episodes of post-ERCP pancreatitis, 1 wound infection, 1 retroperitoneal perforation, and 1 abdominal wall hematoma. They concluded that this approach has a high success rate in cannulation of the common bile duct, low complication rates, and the added benefit of exploration for other intra-abdominal disorders including internal hernia defects.

Patients who have undergone adjustable gastric banding, vertical banded gastroplasty, or sleeve gastrectomy have preserved normal anatomic access to the duodenum allowing standard transoral ERCP.

SUMMARY

Rates of morbid obesity continue to increase in the United States and in most areas of the world. Bariatric surgery is currently the only successful long-term treatment option for these patients. Substantial weight loss after bariatric surgery improves control of many diseases, including diabetes, heart disease, obstructive sleep apnea, hyperlipidemia, arthritis, and infertility, and it may even reduce the risk of many cancers. Biliary disease is one of the few problems with a higher incidence after bariatric surgery. Although there is currently no consensus on the proper management of the gallbladder and related diseases, successful strategies have been used. At our institution, our practice is to perform a cholecystectomy only for patients with documented disease and symptoms. Outside of study protocols, we do not routinely image the gall-bladder to look for asymptomatic disease. For those who still have a gallbladder, we prescribe 300 mg of ursodiol twice daily for the first 6 months after surgery to decrease the risk of developing cholelithiasis during the rapid weight loss phase. We have found an acceptably low rate of subsequent cholecystectomy in our patients. For those who eventually need a cholecystectomy, we find the technical aspects of the operation easier after substantial weight loss. For patients who have had RYGBP and who need an ERCP, laparoscopic-assisted percutaneous transgastric ERCP is our access modality of choice. Official best-practice guidelines may never be instituted for the management of biliary disease in the bariatric patient. Thus, it is the responsibility of each bariatric surgeon to assess the available resources and to use the methods that will provide the best outcomes for patients.

REFERENCES

1. Buchwald H, Williams SE. Bariatric surgery worldwide 2003. Obes Surg 2004; 14:1157–64.
2. Urbach DR, Stukel TA. Rate of elective cholecystectomy and the incidence of severe gallstone disease. CMAJ 2005;172:1015–9.
3. Kodama H, Kono S, Todoroki I, et al. Gallstone disease risk in relation to body mass index and waist-to-hip ratio in Japanese men. Int J Obes 1999;23: 211–6.
4. Kono S, Shinchi K, Ikeda N, et al. Prevalence of gallstone disease in relation to smoking, alcohol use, obesity, and glucose intolerance: a study of self-defense officials in Japan. Am J Epidemiol 1992;136:787–94.
5. Barbara L, Sama C, Morselli Labate AM, et al. A population study on the prevalence of gallstone disease: the Sirmione Study. Hepatology 1987;7:913–7.
6. Gonzalez Villalpando C, Rivera Martinez D, Arredondo Perez B, et al. High prevalence of cholelithiasis in a low income Mexican population: an ultrasonographic survey. Arch Med Res 1997;28:543–7.
7. Rome Group for Epidemiology and Prevention of Cholelithiasis (GREPCO). The epidemiology of gallstone disease in Rome, Italy. Part I. Prevalence data in men. Hepatology 1988;8:904–6.
8. Scragg RK, McMichael AJ, Seamark RF. Oral contraceptives, pregnancy, and endogenous oestrogen in gall stone disease–a case-control study. Br Med J (Clin Res Ed) 1984;288:1795–9.
9. De Santis A, Attili AF, Ginanni Corradini S, et al. Gallstones and diabetes: a case-control study in a free-living population sample. Hepatology 1997;25: 787–90.
10. Sarin SK, Negi VS, Dewan R, et al. High familial prevalence of gallstones in the first-degree relatives of gallstone patients. Hepatology 1995;22:138–41.
11. LaMorte WW, Matolo NM, Birkett DH, et al. Pathogenesis of cholesterol gallstones. Surg Clin North Am 1981;61:765–74.
12. Amaral JF, Thompson WR. Gallbladder disease in the morbidly obese. Am J Surg 1985;149:551–7.
13. Aidonopoulos AP, Papavramidis ST, Zaraboukas TG, et al. Gallbladder findings after cholecystectomy in morbidly obese patients. Obes Surg 1994;4:8–12.
14. Calhoun RC, Willbanks O. Coexistence of gallbladder disease and morbid obesity. Am J Surg 1987;154:655–8.
15. Fobi M, Lee H, Igwe D, et al. Prophylactic cholecystectomy with gastric bypass operation: incidence of gallbladder disease. Obes Surg 2002;12:350–3.

16. Hamad GG, Ikramuddin S, Gourash WF, et al. Elective cholecystectomy during laparoscopic Roux-en-Y gastric bypass: is it worth the wait? Obes Surg 2003; 13:76–81.
17. Iglézias Brandão de Oliveira C, Adami Chaim E, da Silva BB. Impact of rapid weight reduction on risk of cholelithiasis after bariatric surgery. Obes Surg 2003;13:625–8.
18. Griffen WO, Young VL, Stevenson CC. Prospective comparison of gastric and jejunoileal bypass procedures for morbid obesity. Ann Surg 1977;186:500–7.
19. Wattchow DA, Hall JC, Whiting MJ, et al. Prevalence and treatment of gall stones after gastric bypass surgery for morbid obesity. Br Med J 1983; 286:763.
20. Shiffman ML, Sugerman HJ, Kellum JH, et al. Gallstones in patients with morbid obesity: relationship to body weight, weight loss and gallbladder bile cholesterol solubility. Int J Obes Relat Metab Disord 1993;17:153–8.
21. Sugerman HJ, Brewer WH, Shiffman ML. A multicenter, placebo-controlled, randomized, double-blind, prospective trial of prophylactic ursodiol for the prevention of gallstone formation following gastric-bypass-induced rapid weight loss. Am J Surg 1995;169:91–7.
22. Bastouly M, Arasaki CH, Ferreira JB, et al. Early changes in postprandial gallbladder emptying in morbidly obese patients undergoing Roux-en-Y gastric bypass: correlation with the occurrence of biliary sludge and gallstones. Obes Surg 2009;19:22–8.
23. Carey MC. Pathogenesis of gallstones. Am J Surg 1993;165:410–9.
24. Desbeaux A, Hec F, Andrieux S, et al. Risk of biliary complications in bariatric surgery. J Visc Surg 2010;147:e217–20.
25. Jones KB Jr. Simultaneous cholecystectomy: to be or not to be. Obes Surg 1995;5:52–4.
26. Guadalajara H, Sanz Baro R, Pascual I, et al. Is prophylactic cholecystectomy useful in obese patients undergoing gastric bypass? Obes Surg 2006;16: 883–5.
27. Liem RK, Niloff PH. Prophylactic cholecystectomy with open gastric bypass operation. Obes Surg 2004;14:763–5.
28. Oria HE. Gallbladder disease in obesity and during weight loss. In: Deitel M, Cowan GS, editors. Update: surgery for the morbidly obese patient. Toronto: FD Communications; 2000. p. 451–80.
29. Mason EE, Renquist KE. Gallbladder management in obesity surgery. Obes Surg 2002;12:222–9.
30. Dhabuwala A, Cannan RJ, Stubbs RS. Improvement in comorbidities following weight loss from gastric bypass surgery. Obes Surg 2000;10:428–35.
31. Escalona A, Boza C, Munoz R, et al. Routine preoperative ultrasonography and selective cholecystectomy in laparoscopic Roux-en-Y gastric bypass. Why not? Obes Surg 2008;18:47–51.
32. Nagem R, Lazaro-da-Silva A. Cholecystolithiasis after gastric bypass: a clinical, biochemical, and ultrasonographic 3-year follow-up study. Obes Surg 2012;22: 1594–9.
33. Deitel M, Smith L, Harmantas A. Laparoscopic cholecystectomy after vertical banded gastroplasty. Obes Surg 1994;4:13–5.
34. Kothari SN, Obinwanne KM, Baker MT, et al. A prospective, blinded comparison of laparoscopic ultrasound with transabdominal ultrasound for the detection of gallbladder pathology in morbidly obese patients. J Am Coll Surg 2013;216: 1057–62.

35. Portenier DD, Grant JP, Blackwood HS, et al. Expectant management of the asymptomatic gallbladder at Roux-en-Y gastric bypass. Surg Obes Relat Dis 2007;3:476–9.

36. Garra BS, Davros WJ, Lack EE, et al. Visibility of gallstone fragments at US and fluoroscopy: implications for monitoring gallstone lithotripsy. Radiology 1990;174:343–7.

37. Wermke W. Ultrasonic diagnosis of gallstone diseases. Z Gesamte Inn Med 1989;44:377–82.

38. Klingensmith WC 3rd, Eckhout GV. Cholelithiasis in the morbidly obese: diagnosis by US and oral cholecystography. Radiology 1986;160:27–8.

39. Silidker MS, Cronan JJ, Scola FH, et al. Ultrasound evaluation of cholelithiasis in the morbidly obese. Gastrointest Radiol 1988;13:345–6.

40. Neitlich T, Neitlich J. The imaging evaluation of cholelithiasis in the obese patient-ultrasound vs CT cholecystography: our experience with the bariatric surgery population. Obes Surg 2009;19:207–10.

41. Erlinger S. Gallstones in obesity and weight loss. Eur J Gastroenterol Hepatol 2000;12:1347–52.

42. Shiffman ML, Sugerman HJ, Kellum JM, et al. Gallstone formation after rapid weight loss: a prospective study in patients undergoing gastric bypass surgery for treatment of morbid obesity. Am J Gastroenterol 1991;86:1000–5.

43. Uy MC, Talingdan-Te MC, Espinosa WZ, et al. Ursodeoxycholic acid in the prevention of gallstone formation after bariatric surgery: a meta-analysis. Obes Surg 2008;18:1532–8.

44. Miller K, Hell E, Lang B, et al. Gallstone formation prophylaxis after gastric restrictive procedures for weight loss: a randomized double-blind placebo-controlled trial. Ann Surg 2003;238:697–702.

45. Worobetz LJ, Inglis FG, Shaffer EA. The effect of ursodeoxycholic acid therapy on gallstone formation in the morbidly obese during rapid weight loss. Am J Gastroenterol 1993;88:1705–10.

46. Williams C, Gowan R, Perey BJ. A double-blind placebo-controlled trial of ursodeoxycholic acid in the prevention of gallstones during weight loss after vertical banded gastroplasty. Obes Surg 1993;3:257–9.

47. Wudel LJ Jr, Wright JK, Debelak JP, et al. Prevention of gallstone formation in morbidly obese patients undergoing rapid weight loss: results of a randomized controlled pilot study. J Surg Res 2002;102:50–6.

48. Caruana JA, McCabe MN, Smith AD, et al. Incidence of symptomatic gallstones after gastric bypass: is prophylactic treatment really necessary? Surg Obes Relat Dis 2005;1:564–7.

49. Villegas L, Schneider B, Provost D, et al. Is routine cholecystectomy required during laparoscopic gastric bypass? Obes Surg 2004;14:206–11.

50. Kothari SN. Bariatric surgery and postoperative imaging. Surg Clin North Am 2011;91:155–72.

51. Kavanagh PV, vanSonnenberg E, Wittich GR, et al. Interventional radiology of the biliary tract. Endoscopy 1997;29:570–6.

52. Ozden I, Tekant Y, Bilge O, et al. Endoscopic and radiologic interventions as the leading causes of severe cholangitis in a tertiary referral center. Am J Surg 2005;189:702–6.

53. Choi SH, Gwon DI, Ko GY, et al. Hepatic arterial injuries in 3110 patients following percutaneous transhepatic biliary drainage. Radiology 2011;261:969–75.

54. Lennon AM, Kapoor S, Khashab M, et al. Spiral assisted ERCP is equivalent to single balloon assisted ERCP in patients with Roux-en-Y anatomy. Dig Dis Sci 2012;57:1391–8.

55. Itoi T, Ishii K, Sofuni A, et al. Long- and short-type double-balloon enteroscopy-assisted therapeutic ERCP for intact papilla in patients with a Roux-en-Y anastomosis. Surg Endosc 2011;25:713–21.

56. Wright BE, Cass OW, Freeman ML. ERCP in patients with long-limb Roux-en-Y gastrojejunostomy and intact papilla. Gastrointest Endosc 2002;56:225–32.

57. Fobi MA, Chicola K, Lee H. Access to the bypassed stomach after gastric bypass. Obes Surg 1998;8:289–95.

58. Richardson JF, Lee JG, Smith BR, et al. Laparoscopic transgastric endoscopy after Roux-en-Y gastric bypass: case series and review of the literature. Am Surg 2012;78:1182–6.

59. Pimentel RR, Mehran A, Szomstein S, et al. Laparoscopy-assisted transgastrostomy ERCP after bariatric surgery: case report of a novel approach. Gastrointest Endosc 2004;59:325–8.

60. Ceppa FA, Gagne DJ, Papasavas PK, et al. Laparoscopic transgastric endoscopy after Roux-en-Y gastric bypass. Surg Obes Relat Dis 2007;3:21–4.

61. Nakao FS, Mendes CJ, Szego T, et al. Intraoperative transgastric ERCP after a Roux-en-Y gastric bypass. Endoscopy 2007;39(Suppl 1):E219–20.

62. Patel JA, Patel NA, Shinde T, et al. Endoscopic retrograde cholangiopancreatography after laparoscopic Roux-en-Y gastric bypass: a case series and review of the literature. Am Surg 2008;74:689–93.

63. Roberts KE, Panait L, Duffy AJ, et al. Laparoscopic-assisted transgastric endoscopy: current indications and future implications. JSLS 2008;12:30–6.

64. Dapri G, Himpens J, Buset M, et al. Video. Laparoscopic transgastric access to the common bile duct after Roux-en-Y gastric bypass. Surg Endosc 2009;23:1646–8.

65. Gutierrez JM, Lederer H, Krook JC, et al. Surgical gastrostomy for pancreatobiliary and duodenal access following Roux-en-Y gastric bypass. J Gastrointest Surg 2009;13:2170–5.

66. Peeters G, Himpens J. A hybrid endo-laparoscopic therapy for common bile duct stenosis of a choledocho-duodenostomy after a Roux-en-Y gastric bypass. Obes Surg 2009;19:806–8.

67. Sebastian JJ, Resa JJ, Pena E, et al. Laparoscopically assisted ERCP in a case of acute cholangitis in a patient with biliopancreatic diversion with distal gastric preservation. Obes Surg 2009;19:250–2.

68. Badaoui A, Malherbe V, Rosiere A, et al. ERCP by laparoscopic transgastric access and cholecystectomy at the same time in a patient with gastric bypass who was seen with choledocholithiasis. Gastrointest Endosc 2010;71:212–4.

69. Bertin PM, Singh K, Arregui ME. Laparoscopic transgastric endoscopic retrograde cholangiopancreatography (ERCP) after gastric bypass: case series and a description of technique. Surg Endosc 2011;25:2592–6.

70. Saleem A, Levy MJ, Petersen BT, et al. Laparoscopic assisted ERCP in Roux-en-Y gastric bypass (RYGB) surgery patients. J Gastrointest Surg 2012;16:203–8.

Technical Aspects of Cholecystectomy

Alberto R. Ferreres, MD, PhD[a], Horacio J. Asbun, MD[b],*

KEYWORDS

- Cholecystectomy • Laparoscopy • Alternative approaches
- Single-incision laparoscopy • Natural orifice transluminal endoscopic surgery

KEY POINTS

- Laparoscopic cholecystectomy (LC), introduced in the late 1980s and popularized in the early 1990s, is considered the gold standard for the treatment of symptomatic cholelithiasis.
- Even though LC is a very safe operation, the reported incidence of major bile duct injuries remains higher than that for open cholecystectomy. Safety steps should be routinely practiced during LC to prevent bile duct injuries.
- Adherence to sound surgical judgment and technique will result in better outcomes.
- Open cholecystectomy is mostly the result of conversion during LC, and conversion to open surgery should not be implicitly considered as a complication. Surgical trainees and young surgeons should also be adequately trained to complete a cholecystectomy in an open fashion.
- New approaches to even minimize LC have been proposed lately, including NOTES (Natural Orifice Transluminal Surgery), both transgastric and transvaginal, and single-incision laparoscopic surgery, but the benefits of these techniques over the traditional laparoscopic approach have yet to be proved.
- Special attention must be paid to intraoperative and postoperative complications so as to achieve early detection and management if a complication occurs.

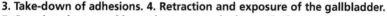
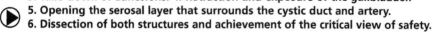

The following videos: 1. Creation of pneumoperitoneum. 2. Insertion of trocars. 3. Take-down of adhesions. 4. Retraction and exposure of the gallbladder. 5. Opening the serosal layer that surrounds the cystic duct and artery. 6. Dissection of both structures and achievement of the critical view of safety. 7. Intraoperative cholangiogram. 8. Dissection clipping and section of the cystic duct and artery. 9. Dissection of the gallbladder from the liver bed. 10. Irrigation

The authors have nothing to disclose.
[a] Division of Gastrointestinal Surgery, University of Buenos Aires, Vicente Lopez 1831 PB, Buenos Aires 1128, Argentina; [b] Hepatobiliary and Pancreas Program, General Surgery, Mayo College of Medicine, Mayo Clinic, 4500 San Pablo Road, Jacksonville, FL 32224, USA
* Corresponding author.
E-mail address: asbun.horacio@mayo.edu

Surg Clin N Am 94 (2014) 427–454
http://dx.doi.org/10.1016/j.suc.2014.01.007
0039-6109/14/$ – see front matter © 2014 Elsevier Inc. All rights reserved.

and final assurance of hemostasis. 11. Extraction of the gallbladder. 12. Trocar retrieval and closure of incisions. 13. Umbilical laparoscopic approach. 14. Transvaginal access. 15. Gallbladder retraction. 16. Gallbladder retraction. 17. Dissection of the hepatic hilum and triangle of Calot. 18. Dissection of gallbladder from the liver bed. 19. Extraction of the gallbladder. 20. Vaginal Closure. 21. Incision and trocar placement. 22. Gallbladder retraction and exposure. 23. Dissection of the hepatic hilum. 24. Dissection of the gallbladder from the liver bed and control. 25. Extraction of the gallbladder. 26. Wound closure accompany this article at http://www.surgical.theclinics.com/

INTRODUCTION

Carl Langenbuch is credited as the first surgeon to perform an open cholecystectomy (OC) in 1882. He had done his research in animals and cadavers before performing the first human procedure. Langenbuch postulated that removal of the gallbladder would result in extraction of the gallstones and of the organ that produced them.[1] In 1985, E. Muhe from Boblingen, Germany performed the first laparoscopic cholecystectomy (LC), but was confronted by great opposition from his colleagues.[2] Three years later a French gynecologist, P. Mouret, performed an LC, which influenced F. Dubois and J. Perissat in developing their technique for this approach. The popularization of this technique in the United States should be credited to E.J. Reddick and D.O. Olsen from Nashville, Tennessee, who performed their first case in 1988 and established the principles of the operation as it is presently known.[3]

During the 1990s, attempts were described to further reduce the laparoscopic minimally invasive approach to a single incision.[4,5] The use of small-diameter 2- to 3-mm trocars and instruments, known as the needlescopic technique, was also tried. Neither of these techniques gained general acceptance because of the lack of proven benefit.

LC became the first procedure in a revolution that changed the way in which abdominal surgery was being performed. In the ensuing 15 years, a laparoscopic approach was reported as feasible for almost every abdominal procedure. This advance resulted in a significant benefit to the patient for most of the procedures, owing to the inherent advantages of the laparoscopic technique. For LC, however, there is still an increased risk of bile duct injury (BDI) in comparison with the now historical OC. The common denominator in the occurrence of BDI is a failure to clearly identify the anatomy of the triangle of Calot (**Fig. 1**). Although this lingering disadvantage to LC does not justify performing an OC, it needs to be continuously attended to. Steps to prevent BDI were described in the early years of LC,[6] and in 1995 Strassberg[7] described the term "critical view of safety" as the most important step in the avoidance of BDI during the procedure (**Fig. 2**).

NOTES stands for Natural Orifice Transluminal Endoscopic Surgery, and owes part of its development to Anthony Kalloo, a gastrointestinal endoscopist from Johns Hopkins, and Paul Swain, a British gastroenterologist. Both of these investigators favored a transgastric approach to NOTES endoscopic cholecystectomy, which, though initially embraced, showed potential disadvantages and difficulties for the performance of cholecystectomy. The proof-leak closure of the gastric opening, the retroflexion required to achieve good visualization to the Calot triangle and cystic structures, the technical challenges and the hazards in extracting the gallbladder through the gastric opening, and the esophageal junction all conspired against the adoption of this technique.[8] After an initial experience in transgastric cholecystectomy by one of the authors (A.R.F.), this approach was abandoned in favor of the

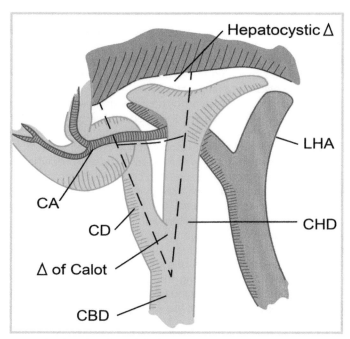

Fig. 1. Anatomy of Calot triangle and the hepatocystic triangle. CA, cystic artery; CBD, common bile duct; CD, cystic duct; LHA, left hepatic artery.

transvaginal approach. A prospective, randomized series of NOTES transvaginal cholecystectomy was performed (World Congress of Endoscopic Surgery 2010, Washington, DC) showing the feasibility of the procedure, but its advantages over LC were limited.

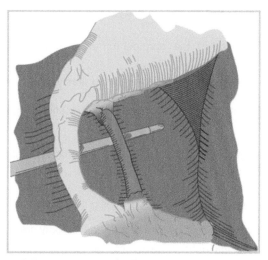

Fig. 2. Achievement of the critical view of safety.

Although the transvaginal approach seems to be a recent development, transvaginal endoscopy, or culdoscopy, was previously described by Senn in the United States and von Ott in Russia.[9,10] Vaginal surgery is one of the oldest procedures ever described in surgical history, having been performed by gynecologists for decades; there is robust literature supporting the efficacy and safety of this approach, which is associated with few risks and complications.[8]

In 1946, Palmer described transvaginal culdoscopy using the dorsal decubitus position, and 1 year later Decker and Cherry described rigid culdoscopy in the genupectoral position, which allowed for spontaneous pneumoperitoneum. In 2003, Tsin[11] reported the first case of a culdolaparoscopic cholecystectomy in a patient who also underwent vaginal hysterectomy, with removal of the gallbladder through the vagina. During 2007, different groups presumed to be the first ones to perform NOTES cholecystectomy, either transvaginal or transgastric, with a pure NOTES approach or assisted with laparoscopic instruments.[12–15] This last technique is known as the or laparoscopically assisted or hybrid technique.

Nevertheless, the inherent difficulties and the lack of optimal technical devices for the performance of NOTES cholecystectomy led many groups to reconsider the utility of this technique. Subsequently, much of the instrumentation developed and skills learned in NOTES evolved into revisiting the adoption of a previously abandoned approach: single-incision LC. This technique has evolved further than NOTES and is currently adopted by more surgeons, but has yet to prove its benefits over the laparoscopic counterpart.

PREOPERATIVE PLANNING

The indications for cholecystectomy include the following conditions[16]:

- Symptomatic cholelithiasis (biliary colic, chronic cholecystitis)
- Asymptomatic cholelithiasis (mainly in countries with a high incidence of gallbladder cancer)
- Complications of cholelithiasis: acute cholecystitis, gallstone pancreatitis (once subsided), choledocholithiasis
- Biliary dyskinesia
- Acute acalculous cholecystitis
- Gallbladder polyps larger than 1 cm

The expected benefits of the surgical removal of the gallbladder are the following:

- Remission of symptoms and improvement of lifestyle because biliary colic will most likely recur
- Prevention of complications secondary to the presence of gallstones:
  - Biliary pancreatitis
  - Biliary obstruction caused by choledocholithiasis
  - Acute cholecystitis, which may progress to necrosis and sepsis unless cholecystectomy is performed

SURGICAL TECHNIQUES

The different techniques used to perform a cholecystectomy are:

- LC: Regarded as the gold standard and by far the most routinely practiced worldwide.

- OC: Currently done only when the procedure is converted to open during LC or because LC is contraindicated, or as part of another open abdominal procedure.
- NOTES approach, including transgastric and transvaginal access: A procedure that had initially been received with enthusiasm by some surgeons, but at present is being practiced by very few.
- Single-incision cholecystectomy: A procedure that still needs to prove its advantages over the traditional LC. However, it is being performed in some centers, and only time will determine its place in the armamentarium of the surgical treatment of the gallbladder.

In this article, all of these techniques are addressed because the purpose is to describe the technical aspects of cholecystectomy as practiced today. The reader is encouraged to bear in mind that the description of the latter 2 techniques does not implicitly endorse their performance.

LAPAROSCOPIC CHOLECYSTECTOMY

LC is usually performed under general anesthesia on an outpatient basis or with overnight stay.

Absolute contraindication is represented by the inability to tolerate CO_2 abdominal insufflation.

Relative contraindications include:

- Suspicion of gallbladder cancer
- Cirrhosis, portal hypertension, or bleeding disorders
- Previous abdominal operations precluding minimal invasive approach
- Pregnancy (first or third trimester)

Patient positioning will depend on the operative technique (American or French). In the American technique, the surgeon is placed to the left of the patient, whereas in the French technique the patient is placed in a split-leg position with the surgeon standing between the patient's legs. The American approach to the procedure is described here.

The equipment required for the performance of the operation is as follows.

- Standard laparoscopic equipment: high-definition camera, monitor, light source, and automatic 40-L insufflator
- Laparoscopic instruments:
  - A total of 4 trocars are used. The most common approach includes two 5-mm and two 10-mm trocars. Depending on the patient's body habitus and disease process, the trocar size can vary to three 5-mm trocars and only one 10-mm trocar for the camera and extraction of the specimen. Alternatively, one may use two 3.5-mm trocars, one 5-mm trocar for the subxiphoid port, and one 10-mm trocar
  - A 30° scope, which allows a better view of the cystic pedicle and main hepatic duct or standard zero-degree scope
  - Electrocautery (hook-spatula)
  - Maryland dissector
  - Clip applier
  - Scissors
  - Atraumatic forceps (different types)

LC comprises the following steps/phases:

1. Creation of pneumoperitoneum (Video 1)

2. Insertion of trocars (Video 2)

3. Take-down of adhesions, if present (Video 3)

4. Retraction and exposure of the gallbladder (Video 4)

5. Opening the serosal layer that surrounds the cystic duct and artery (Video 5)

6. Dissection of both structures and achievement of the critical view of safety (Video 6)

7. Intraoperative cholangiogram (Video 7)

8. Dissection, clipping, and section of the cystic duct and artery (Video 8)

9. Dissection of the gallbladder from the liver bed (Video 9)

10. Irrigation and assurance of hemostasis (Video 10)

11. Extraction of the gallbladder (Video 11)

12. Trocar retrieval and closure of incisions (Video 12)

Creation of Pneumoperitoneum

A small periumbilical incision is made, depending on its location, orientation, and extent on the patient's body habitus, and based on cosmetic considerations. Options are the following:

- Closed technique using a Veress needle; after achieving pneumoperitoneum with a pressure of 15 mm Hg, the 10-mm umbilical trocar is introduced in a blind fashion.
- Open technique using a 10-mm Hasson trocar. After dissection and insertion, the abdomen is insufflated and the camera is placed through this port.
- Introduction of an Optiview trocar with the scope, the preferred choice in obese patients.

Insertion of Trocars

After placement of the first periumbilical port, a pneumoperitoneum is obtained and a laparoscope is introduced. The entry site is inspected and the other 3 accessory ports are placed under direct laparoscopic visualization. According to the American technique, the two 5-mm trocars are inserted next. One is placed 2 finger breadths below the costal margin close to the anterior axillary line, and the second 2 finger breadths below the costal margin at the level of the midclavicular line. The main function of the grasper introduced through the first trocar is to displace the fundus of the gallbladder cephalad, and this is best done from as lateral a position as possible. After retraction of the gallbladder has been achieved, the operating 10-mm trocar is inserted. A needle can be used as a guide to plan the angle placement and location, to facilitate access to the dissection of the triangle of Calot. This port is usually placed at a slight angle to enter the abdomen, immediately to the right of the insertion of the falciform ligament. This positioning of the port sites is based on the position of the surgeon standing to the left of the patient. In the French technique, with the surgeon standing between both legs, the operating 10-mm trocar is usually positioned in the left supraumbilical area.

Dissection of Adhesions

Inspection of the entry sites and visual laparoscopic exploration of the abdomen is recommended to assess for adhesions and/or potential injuries or bleeding resulting from the port placement. Adhesions to the gallbladder are released using blunt or sharp dissection, in some cases with the aid of monopolar electrocautery. It is recommended that a two-handed technique be used to aid using traction and countertraction.

Retraction and Exposure of Gallbladder

Retraction of the gallbladder should achieve the following aims:

- Maximum cephalad traction, providing reduction of redundancies in the gallbladder infundibulum and better visualization of the region of the Calot triangle.
- Lateral and inferior retraction of the Hartmann pouch of the gallbladder. During this retraction it is important to avoid aligning the cystic duct with the common duct (**Fig. 3**). The lateral and inferior direction of retraction of the Hartmann pouch facilitates the creation of a more distinct angle between the cystic duct and the common duct. This retraction is achieved with the graspers inserted through the two 5-mm lateral ports.

In some situations the gallbladder retraction can be difficult:

- A grossly distended gallbladder may be difficult to grasp and is prone to rupture; therefore, percutaneous puncture and aspiration is recommended. Bile leak from the puncture site may be prevented by occluding the puncture site with the fundus-grasping forceps.
- Adhesions between the liver and the anterior abdominal wall or to the retroperitoneum may cause difficulty in the retraction, so the recommendation is to free them before starting the cholecystectomy.

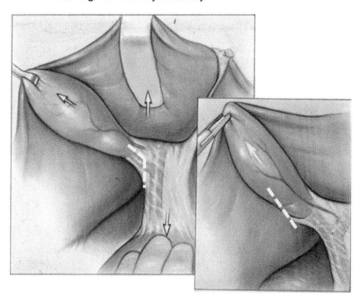

Fig. 3. Prevention of bile duct injury (BDI). In open surgery, the lines of traction create an angle between the cystic duct and common bile duct. In laparoscopic surgery, care should be taken to avoid alignment of the cystic duct with the common bile duct. (*Courtesy of* The Lahey Hospital & Medical Center, Burlington, MA.)

- A scleroatrophic gallbladder may not permit grasping the fundus; sometimes an additional trocar must be placed to retract the liver. Alternatively, placing a percutaneous suture to lift and retract the gallbladder can be useful.
- A thick wall (acute cholecystitis with days of evolution) may require a toothed grasper for retraction.
- An impacted stone in the gallbladder neck is a major obstacle to grasping and retractions.

Retraction of the gallbladder using a blunt grasper with the jaws opened can be useful in any of the latter 3 situations.

Opening of the Serosal Layer that Surrounds the Cystic Duct and Artery

Contrary to the teachings of OC, whereby the dissection was advocated to be close to the junction of the cystic duct and common bile duct, in LC the dissection is initiated high in the cystic duct to identify its junction with the gallbladder neck. The cystic duct lymph node is a good landmark to start the dissection.

A hook cautery is used to carefully dissect, coagulate, and cut the peritoneum covering the triangle of Calot, continuing upward along the two faces of the gall-bladder neck.

The dissection is then carried from lateral to medial. In this direction the cystic duct will be the first tubular structure to be identified. Then the connective tissue is dissected using blunt dissection (with a Maryland dissector) or with hook cautery (the authors' preference) to carefully surround the cystic duct in 360°. The goal is to create a window between the gallbladder neck and the liver (**Fig. 4**). The creation of this window is facilitated by turning the Hartmann pouch medially for posterolateral dissections with the left hand lifting the Hartmann pouch cephalad and to the left; the posterior aspect of Hartmann pouch is displayed. The posterior aspect of the junction of the gallbladder to the cystic duct is defined with the help of a hook cautery. The cystic duct junction is identified posteriorly. This dissection will facilitate the

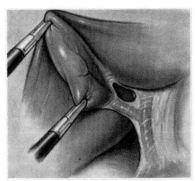
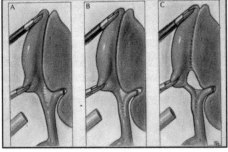

Fig. 4. Prevention of BDI. Create a window between the neck of the gallbladder and the liver bed, clearly visualizing the gallbladder–cystic duct junction; this allows one to obtain what is designated as the "critical view of safety." (*Courtesy of* The Lahey Hospital & Medical Center, Burlington, MA.)

completion of the window through further anterior dissection. In several patients, a posterior window may be completed by pursuing the posterior blunt dissection until the liver can be seen through this window. If this technique is used, care should be taken to avoid directing the dissection toward the hepatic hilum or the area of the right hepatic duct.

The creation of the window between the gallbladder neck and the liver bed is the basis for obtaining the critical view, as described by Strasberg and Brunt.[17]

The triangle of Calot is bordered by the cystic duct, the common hepatic duct, and the cystic artery; meanwhile, the hepatocystic triangle is defined by the cystic duct, the common hepatic duct, and the liver (see **Fig. 1**).

Dissection of Both Structures and Achievement of the Critical View of Safety

After clear identification of the cystic duct–gallbladder junction, anterior dissection is continued with lateral and downward traction on the gallbladder neck. As mentioned, it is paramount to perform a circumferential dissection around the gallbladder and cystic duct junction. The more the adhesions or the more uncertain the anatomy, the more the dissection should move further up the neck of the gallbladder so that the entire circumference of the gallbladder is dissected, creating a larger window between the gallbladder and the liver bed to clearly expose the anatomy of the triangle of Calot (see **Fig. 1**). At this point, only 2 tubular structures (the cystic duct and the cystic artery) remain connected to the proximal gallbladder, representing the critical view of safety.[7] Sometimes hydrodissection can be useful to render a safe dissection of the area.

Intraoperative Cholangiogram

Intraoperative cholangiography is performed (**Fig. 5**)[18]:

- Even though it may not necessarily prevent a BDI, it allows for prompt recognition if it occurs.
- Offers a detailed study of the biliary anatomy, visualizing the biliary tree proximal to the biliary bifurcation (revealing both right and left hepatic ducts), as well as passage of the contrast material into the duodenum through the papilla.

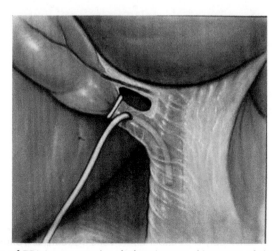

Fig. 5. Prevention of BDI. Intraoperative cholangiogram. (*Courtesy of* The Lahey Hospital & Medical Center, Burlington, MA.)

- Allows detection of unsuspected stones in the common bile duct (5% incidence). If stones are detected in the common bile duct, they can be managed by means of a laparoscopic bile duct exploration or postoperatively with endoscopic retrograde cholangiopancreatography (ERCP), depending on the surgeon's experience and preference, institutional guidelines, and/or availability of resources.

For this purpose a clip is applied on the cystic duct close to the infundibulum, and an anterolateral cystic ductotomy is made distal to the clip. A cholangiogram catheter is inserted through the cystic opening and secured in place using either clips or ad hoc clamps. Another possibility is to perform a cholecystogram, by puncture of the gallbladder and injection of the contrast. Alternatively, an intraoperative ultrasonogram can be very useful in experienced hands.

Clipping and Section of Cystic Duct and Artery

After removing the cholangiography catheter, the cystic duct is double clipped proximal to the previous opening, away from the common bile duct, and divided (**Fig. 6**). The cystic artery is similarly divided between the clips. Sometimes it is easy to clip and section the cystic artery before the performance of the cholangiography. Careful examination of each stump is recommended.

Dissection of the Gallbladder from the Liver Bed

Once freed from the cystic duct and artery, one of the forceps is placed in the infundibulum to aid in the retraction and enhance visualization of the posterior wall of the gallbladder. Then the dissection is continued with hook cautery and care is taken to keep dissection in the right plane, close to the gallbladder wall. The electrocautery setting for this portion of the procedure is at a power of 20 to avoid perforation of the gallbladder. If a perforation occurs, steps should be immediately taken to avoid any significant spillage. Aspiration of bile and stones is done. One of the grasping forceps may be placed at the site of the perforation or, if possible, an endoloop or a clip is used to close the perforation. In several instances, further dissection of the gallbladder

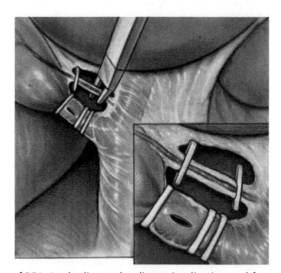

Fig. 6. Prevention of BDI. Apply clips under direct visualization and from medial to lateral. The clips are safely placed with the tips of the applier facing laterally. (*Courtesy of* The Lahey Hospital & Medical Center, Burlington, MA.)

wall off the liver bed is necessary to better expose the edges of the opening before placing an endoloop or clip. In cirrhotic patients or when there is no plane of dissection between the liver and the gallbladder, the posterior wall of the gallbladder may be left attached to the liver and its mucosa be ablated with electrocautery. Though uncommon this is a useful technique, when needed, requiring careful collection of stones and debris from the gallbladder to avoid any significant spillage. In selected cases, anterograde dissection of the gallbladder from the fundus down may be performed more easily. Bleeding from the gallbladder bed usually can be prevented by keeping the dissection in the right plane.

Irrigation and Control of Hemostasis

All bleeding must be checked and controlled, and irrigation and suction are recommended. Careful examination of the abdomen, including the Winslow hiatus and subhepatic and subdiaphragmatic spaces, is done.

Extraction of the Gallbladder

The gallbladder is preferably placed in an endoscopic removal bag, and removed from the abdominal cavity. Most commonly the umbilical port is used for the extraction site, but some surgeons remove it through the subxiphoid site depending on the gallbladder and stone size. When the gallbladder is not distended or severely inflamed and the stones are of relatively small size, extraction is not difficult. When stones are larger, there is an option to crush the stones from outside with forceps under laparoscopic view once the neck of the gallbladder is extracted. The gallbladder is kept in an endoscopic retrieval bag while crushing the stones to avoid any spillage. Drains are seldom used, and their use depends on the surgeon's preference.

Trocar Retrieval and Closure of Incisions

The ports are removed under direct vision to evaluate possible bleeding. The fascial defects in the 10-mm umbilical port are closed with interrupted 0 Vicryl sutures. Cleaning and dressing of the incisions is performed.

Tips and Tricks for Avoiding Complications

- Assume every case has a short cystic duct and/or other anatomic abnormalities. The goal is dissection of the cystic duct starting at the junction with the gallbladder.[19]
- Use the critical view of safety technique to clear the Calot triangle, and completely individualize, identify, and isolate the cystic duct and artery before dividing them.[7]
- During the whole operation, always bear in mind that your interpretation of anatomy may be wrong or mistaken; this is a safeguard to prevent BDIs.
- A panicked reaction to bleeding, resulting in bulk clip application or cautery, leads to disaster. Compression, irrigation, and suction and the use of a duck-beak forceps to pick up the bleeding point is recommended. Be aware of the $16\times$ magnification of the laparoscopic view.
- Beware of excessive retraction of the Hartmann pouch, which can lead to misinterpretation of the common bile duct for the cystic duct.

When confronted with a wide cystic duct, cholangiography is mandatory to ensure that it is the cystic duct and not the common bile duct. For closure, 2 endoloop sutures may be placed instead of regular titanium clips.

Important Steps in Avoiding Bile Duct Injury

From the surgical technique described, the main steps to avoid BDI are[6]:

1. Maximum cephalic traction of the gallbladder fundus
2. Lateral and inferior retraction (toward right foot) of the Hartmann pouch, pulling it away from the liver and avoiding alignment of the cystic duct with the common bile duct
3. Start the dissection high in the gallbladder neck and carry it from lateral to medial
4. Turn Hartmann pouch medially for a posterolateral dissection of the serosa of the gallbladder
5. Free the neck of the gallbladder from the liver bed, creating a window that would be as large as necessary to clearly expose the anatomy of the triangle of Calot, and obtain a critical view of safety.
6. Place the clips under direct visualization of both limbs in a medial to lateral direction, from the subxyphoid port.
7. Perform intraoperative cholangiography if there are any questions with the biliary anatomy.
8. When starting the subsequent detachment of the gallbladder from the liver bed, keep the dissection close to the gallbladder wall and away from the structures of the hilum of the liver. Judicious use of electrocautery is recommended.

Postoperative Management

- The orogastric tube is removed at the end of the procedure before waking the patient from anesthesia.
- Analgesic medication is prescribed.
- Diet is started after 4 to 6 hours, and advanced as tolerated.
- Ambulation should be started as soon as possible.
- Severe pain is uncommon, and should be seriously taken into consideration as a sign of a possible complication if it occurs or persists.

Complications

- Hollow viscus injury should be recognized early and repaired.
- Bile leak may be from the cystic duct stump, an aberrant Lushka duct, or a BDI. Its management will depend on the presence of abdominal drainage and if intraoperative cholangiography was performed. Ultrasonography or computed tomography scan of the abdomen is required for evaluation of free abdominal fluid and collections. ERCP with stenting, sphincterotomy, or both should be considered early. Placement of a percutaneous abdominal drain should be used for drainage of bilomas.
- BDI most frequently results from a failure to recognize the anatomy of the triangle of Calot (eg, common bile duct or right hepatic duct mistaken for the cystic duct), but may also result from excessive use of electrocautery or clips to control bleeding in the porta hepatis, or excessive traction on the cystic duct and common bile duct during dissection.[20]
- Management depends on the timing of recognition (intraoperative vs postoperative), nature, and severity of the injury.
- Retained spilled stones: every effort should be made to profusely irrigate the operative area and to recover spilled stones when they occur.
- Retained CBD stones can usually be managed endoscopically if identified in the postoperative period.

It is important to emphasize that LC is a surgical procedure that should have a low incidence of complications, and the main effort should be concentrated on prevention rather than treatment.

OPEN CHOLECYSTECTOMY

Most OC are the result of conversions during laparoscopic procedures[21] or are performed as part of another major open abdominal procedure. Surgeons-in-training and most young practicing surgeons have had very limited exposure to OC. This issue creates significant concern because well-trained surgeons in the laparoscopic approach with limited experience in the open approach may find themselves converting a difficult LC without having someone with experience in the open approach available to assist.[22] Therefore, surgeons-in-training should take any opportunity to participate in OC when performed as part of another open procedure.

Conversion to open may occur because of:

- Technical difficulties
- Inability to keep CO_2 insufflation (eg, patients with severe cardiopulmonary disease)
- Anatomic findings that preclude clear identification of the anatomy within the area of the Calot triangle
- Bleeding
- Difficult LC with the following predicting factors[23]
  ○ Age greater than 60 years
  ○ Male sex
  ○ Weight greater than 65 kg
  ○ Presence of acute cholecystitis
  ○ History of prior upper abdominal surgery
  ○ Diabetic patients
  ○ Less experienced surgeon

OC can be the first choice for a certain subset of patients:

- Gallbladder mass or porcelain gallbladder
- Suspicion of malignancy
- Mirizzi syndrome diagnosed in the preoperative stage
- Extensive upper abdominal surgery
- Third trimester of pregnancy
- Contraindication to CO_2 abdominal insufflation
- Cirrhosis

OC are also performed during several major open operations such as pancreatico-duodenectomy, liver resections, and choledochal cyst excision. Cholecystectomy should not be attempted during emergency operation for gallstone ileus.

OC is usually performed through a right subcostal incision or a midline upper abdominal incision. When it is the result of conversion, the subcostal approach is most commonly used and usually the incision encompasses the previously made trocar incisions.[24] The surgeon usually stands to the right side of the patient.

Once in the abdominal cavity, the overall principles of the technique are similar to the one described for the laparoscopic approach, but the following are steps that are particular to the open approach:

- The Teres ligament is divided between clamps, and ligated in most cases.

- In cases where the liver and gallbladder are located under the costal margin, a hand is passed over the dome of the liver, allowing air to enter between the diaphragm and the liver to aid in the downward retraction of the liver. If necessary, it is helpful to place 1 to 2 rolled moist laps superior to the dome of the liver for downward retraction and 1 to 2 rolled laps posterolateral to the right lobe of the liver for medial and anterior retraction. This maneuver will bring the gallbladder and hilum of the liver more into the operative field.
- A clamp is used in the fundus of the gallbladder for the cephalad retraction, and 1 in the Hartmann pouch for lateral and inferior retraction, as described for LC.
- The assistant surgeon exerts downward traction on the colon and duodenum with a moist rolled lap. This maneuver maintains exposure throughout the dissection of the triangle of Calot, and it is important to accentuate the angle between the cystic duct and the common bile duct because it also indirectly retracts the duct downward (see **Fig. 3**).
- As for LC, the serosal layer surrounding the cystic duct and artery is carefully opened, after which a Kittner (peanut) dissection is useful for the exposure of the cystic duct and artery. Short, partially pushing, and rotating motions are used with the Kittner from the gallbladder toward the common bile duct. The cystic duct and artery are gradually uncovered.
- The dissection clipping and division of the duct and artery are done in a fashion similar to that in LC, but using open instruments.
- The separation of the gallbladder from the liver bed is done with electrocautery and can be done from the fundus down or from the neck upward in accordance with the surgeon's preference. The retrograde, fundus-down technique is standard for many experienced surgeons, and is particularly indicated when severe inflammation is present.

NATURAL ORIFICE TRANSLUMINAL ENDOSCOPIC SURGERY TRANSVAGINAL CHOLECYSTECTOMY

As mentioned earlier, few surgeons worldwide are practicing NOTES transvaginal cholecystectomy, and many investigators who were initially enthusiastic about the technique have reconsidered its adoption. It is not the goal of this article to discuss the merits of the procedure, but rather to describe the technical steps. This section represents the significant experience in the procedure by one of the authors (A.R.F.).

NOTES transvaginal cholecystectomy can be performed in a totally pure fashion or with a hybrid technique (with laparoscopic support by means of a 5-mm umbilical port), which is the standard option.[8]

The advantages of the hybrid technique are:

- The umbilical 5-mm port allows visualization and control of the transvaginal access
- Prevention of rectal and/or vascular injuries
- Better control of CO_2 intra-abdominal insufflation
- Use of standard 5-mm laparoscopic instruments
- Requirement of standard laparoscopic titanium clips for management and occlusion of the cystic duct and artery (instead of endoscopic ones)
- Introduction of retraction devices through the umbilical port
- Laparoscopic-view backup, essential when surgeons are performing their first cases (endoscopic transvaginal view is down-upward, whereas laparoscopic view is lateral)

Patient Selection

Patients should fulfill the following inclusion criteria for the performance of a NOTES transvaginal cholecystectomy[8]:

- Women between 18 and 65 years
- Symptomatic gallbladder stones
- Absence of symptoms that would suggest the presence of common bile duct stones
- Normal liver function tests
- Nonrelevant ultrasonography findings, other than the presence of gallstones
- Body mass index of 30 kg/m^2 or less
- Previous pregnancy
- Negative pregnancy tests
- Normal cardiovascular preoperative evaluation
- American Society of Anesthesiologists risk grades I and II
- Mini-Mental State Evaluation (for cognitive status) of 14 or higher
- Compliance with the following process of surgical informed consent: 2 individual interviews (patient and relatives) and 1 group meeting, printed information with pictures and figures, explanation of doubts and further inquiries. Final decision is documented with the following points: (1) nature of disease and of the proposed operation, (2) knowledge that LC is the accepted gold standard and that NOTES transvaginal cholecystectomy represents a surgical innovation, (3) potential benefits, (4) risks and complications, and (5) alternative treatments
- Gynecologic evaluation, including:
  - Detailed interrogation
  - Physical examination including colposcopy
  - Pelvic and transvaginal ultrasonography

The exclusion criteria for the performance of a NOTES transvaginal cholecystectomy are:

- Failure to fulfill the above inclusion criteria
- Pregnancy
- Gynecologic conditions: endometriosis, inflammatory pelvic disease, myomatosis
- Previous pelvic or abdominal operations (cesarean section and appendectomy are not considered absolute contraindications)
- Severe comorbidities

Surgical Technique

The preoperative workup and preparation includes:

- Patient selection
- Compliance with inclusion and exclusion requirements
- Surgical informed consent process
- Negative pregnancy test at admission (for fertile patients)
- When intrauterine device is present, the patient must agree to its removal before surgery
- Vaginal hygiene: preoperative local metronidazole tablets for 3 days, local iodopovidone, and antibiotic prophylaxis (cefazoline or similar) during the anesthetic induction. An indwelling urinary bladder catheter is placed and removed before recovery.
- All procedures are performed with general anesthesia and tracheal intubation.

The NOTES transvaginal hybrid cholecystectomy can be summarized in the following steps:

1. Umbilical laparoscopic approach (Video 13)

2. Transvaginal access (Video 14)

3. Gallbladder retraction (Videos 15 and 16)

4. Dissection of the hepatic hilum and triangle of Calot (Video 17)

5. Dissection of gallbladder from the liver bed (Video 18)

6. Extraction of the gallbladder (Video 19)

7. Vaginal closure (Video 20)

Umbilical laparoscopic access

Because the authors' preference is the NOTES hybrid transvaginal approach, a 5-mm umbilical trocar is placed in an open fashion, and insufflation with CO_2 to a maximum abdominal pressure of 15 mm Hg is attained with the patient in Trendelenburg position (**Fig. 7**).

Transvaginal access

After speculoscopy, hysterometry, and cervix dilatation, a uterine disposable manipulator is placed to mobilize the uterus and facilitate the laparoscopic control of the vaginal entrance (**Figs. 8–13**). A 2-channel trocar (width 18 mm, length 22 cm) is inserted through the right posterior vaginal cul-de-sac with gentle maneuvers and under direct laparoscopic visualization. A flexible videoendoscope, a long forceps, and diverse rotating instruments are inserted through the dual-lumen trocar. On some occasions, a rigid laparoscope or one with a flexible tip is used.[25] The instruments are used to grasp the gallbladder neck, and may be managed by the surgeon or the assistant.

Gallbladder retraction

The retraction of the gallbladder fundus is mandatory to attain a good view and achieve the critical view of safety; this can be done in the following fashion (**Figs. 14–16**):

- Magnetic retraction, which up to now has proved difficult to handle because of the variable intensity of the attraction of the external magnet

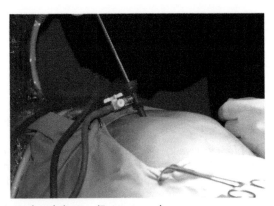

Fig. 7. Open access to the abdomen (5-mm trocar).

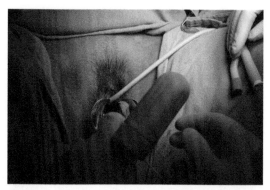

Fig. 8. Placement of uterine manipulators after speculoscopy, hysterometry, and cervical dilatation.

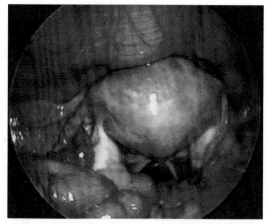

Fig. 9. Laparoscopic view of the posterior wall of the fornix (with uterine manipulator in place).

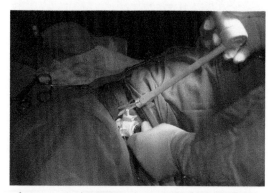

Fig. 10. Placement of transvaginal trocar and removal of manipulator.

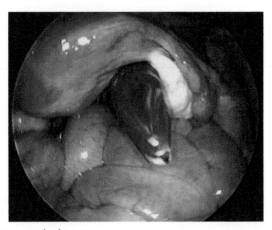

Fig. 11. Detail of transvaginal trocar.

- Endocavitary retraction devices (eg, Endograb, Virtual Ports, Boulder, CO), which are very useful, but expensive and difficult to relocate and displace after use
- External percutaneous sutures in the gallbladder fundus and neck, which is the authors' method of choice
- Additional 2.5-mm grasping forceps, placed in the right subcostal position

Dissection of the hepatic hilum and triangle of Calot

The dissection of the cystic elements (duct and artery) and the Calot triangle is performed with electrocautery, scissors, and/or Maryland forceps through the umbilical port, in a laparoscopic fashion, while the fundus is retracted by means of the rotating transvaginal forceps (**Fig. 17**). The endoscopic view provided is upside-down, and the gallbladder tends to be retracted longitudinally and not laterally. The possibility to switch to a traditional laparoscopic view, through the umbilical trocar, is very useful for guiding surgeons during their first cases, and adds to the safety of the procedure.

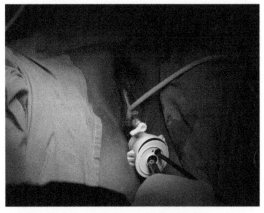

Fig. 12. External view of the endoscope and rotating forceps.

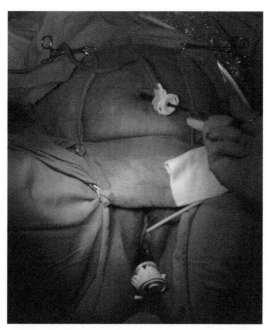

Fig. 13. Surgeon using his hands to manipulate the transvaginal forceps and the laparoscopic instrument through the umbilicus.

In cases of any difficulty, additional trocars can be placed in a standard fashion to aid in the retraction and improve the exposure of the anatomic structures. Intraoperative cholangiography can and should be performed routinely, by either cystic catheterization or percutaneous puncture of the gallbladder fundus.

Control of the cystic artery and duct is achieved by the placement of titanium clips with a 5-mm disposable clip applier, introduced through the umbilical port. Endoscopic clips offer only a partial bite of the structures.

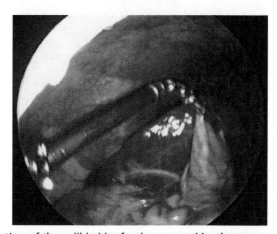

Fig. 14. Identification of the gallbladder fundus, grasped by the transvaginal forceps.

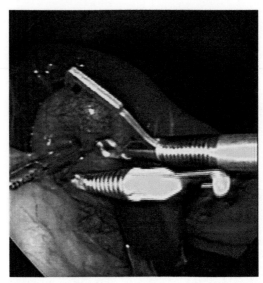

Fig. 15. Placement of retraction devices.

Dissection of gallbladder from the liver bed

The separation of the gallbladder from the liver bed is performed in a standard way with the use of 5-mm electrocautery (**Fig. 18**). The authors systematically perform the cholecystectomy after clipping and cutting the cystic duct and artery; nonetheless, in select cases a retrograde cholecystectomy may be used, according to the anatomic findings.

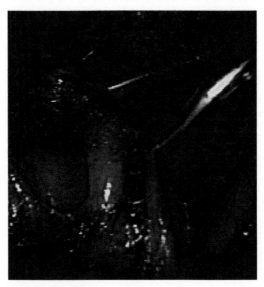

Fig. 16. Dissection of cystic structures.

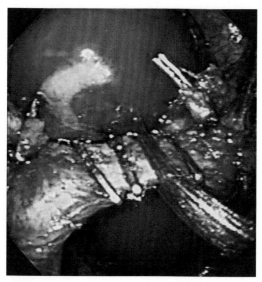

Fig. 17. Cutting the cystic duct.

Extraction of the gallbladder

Once the gallbladder is divided from its liver attachments, a polypectomy forceps is introduced through the endoscope and placed in the gallbladder neck, close to the junction with the cystic duct (**Figs. 19–21**). The laparoscope is placed in the umbilical trocar to aid the view of the specimen on the tip of the endoscope. The transvaginal trocar is removed together with the endoscope and the gallbladder. Very seldom it is necessary to enlarge the vaginal cul-de-sac opening to help in the removal of the specimen.

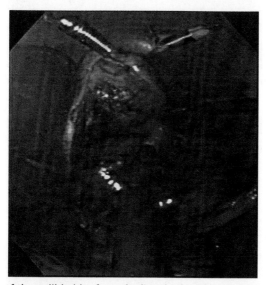

Fig. 18. Dissection of the gallbladder from the liver bed, with retraction of the gallbladder from the liver bed with endograbs and transvaginal forceps.

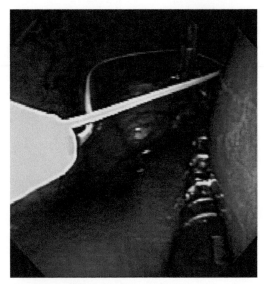

Fig. 19. Placement of endoscopic loop in the gallbladder neck.

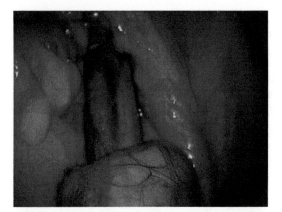

Fig. 20. Laparoscopic view of endoscopic withdrawal of the gallbladder.

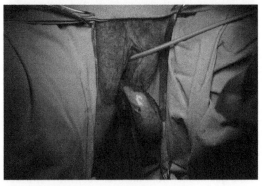

Fig. 21. Extraction of the gallbladder through the vagina.

Vaginal closure

After placing retractors, the hemostasis of the vaginal opening is checked and then closed with a running suture of absorbable 2-0 material (**Fig. 22**).

Postoperative care includes analgesic medications on demand, antiemetics, resumption of diet after 4 hours, and early ambulation. No tampons, topical estrogens, or healing creams or tablets are prescribed; patients are required to refrain from sexual activity for 3 weeks. The postoperative follow-up is performed at postoperative days 7, 30, 60, 120, 180, and 360 for general evaluation and gynecologic assessment (guided questionnaire, physical examination, and colposcopy).

Results

Between August 2007 and July 2013, 320 patients have had a NOTES transvaginal hybrid cholecystectomy at the institution of one of the authors (A.R.F.) (NOSCAR Summit, 2013 Chicago), with the following results.

- The mean time to achieve entrance in the abdominal cavity was 12 ± 4 minutes.
- Average operative time was 62 ± 16.34 minutes.
- The procedure was completed with transvaginal extraction and without complications in 273 patients (95%). In 13 cases, conversion to conventional laparoscopic surgery was required (in 3 owing to impossibility to achieve a transvaginal entrance); in 1 (case 6) a mini-laparotomy was required.
- In 28 cases (10%), an additional 2-mm trocar was placed to aid with retraction of the gallbladder in the right upper quadrant.
- Average pain (analogue visual scale) was 0.7 (for a maximum of 5).
- Length of stay was 20 ± 5.6 hours.
- Return to work was 4.5 days.
- Cosmetic results were considered to be very good.

Complications

The complication rate of the transvaginal approach is low. In this series, no significant complications occurred that can be attributed to the technique, except for 1 case early in the experience. In this patient, case 6, the authors performed a mini-laparotomy for checking hemostasis of the Douglas cul-de-sac.

Regarding the transvaginal removal of the gallbladder, no difficulties were encountered, independent of the size and characteristics of the gallbladder. The authors

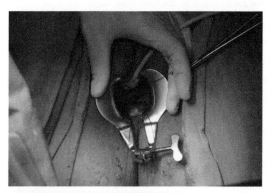

Fig. 22. Closure of the transvaginal opening (detail).

preferred to use an endoscopic polypectomy forceps instead of an endoscopic endo-loop or a transvaginal forceps.

Regarding the functional impact of the transvaginal approach, no dyspareunia or fertility issues were encountered. After complete recovery from the transvaginal procedure and discharge from care, 7 patients became pregnant with normal deliveries. The potential risk of infection may be a disadvantage of this access, but no infections related to the access or to the extraction of the gallbladder through the vaginal opening occurred. This finding is in concordance with those of other investigators.[26] It is clear, however, that this is not an operation appropriate for every surgeon, institution, or patient. Each group should define its goals, and a multidisciplinary team with expertise in laparoscopic surgery, gynecology, and flexible endoscopy must be gathered before any clinical activity.[27]

SINGLE-INCISION LAPAROSCOPIC CHOLECYSTECTOMY

The inherent difficulties encountered with the NOTES access provided the groundwork and served as a bridge for the adoption of single-incision LC.[27] Despite being adopted more widely than NOTES, recent reviews show that there is little evidence to support the enthusiasm for the adoption of single-incision cholecystectomy.[28] Only a few series document and support the clinical benefits of this approach, and it appears that the procedure is associated with a higher rate of incisional hernias.[29] Some centers have been performing robotic-assisted single-incision laparoscopic cholecystectomy. Such an approach seems difficult to justify, given the expense involved and the lack of evidence supporting its benefits.

This technique encompasses basically 2 types of approach: (1) single-incision with insertion of 3 ports, and (2) single port access with a multiport device.[30]

Different acronyms have been used in the literature to define this approach:

- NOTUS: Natural Orifice TransUmbilical Surgery
- SILS: Single-Incision Laparoscopic Surgery
- SIS: Single-Incision Surgery
- LESS: LaparoEndoscopic Single-Site Surgery
- TUES: TransUmbilical Endoscopic Surgery
- Monotrocar/Single-Port Surgery
- OPUS: One-Port Umbilical Surgery
- SPA: Single-Port Access

The procedure can be summarized in the following steps:

1. Incision and trocar placement (Video 21)

2. Gallbladder retraction and exposure (Video 22)

3. Dissection of the hepatic hilum and triangle of Calot (Video 23)

4. Dissection of the gallbladder from the liver bed and control of hemostasis (Video 24)

5. Extraction of the gallbladder (Video 25)

6. Wound closure (Video 26)

Incision and Trocar Placement

- Transumbilical or infraumbilical 2-cm incision after CO_2 insufflation through a Veress needle (Video 21). Three 5-mm trocars are inserted after dissecting both lateral spaces, according to the angles of an upward triangle, in a fashion known as the Mickey Mouse technique. Some prefer to use a 10-mm trocar, which allows the use of a reusable clip applier and the extraction of the gall-bladder. It is recommended to use low-profile trocars to prevent outside crowding, or even a flexible port on the right side of the patient (**Figs. 23 and 24**).

- Transumbilical or infraumbilical 2.5- to 3-cm incision of the fascia and use of different devices with a connecting channel for CO_2 insufflation. One of the less expensive methods consists of the placement of an XS Alexis retractor (Applied Medical, Rancho Santa Margarita, CA, USA) with a glove attached to it. In 3 fingers, 5-mm trocars are fixed and then inserted in the abdomen (**Fig. 25**).
- A third option is to use a commercially available triangulating surgical platform (**Fig. 26**).

Gallbladder Retraction and Exposure

This step is performed in the same fashion as described for the NOTES approach (Video 22).

Dissection of the Hepatic Hilum and Triangle of Calot

These steps can be helped by the use of flexible or reticulating instruments, but can also be performed with standard laparoscopic instruments (Video 23). The authors routinely use a rigid 30° scope, but a flexible-tip scope is useful. The use of 5-mm trocars makes mandatory the use of a 5-mm clip applier.

Dissection of the Gallbladder from the Liver Bed and Control of Hemostasis

This step follows the same rules as apply for the conventional laparoscopic approach (Videos 6 and 24).

Extraction of the Gallbladder

If a 3-trocar approach is used, this step will depend on the use of 10- or 5-mm trocars (Video 25). Sometimes 2 of the trocars' openings need to be connected to allow the extraction of the specimen. With the use of a device, one simply opens it wide enough to allow this step, and performs the extraction through it.

Wound Closure

Particular attention should be paid to this step, to prevent surgical-site infection and/or incisional hernias (Video 26).

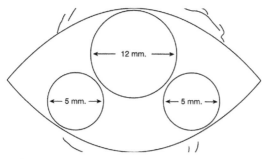

Fig. 23. Positioning of trocars with the Mickey Mouse technique.

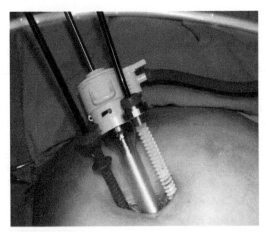

Fig. 24. Single-incision laparoscopic surgery (SILS) technique with one 10-mm trocar, one 5-mm trocar, and one flexible 5-mm trocar.

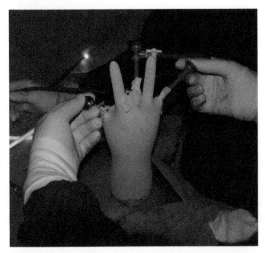

Fig. 25. Poor surgeon's SILS device (I).

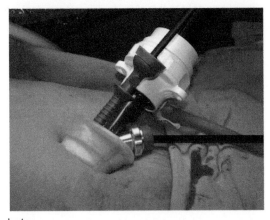

Fig. 26. SILS type device.

SUMMARY

- The gold standard for the surgical treatment of symptomatic cholelithiasis is conventional LC.
- Despite being associated with a slightly higher incidence of BDI in comparison with OC, LC is considered a very safe operation.
- Steps to prevent BDI should be routinely performed in every LC.
- Recent trends include the performance of cholecystectomy through a single incision and NOTES. Although it has been demonstrated that both are feasible approaches, lack of evidence of clinical advantage prevents its widespread adoption, and more data are needed to assess whether its use is warranted.
- OC is mostly reserved for conversions or as part of other major procedures. Training of young surgeons in this approach poses limitations, but the need for adequate training should be stressed.

ACKNOWLEDGMENTS

The authors would like to thank Dr Anibal Rondan (Hospital Carlos Bocalandro, Buenos Aires, Argentina) for his assistance in this article.

SUPPLEMENTARY DATA

Supplementary data related to this article can be found online at http://dx.doi.org/10.1016/j.suc.2014.01.007.

REFERENCES

1. Langenbuch C. Ein fall von exstirpation der gallenblase wegen chronischer cholelithiasis: heilung. Berliner Klin Wochenschr 1882;19:725–7.
2. Muhe E. Die erste cholecystektomie durch das laparoskop. Langenbecks Arch Klin Chir 1986;369:804.
3. Reddick EJ, Olsen DO. Laparoscopic laser cholecystectomy: a comparison with minilap cholecystectomy. Surg Endosc 1989;3:131–3.
4. Navarra G, Pozza E, Occhionorelli S, et al. One-wound laparoscopic cholecystectomy. Br J Surg 1997;84:695.
5. Wg WT, Kong CK, Wong YT. One wound laparoscopic cholecystectomy. Br J Surg 1997;84:1627.
6. Asbun HJ, Rossi RL, Lowell JA, et al. Bile duct injury during laparoscopic cholecystectomy: mechanisms of injury, prevention and management. World J Surg 1993;17:547–52.
7. Strasberg SM, Hertl M, Soper NJ. An analysis of the problem of biliary duct injury during laparoscopic cholecystectomy. J Am Coll Surg 1995;180:101–25.
8. Horgan S, Cullen JP, Talamini M, et al. Natural orifice surgery: initial clinical experience. Surg Endosc 2009;23:1512–8.
9. Senn N. The early history of vaginal hysterectomy. JAMA 1895;XXV(12):476–82.
10. von Ott DO. Die Beleuchtung der Bauchhohle (Ventroskopie) als Methode bei Vaginaler Coeliotomie. Abl Gynakol 1902;231:817–23.
11. Tsin DA, Sequeria RJ, Giannikas G. Culdolaparoscopic cholecystectomy during vaginal hysterectomy. J Soc Laparoendosc Surg 2003;7:171–2.
12. Bessler M, Stevens PD, Milone L, et al. Transvaginal laparoscopically assisted endoscopic cholecystectomy: a hybrid approach to natural orifice surgery. Gastrointest Endosc 2007;66:1243–5.

13. Marescaux J, Dallemagne B, Perretta S, et al. Surgery without scars: report of transluminal cholecystectomy in a human being. Arch Surg 2007;142:823–7.
14. Ramos AC, Murakami A, Galvao Neto M, et al. NOTES transvaginal video-assisted cholecystectomy: first series. Endoscopy 2008;40:572–5.
15. Zorron R, Filgueiras M, Maggioni LC, et al. NOTES transvaginal cholecystectomy: report of the first case. Surg Innov 2007;14:279–83.
16. Ponsky TA, Desagun R, Brody F. Surgical therapy for biliary dyskinesia: a meta-analysis and review of the literature. J Laparoendosc Adv Surg Tech 2005;15: 439–42.
17. Strasberg SM, Brunt LM. Rationale and use of the critical view of safety in laparoscopic cholecystectomy. J Am Coll Surg 2010;211:132–8.
18. Mirizzi PL. La colangiografía durante las operaciones de las vías biliares. Bol Soc Cir Buenos Aires 1932;16:1133–5.
19. Asbun HJ, Rossi RL. Techniques of laparoscopic cholecystectomy: the difficult operation. Surg Clin North Am 1994;74:755–75.
20. Deziel DJ, Millikan KW, Economou SG, et al. Complications of laparoscopic cholecystectomy: a national survey of 4292 hospitals and an analysis of 77604 cases. Am J Surg 1993;165:9–14.
21. Visser BC, Parks RW, Garden OJ. Open cholecystectomy in the laparoscopic era. Am J Surg 2008;195:108–14.
22. McAneny D. Open cholecystectomy. Surg Clin North Am 2008;88:1273–94.
23. Ibrahim S, Hean TK, Ho LS, et al. Risk factors for conversion to open surgery in patients undergoing laparoscopic cholecystectomy. World J Surg 2006;134: 308–10.
24. Dunham R, Sackier JM. Is there a dilemma in adequately training surgeons in both open and laparoscopic biliary surgery. Surg Clin North Am 1994;74:913–21.
25. Lehmann KS, Ritz JP, Wibmer A, et al. The German registry for natural orifice translumenal endoscopic surgery: report of the first 551 patients. Ann Surg 2010;252:263–70.
26. Lomanto D, Chua HC, Myat MM, et al. Microbiological contamination during transgastric and transvaginal technique. J Laparoendosc Adv Surg Tech 2009; 19:465–9.
27. Horgan S, Meireles OR, Jacobsen GR, et al. Broad clinical utilization of NOTES: is it safe? Surg Endosc 2013;27:1872–80.
28. Pfluke JM, Parker M, Stauffer JA, et al. Laparoscopic surgery performed through a single incision: a systematic review of the current literature. J Am Coll Surg 2011;212:113–8.
29. Marks JM, Philips MS, Tacchino R. Single-incision laparoscopic cholecystectomy is associated with improved cosmesis scoring at the cost of significantly higher hernia rates: 1-year results of a prospective, randomized, multicenter single-blinded trial of traditional multiport laparoscopic cholecystectomy vs. single-incision laparoscopic cholecystectomy. J Am Coll Surg 2013;216:1037–48.
30. Curcillo PG, Wu AS, Podolsky ER, et al. Single-port access (SPA) cholecystectomy: a multi-institutional report of the first 297 cases. Surg Endosc 2010;24: 1854–60.

Cholecystitis

Lawrence M. Knab, MD[a], Anne-Marie Boller, MD[b],
David M. Mahvi, MD[b],*

KEYWORDS

- Acute cholecystitis • Chronic cholecystitis • Acalculous cholecystitis • Gallstones
- Cholecystectomy

KEY POINTS

- Disorders of the gallbladder are the most common surgical diseases treated by the general surgeon.
- Risk factors for gallstones include advanced age, female gender, obesity, and certain ethnicities, including North American Indian.
- The gold standard treatment of acute cholecystitis is a laparoscopic cholecystectomy.
- Operating early in the disease course decreases overall hospital days and does not lead to increased complications, conversion to open procedures, or mortality.
- Cholecystitis during pregnancy is a challenging problem for surgeons. Operative intervention is generally safe for both mother and fetus, given the improved morbidity of the laparoscopic approach compared with open, although increased caution should be exercised in women with gallstone pancreatitis.

OVERVIEW

Gallstone disease is an ancient problem. Autopsies on Egyptian mummies have shown gallstones from at least 3500 years ago.[1] Disorders of the gallbladder are the most common surgical diseases treated by a general surgeon. More than 700,000 cholecystectomies are performed in the United States every year, costing about 6.5 billion dollars. This situation makes gallbladder disease the most costly digestive disorder.[2] This article focuses specifically on the pathophysiology, diagnosis, and treatment of acute cholecystitis (calculous and acalculous), as well as chronic cholecystitis.

EPIDEMIOLOGY

It is estimated that 20 to 25 million Americans (10%–15% of the population) have gallstones.[2] Most people with gallstones are asymptomatic.[3] Population-based studies

[a] Department of Surgery, Northwestern University Feinberg School of Medicine, Lurie Building Room 3-250, 303 East Superior Street, Chicago, IL 60611, USA; [b] Department of Surgery, Northwestern University Feinberg School of Medicine, NMH/Arkes Family Pavilion Suite 650, 676 North Saint Clair, Chicago, IL 60611, USA
* Corresponding author. Department of Surgery, Northwestern University Feinberg School of Medicine, NMH/Arkes Family Pavilion Suite 650, 676 North Saint Clair, Chicago, IL 60611.
E-mail address: dmahvi@nmh.org

Surg Clin N Am 94 (2014) 455–470
http://dx.doi.org/10.1016/j.suc.2014.01.005
0039-6109/14/$ – see front matter © 2014 Elsevier Inc. All rights reserved.

suggest that 10% to 18% of those with silent gallstones develop biliary pain and 7% require operative intervention.[4,5] One percent to 4% of those with gallstones develop complications such as acute cholecystitis, gallstone pancreatitis, and choledocholithiasis.[6]

The prevalence of cholelithiasis in North America varies widely depending on ethnicity. North American Indians have a prevalence as high as 73% in women older than 30 years. White Americans have a lower prevalence of gallstones, at 16.6% in women and 7.9% in men. Asian populations have intermediate rates of 5% to 20%, black African Americans have rates of about 14%, and black Africans have low rates, at less than 5%.[2]

Incidence of gallbladder disease increases with age, making this an important issue in our aging population. A study of gallstone prevalence at necropsy in the United Kingdom reported an incidence of gallstones of 24% in women 50 to 59 years old, increasing to 30% in the ninth decade. The rates for men are 18% in the 50-year-old to 59-year-old range, with an increase to 29% in the ninth decade.[7]

RISK FACTORS

The development of cholelithiasis is multifactorial. Advancing age is a risk factor for gallstone development in all ethnic groups. Gallstones are rarely reported in infants and children, but prevalence markedly increases in individuals older than 20 years, particularly in women. Female gender is also a risk factor. Women are at a greater risk of having gallstones as well as undergoing operative intervention. Estrogen seems to play a critical role in this increased risk, because pregnancy, parity, and estrogen replacement therapy all increase the risk of gallstones.[2] Obesity is another risk factor for gallstone development, likely caused by increased hepatic secretion of cholesterol. This risk factor is stronger in women than men. Obese women have a 7-fold increase of developing gallstones compared with their normal weight female counterparts. Ironically, rapid weight loss is also a risk factor for gallstone development and occurs as in as many as 25% to 30% of patients after bariatric surgery.[2]

GALLSTONE FORMATION

The type of gallstone and location in the biliary system vary depending on ethnicity. Most of the gallstones encountered in developed countries are cholesterol stones (about 80%) with a few being pigmented (black stones).

The pathogenesis of cholesterol gallstones is dependent on multiple factors: cholesterol supersaturation in the bile, crystal nucleation, gallbladder dysmotility, and gallbladder absorption.

Pigmented gallstones can be divided into black stones and brown stones. Black stones consist of calcium bilirubinate and mucin glycoproteins.[2] Black stones are generally associated with hemolytic conditions or cirrhosis, which cause increased levels of unconjugated bilirubin.[8] These stones are usually located in the gallbladder. Brown stones are typically associated with bacterial infection, are more prevalent in Asian populations, and are usually located elsewhere in the biliary tree as opposed to the gallbladder.[8]

ACUTE CHOLECYSTITIS

Acute cholecystitis accounts for 14% to 30% of cholecystectomies.[9–11]

Pathophysiology

Acute cholecystitis is defined as inflammation of the gallbladder, generally caused by obstruction of the cystic duct. The most common causes of cystic duct obstruction are gallstones or biliary sludge, although other less common causes include a mass (primary tumor or gallbladder polyp), parasites, or foreign bodies (bullets have been described).[12] Cholecystitis can also occur in the absence of gallstones and is known as acalculous cholecystitis, which is reviewed in a later section.

When the cystic duct is obstructed, the gallbladder mucosa continues to produce mucus but has no outlet for drainage, leading to increased gallbladder pressure, venous stasis, followed by arterial stasis and gallbladder ischemia and necrosis (**Fig. 1**). Necrotic tissue can then lead to complications such as gallbladder perforation and empyema.

Clinical Presentation

Most patients who present with acute cholecystitis have symptoms of right upper quadrant or epigastric abdominal pain. Often, this pain starts as diffuse epigastric abdominal pain and develops a bandlike quality radiating around the back. As gallbladder inflammation worsens, the pain tends to localize in the right upper quadrant. Patients may also describe previous episodes of biliary colic, in which the pain comes in waves (hence the term colic) and is sometimes postprandial, particularly after high-fat meals. Patients often describe being awakened in the middle of the night by the pain. Nausea, vomiting, and anorexia are commonly associated with acute cholecystitis.

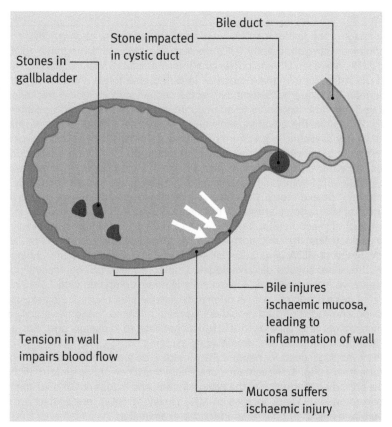

Fig. 1. Pathogenesis of acute cholecystitis secondary to impacted gallstone in the cystic duct. *Arrows* indicate interaction of the ischemic mucosa with bile resulting in inflammation. (*From* Sethi H, Johnson CD. Gallstones. Medicine 2011;39(10):625; with permission.)

Physical examination can show tachycardia and a fever. Patients generally have tenderness to palpation in the epigastric region or right upper quadrant. Some patients may have a Murphy's sign, which is cessation of inspiration with palpation in the right upper quadrant over the gallbladder.

As with most inflammatory conditions, acute cholecystitis is usually associated with leukocytosis, although the presentation can be variable. Only 32% to 53% of patients have a fever on presentation, and 51% to 53% have leukocytosis.[13,14] Evaluation of a group of 103 patients with acute cholecystitis showed that most patients (71%) do not present with a fever within the first 8 hours of arrival to the hospital.[15] Sixty-eight percent of those patients did have a leukocytosis (white blood cells >12,000), and 25% had both a fever and leukocytosis.[15] Of the patients with gangrenous cholecystitis, 41% presented with fever and 73% with leukocytosis.[15] The diagnosis must always be made based on a combination of history, physical findings, laboratory values, and diagnostic imaging if needed.

When a patient presents with symptoms consistent with acute cholecystitis, the possibility of choledocholithiasis must also be entertained, because this can alter operative plans. Relevant clinical findings such as clay-colored stools or dark urine can provide clues. Increased bilirubin and liver enzyme levels and dilated common bile duct on imaging can also indicate choledocholithiasis.

Imaging

Multiple imaging modalities can be used to diagnose acute cholecystitis including transabdominal ultrasonography (US), cholescintigraphy, and magnetic resonance imaging (MRI); however, US and cholescintigraphy are used most frequently. Transabdominal US is the ideal imaging modality to detect gallstones and measure the bile duct diameter. Findings consistent with acute cholecystitis include a thickened gallbladder wall (>4 mm) secondary to edema, gallstones or sludge, and pericholecystic fluid (**Fig. 2**). US has the advantages of being noninvasive, quick, relatively inexpensive, and widely available, even after hours. One major limitation of US is poor visualization when intraluminal gas is present between the probe and the gallbladder.

Cholescintigraphy is an alternative method of imaging and uses technetium-labeled hepatic 2,6-dimethyl-iminodiacetic acid (HIDA). HIDA is injected intravenously, taken up by the liver, and excreted in the bile and is therefore able to visualize the biliary system. A normal scan shows uptake in the liver, gallbladder, bile duct, and duodenum within an hour of injection (**Fig. 3**A). If the cystic duct is obstructed, as typically found in acute cholecystitis, the gallbladder is not visualized on this scan (see **Fig. 3**B). The main advantage of HIDA is its superior sensitivity in diagnosing acute cholecystitis. However, there are several disadvantages. Compared with US, cholescintigraphy is more expensive, time intensive (it takes several hours compared with 10–15 minutes for US), requires skilled staff, and is often not available after hours. It also exposes patients to ionizing radiation and provides information limited to the hepatobiliary system, whereas US and MRI do not expose patients to radiation and can provide added information outside the hepatobiliary system.

MRI is increasingly used for hepatobiliary imaging as the technology and diagnostic accuracy improve (**Fig. 4**). Advantages of MRI are that it can provide information about the whole abdomen in addition to the biliary system, and it does not expose the patient to ionizing radiation. Disadvantages of MRI, similar to HIDA, are limited availability after hours and length of time needed for the examination.

Multiple studies have evaluated the sensitivity and specificity of these diagnostic studies in acute cholecystitis.[16–19] A meta-analysis evaluating US, HIDA, and MRI, showed a range of sensitivities in US from 50% to 100%, with a summary estimate

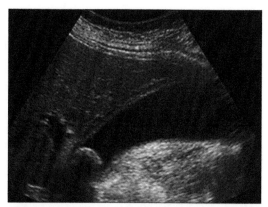

Fig. 2. Acute cholecystitis. Sagittal sonogram showing a single calculus impacted in the neck of the gallbladder. Additional findings include a mildly distended gallbladder and striated wall thickening. (*From* Glanc P, Maxwell C. Acute abdomen in pregnancy: role of sonography. J Ultrasound Med 2010;29(10):1458; with permission.)

of 81%, HIDA with sensitivities from 78% to 100% and a summary estimate of 96%, and MRI with a range of 50% to 91% and a summary estimate of 85%.[16] A head-to-head comparison was evaluated in 11 studies (1199 patients) in the meta-analysis, and again HIDA was found to be significantly superior to US. The sensitivity of HIDA was 94% compared with 80% for US.[16] In most studies, HIDA is significantly more sensitive compared with US and MRI for diagnosing acute cholecystitis.

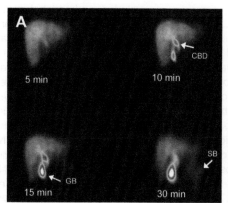
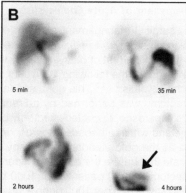

Fig. 3. (*A*) Normal technetium 99m HIDA series. Selected anterior planar images from an HIDA examination show prompt and uniform tracer uptake by the hepatic parenchyma, followed by excretion of activity into the intrahepatic and extrahepatic biliary tree and normal filling of the gallbladder. Activity then proceeds unimpeded into the proximal small bowel. This entire sequence is usually complete within 30 to 60 minutes. CBD, common bile duct; GB, gallbladder; SB, small bowel. (*B*) Acute cholecystitis. Anterior planar images from an HIDA examination show uniform tracer uptake within the hepatic parenchyma followed by rapid clearance of hepatic activity with visualization of the biliary tree and unimpeded flow into the distal small bowel (*arrow*). However, there is nonvisualization of the gallbladder even on delayed imaging up to 4 hours, consistent with acute cholecystitis. (*From* Lambie H, Cook AM, Scarsbrook AF, et al. Tc99m-hepatobiliary iminodiacetic acid (HIDA) scintigraphy in clinical practice. Clin Radiol 2011;66(11):1095–6; with permission.)

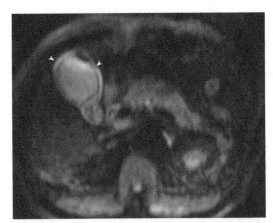

Fig. 4. Diffusion-weighted MRI of abdomen showing acute cholecystitis and pancreatitis; arrowheads indicate gallbladder wall thickening. (*From* Lee NK, Kim S, Kim GH, et al. Diffusion-weighted imaging of biliopancreatic disorders: correlation with conventional magnetic resonance imaging. World J Gastroenterol 2012;18(31):4106; with permission.)

The advantages and disadvantages must be evaluated for each individual patient when deciding which type of imaging to use. If acute cholecystitis is highly suspected, US is likely the ideal choice given its widespread availability, quick administration time, low cost, and patient safety profile. If the diagnosis of acute cholecystitis is in question and 1 imaging study was equivocal, HIDA is likely the better choice, given its superior sensitivity compared with both US and MRI. The role of MRI is emerging as the availability and accuracy both improve.

Management of Acute Cholecystitis

Early surgical management of acute cholecystitis was confined to stone extraction. Cholecystostomy was initially described by Bobbs and Sims and perfected by Kocher and Tait.[20] The first cholecystectomy was performed in 1882 by Carl Langenbuch in Berlin, and for the following 100 years, open cholecystectomy was the gold standard for cholecystitis.[20–22] This gold standard changed after the first laparoscopic cholecystectomy was performed by a French surgeon in 1987. Over the course of a few years, laparoscopic cholecystectomy became more common than open cholecystectomy, and within a decade, laparoscopic cholecystectomy replaced the open equivalent as the gold standard of therapy for acute cholecystitis.[21] Data from Maryland indicate that before the advent of laparoscopy in 1985 the rate of laparoscopic cholecystectomy was 0 patients per 1000 people compared with open cholecystectomy with a rate of 1.65 per 1000 people. Just 7 years later, in 1992, the rate of laparoscopic surgery increased to 1.66 per 1000 people, and the open cholecystectomy rate decreased dramatically to 0.51 per 1000 people.[9] There is little debate that the gold standard treatment of acute cholecystitis is a cholecystectomy, and this has been the case for many years. The laparoscopic approach, as well as the timing of the cholecystectomy, has evolved rapidly over the last 20 years.

Timing of Operation

Two main treatment pathways have been used when dealing with acute cholecystitis. The early cholecystectomy (EC) school of thought endorses performing a cholecystectomy during the initial hospital stay. The idea is to reduce overall hospital stay and prevent subsequent readmissions secondary to cholecystitis or symptomatic cholelithiasis. The delayed cholecystectomy (DC) group endorses treating the patient with antibiotics during the initial hospitalization and performing the cholecystectomy about 4 to 8 weeks after the initial insult. The advantages posited for this approach include operating in a field with less inflammation and therefore less potential for complications and conversion to an open procedure.

Several meta-analyses and randomized control trials have evaluated this question, and most of the data indicate that an EC is safe and results in a shorter overall hospital stay (**Table 1**). The hypothesis that a DC significantly reduces complications and conversion rates has not been validated by existing studies.

One randomized control trial by Lo divided 45 patients into the EC group and 41 patients in the DC group. The EC group underwent a laparoscopic cholecystectomy within 72 hours of admission, and the DC group was managed nonoperatively during the initial hospitalization and readmitted 8 to 12 weeks later for an elective procedure. Twenty percent of the DC group underwent an interval procedure because of failure to respond to initial nonoperative treatment. The EC group had a longer median operative time compared with the DC group (135 minutes vs 105 minutes, respectively) although there was no significant difference in conversion to an open procedure (11% in the EC vs 23% in the DC group).[27] There was no significant difference in morbidity between the 2 groups, although there was a trend toward an increase in complications in the DC group (13% in the EC vs 29% in the DC; $P = .07$). The EC group had a significantly shorter overall hospital stay compared with the DC group (5 days vs 7 days, respectively).[23]

A second randomized control trial by Johansson included 74 patients in the EC group (who underwent operation within 7 days from onset of symptoms) and 71 patients in the DC group (elective operation 6–8 weeks later). In this study, 25% of the DC group underwent an interval procedure because of failure to respond to nonoperative management. There was no significant difference in the operating time or the conversion rates between the 2 groups.[24]

A meta-analysis[28] evaluated 5 randomized control trials with a total of 223 in the EC group and 228 in the DC group. The EC underwent an operation within 1 week of symptom onset, and the DC group underwent an elective operation within 6 to 12 weeks. There was a trend toward increased postoperative bile leak in the EC group compared with the DC group, although no significant difference in postoperative

Table 1
Early versus late cholecystectomy

Reference	Study Type	EC	LC	Operating Room Time (min)	Conversion to Open (%)	Complications (%)	Mortality (%)	Hospital Stay (d)
Lo et al,[23] 1998	RCT	45	41	135 vs 105 ($P = .02$)	11 vs 23 (NS)	13 vs 29 ($P = .07$)	0 vs 0	6 vs 11 ($P<.001$)
Johansson et al,[24] 2003	RCT	74	71	98 vs 100	31 vs 29	No significant difference	0 vs 0	5 vs 8 ($P = .05$)
Lai et al,[25] 1998	RCT	53	51	123 vs 107 ($P = .04$)	-	9 vs 8 (NS)	0 vs 0	7.6 vs 11.6 ($P<.001$)
Kolla et al,[26] 2004	RCT	20	20	104 vs 93 (NS)	25 vs 25 (NS)	20 vs 15 (NS)	0 vs 0	4.1 vs 10.1 ($P = .02$)

Abbreviations: LC, late cholecystectomy; n, number; NS, not significant; RCT, randomized controlled trial.

complications or conversion rate was reported. The overall hospital stay was significantly shorter in the EC group compared with the DC group by 4 days (*P*<.001).

When evaluating these studies, a few trends become apparent. One is that EC in acute cholecystitis is safe and is not associated with a statistically significant increase in complications or conversion rate. Patients who undergo EC also have an overall shorter hospital stay compared with the DC group. In the DC group, there are many patients (about 20%) who require emergency surgery for persistent symptoms and are therefore at increased risk for conversion to an open procedure.

TYPE OF OPERATION
Laparoscopic Cholecystectomy

As mentioned earlier, laparoscopic cholecystectomy is the gold standard treatment of acute cholecystitis. The shift from open to laparoscopic cholecystectomy occurred in the late 1980s. As surgeon training progressed in laparoscopy, many surgeons started using a single-incision approach known as single-incision laparoscopic cholecystectomy (SILC). The advantages of SILC include the advantages of conventional multiport laparoscopic cholecystectomy (CMLC) over the open approach, as well as theoretic improved cosmetic result and decreased postoperative pain secondary to a decreased incision length; however, neither of these parameters has been consistently validated in the literature. The main disadvantages of SILC are increased operative time, which can lead to increased intraoperative blood loss and hospital stay, as well as increased overall costs compared with conventional laparoscopic surgery.

Many studies evaluating SILC exclude patients with acute cholecystitis. The inflammatory condition inherent in acute cholecystitis tends to make an already challenging laparoscopic dissection and critical view of safety even more difficult when facing the added technical considerations of a single port. One study evaluating risk factors for prolonged operating time in SILC using multivariate analysis found that acute cholecystitis and body mass index were independent risk factors.[29] In addition, prolonged operating time was associated with statistically significant intraoperative blood loss and hospital length of stay.[29] A review evaluating 30 studies showed that acute cholecystitis was a significant risk factor for SILC failure, with a success rate of 60% in SILC studies including patients with acute cholecystitis versus 93% success in those studies excluding acute cholecystitis.[30]

A prospective randomized trial with 79 patients (about 25% with acute cholecystitis) who underwent either SILC or CMLC reported a statistically significant increase in overall cost associated with the SILC group compared with the CMLC ($2100 more, on average). Several quality-of-life measures were evaluated, including postoperative pain (followed out to 6 months), body image impact, and satisfaction with cosmetic results, and no statistically significant differences were found.[31]

A meta-analysis[32] that evaluated 12 randomized prospective trials (only 2 included patients with acute cholecystitis) comparing SILC with CMLC reported that mean operating time was significantly increased in the SILC group compared with the CMLC group (63 vs 46 minutes, respectively), and the conversion rate to laparotomy was similar. The pain scores 6 hours and 24 hours postoperatively were not statistically significant between the 2 groups, and although the length of hospital stay for the SILC group trended toward being less than the CMLC group (2.0 days vs 2.2 days), the difference was not significant. There were no significant differences in postoperative morbidity, bleeding, incisional hernias, or surgical site infections. Only 3 studies investigated patient satisfaction with cosmetic outcome, and based on survey results, the SILC patients reported statistically significant improved cosmetic results.

Using SILC in patients with acute cholecystitis should be approached with caution. Although technically possible, SILC often results in increased operative time, blood loss, and overall expense, without a clear advantage in postoperative pain or decreased hospital stay.

Open Cholecystectomy

Laparoscopic cholecystectomy has replaced open cholecystectomy as the gold standard treatment of acute cholecystitis, and many reported studies have repeatedly proved the safety of the procedure after initial skepticism about bile duct injury rates. These studies have reported bile duct injury rates ranging between about 0.3% and 0.4% after accounting for the initial learning curve after the introduction of the laparoscopic cholecystectomy.[33–35] Studies have also shown similar morbidity and mortality between laparoscopic and open surgery and decreased length of hospital stay and postoperative pain.[21,36] We argue that 100% of operations for acute cholecystitis should be initiated laparoscopically. The surgeon must be aware of the variable biliary anatomy (**Fig. 5**) and ensure a critical view of safety. The critical view of safety is a view of the gallbladder after dissection showing only 2 structures entering the gallbladder: the cystic artery and cystic duct (**Fig. 6**). If it is determined that the operation cannot be completed safely and the critical view of safety not obtained via a laparoscopic dissection, conversion to an open operation is always an option. In some of the most experienced hands, conversion to an open procedure occurs in about 1% to 2% of patients undergoing an elective procedure, although the rate increases in acute cholecystitis.[37,38] There is little downside to an attempt at laparoscopy in a patient without previous upper abdominal surgery. A less frequent indication to convert to an open procedure is concern for gallbladder malignancy.

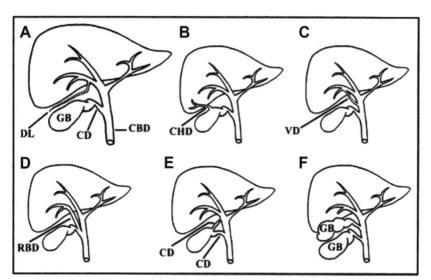

Fig. 5. Schematic view of main variations of the biliary system anatomy in the triangle of Calot and the gallbladder fossa. (*A*) Duct of Luschka (DL), (*B*) cystohepatic duct (CHD), (*C*) vaginali ductuli (VD), (*D*) variant drainage of right posterior sector, (*E*) duplication of cystic duct (CD), (*F*) duplication of gallbladder (GB). CBD, common bile duct; RBD, right bile duct. (*From* Sharif K, de Ville de Goyet J. Bile duct of Luschka leading to bile leak after cholecystectomy–revisiting the biliary anatomy. J Pediatr Surg 2003;38(11):E22; with permission.)

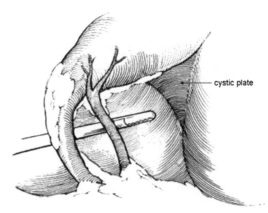

cystic plate

Fig. 6. Critical view of safety, showing only the cystic duct and artery entering directly into the gallbladder with the bottom of the liver bed visible. (*From* Strasberg SM, Hertl M, Soper NJ. An analysis of the problem of biliary injury during laparoscopic cholecystectomy. J Am Coll Surg 1995;180(1):113; with permission.)

Intraoperative Imaging of the Common Bile Duct

Intraoperative imaging of the common bile duct is a widely debated topic among surgeons. Surgeons perform intraoperative cholangiograms routinely, selectively, or not at all. There are 2 main reasons to perform intraoperative imaging of the biliary anatomy: to delineate the relevant anatomy when there is question during the dissection and to evaluate the presence of common bile duct stones. Many surgeons agree that those patients who present with clinical evidence, laboratory values, or imaging consistent with choledocholithiasis, including gallstone pancreatitis, jaundice, increased liver enzyme levels, or a dilated common bile duct, should undergo common bile duct evaluation by some method. There are varying strategies to evaluate the common bile duct perioperatively, including preoperative or postoperative endoscopic retrograde cholangiopancreatography, magnetic resonance cholangiopancreatography, or intraoperative imaging modalities, including cholangiography or US. The most efficient and cost-effective method varies according to the resources available at any given institution and must be individualized.

For those patients with no preoperative evidence of common bile duct stones, the decision to evaluate the common bile duct is controversial. In a series of patients undergoing laparoscopic cholecystectomy with routine intraoperative cholangiography and no preoperative evidence of common bile duct stones, 4% had common bile duct stones.[39,40] The false-positive rate was between 0.8% and 1.6%.[39] In a series of patients undergoing laparoscopic cholecystectomy with selective intraoperative cholangiography and no preoperative evidence of choledocholithiasis, only about 0.6% became symptomatic from retained common bile duct stones.[39] These data suggest that only about 15% of silent retained common duct stones cause symptoms. The decision to proceed with intraoperative biliary imaging should be based on a patient's risk factors and presentation.

ACALCULOUS CHOLECYSTITIS
Pathophysiology

Acalculous cholecystitis (ACC) differs from calculous acute cholecystitis because it is not precipitated by occlusion of the cystic duct by gallstones or biliary sludge. Two percent to 15% of patients with acute cholecystitis do not have stone disease.[41] ACC is generally the result of biliary stasis and gallbladder ischemia, although the pathophysiology has yet to be determined and is likely multifactorial. It is often associated with critical illness, such as septic shock, severe trauma, burns, and major nonbiliary operations.[41] Biliary stasis can also be a precipitating cause as a result of prolonged fasting or hyperalimentation. ACC has been associated with mortality as high as 41%.[42]

ACC is associated with an increased frequency of gallbladder complications, such as gallbladder perforation, gangrenous gallbladder, and emphysematous gallbladder. Reports indicate that 40% to 100% of patients presenting with ACC have one of these complications.[41]

Clinical Presentation

ACC can be difficult to diagnose, because the clinical manifestations are varied and often nondescript. Patients can present in a similar fashion to acute calculous cholecystitis with right upper quadrant abdominal pain, nausea, vomiting, anorexia, and fever, although sometimes, the main complaint is vague abdominal pain. In the critically ill setting, a high index of suspicion must be maintained, because ACC is often a diagnosis of exclusion in a critically ill patient with persistent fevers and leukocytosis. ACC can result in rapid decompensation and mortality.

Imaging

Imaging modalities in ACC are similar to those of acute calculous cholecystitis, with US findings of gallbladder wall thickening, pericholecystic fluid, and a distended gallbladder, although no gallstones or biliary sludge are present. In critically ill patients with cardiac or renal insufficiency, gallbladder wall edema may be secondary to fluid overload, and interpretation of transabdominal US can be difficult. In these scenarios, an HIDA scan can be more efficacious.

TREATMENT

The preferred treatment of ACC is cholecystectomy, although many patients diagnosed with ACC are poor surgical candidates. Often, a temporizing percutaneous cholecystostomy is performed, with the plan for a subsequent cholecystectomy once the patient has improved clinically and is fit to undergo an operation.

There is, of course, debate as to which patients are operative candidates and when cholecystostomy should be used instead of cholecystectomy. The literature on this topic is varied and difficult to analyze, given the disparities between treatment groups and the mixing of patients with calculous cholecystitis and ACC. Some studies show increased perioperative morbidity and complications with cholecystectomy[43] and others with percutaneous cholecystostomy.[44] Most of these studies do not include enough patients to meaningfully determine survival rates. One study evaluated nationwide outcomes of percutaneous cholecystostomy for both calculous cholecystitis and ACC. More than 58,000 ACC cases were included, and multivariate analyses indicated that those who underwent a percutaneous cholecystostomy had decreased odds of complications, although they had increased risk of mortality, length of hospital stay, and overall expense.[45] This study suggests that older patients with increased comorbidities tend to undergo cholecystostomy and that more patients should be considered for cholecystectomy. If the patient is a surgical candidate, a cholecystectomy should be performed, because this generally leads to overall less hospital length of stay, decreased expense, and complication rates, and mortality has not been shown to be increased. If a patient is not a surgical candidate, a percutaneous cholecystostomy is a useful option, but many patients are readmitted with biliary complications and require a cholecystectomy at a later time.

CHRONIC CHOLECYSTITIS

Chronic cholecystitis and biliary colic account for 79% of cholecystectomies.[10]

Pathophysiology

Chronic cholecystitis occurs when a patient develops repeated occurrences of gallbladder inflammation, leading to gradual scarring and gallbladder dysfunction.[46] The most common cause is gallstones intermittently obstructing the cystic duct, leading to biliary colic or episodic waves of epigastric pain and discomfort. The cystic duct is commonly obstructed for some time, leading to gallbladder distention and inflammation, followed by relief of the obstruction (the stone or sludge no longer obstructs the cystic duct) and cessation of pain. This cycle can be repeated for months or years, leading to a chronic gallbladder inflammation and scarring. Histologically, chronic cholecystitis can be characterized by an increase in subepithelial and subserosal fibrosis, as well as a mononuclear cell infiltrate secondary to this chronic inflammation.[46]

Clinical Presentation

Similar to acute cholecystitis, the most common presenting symptom of chronic cholecystitis is pain. As described earlier in the section on pathophysiology, chronic cholecystitis is often caused by repeated inflammatory episodes, and patients often report episodes of biliary colic, which can last for hours at a time followed by a pain-free period. These episodes are generally described as epigastric or right upper quadrant pain, which can radiate to the back. Nausea, vomiting, and anorexia can also be associated with these episodes. Chronic cholecystitis and acute cholecystitis are a spectrum of diseases, and an episode of biliary colic caused by cystic duct obstruction can precipitate acute cholecystitis if the obstruction is not relieved. Many patients who present with chronic cholecystitis do not have pain at the time of presentation but endorse the characteristic history. Physical examination is often unremarkable as well, unless the patient is experiencing pain.

Imaging

Transabdominal US is the main imaging modality used to diagnose chronic cholecystitis. Most patients with chronic cholecystitis have evidence of gallstones on US. These imaging findings combined with a history of abdominal pain consistent with biliary colic are generally diagnostic of biliary colic and chronic cholecystitis.

Management

The treatment of chronic cholecystitis is an elective cholecystectomy. Most patients with typical biliary symptoms and gallstones on imaging have improvement of symptoms after a cholecystectomy.

SPECIAL CONSIDERATIONS: ACUTE CHOLECYSTITIS IN PREGNANCY

Gallstone-related disease remains the second most common nongynecologic condition requiring surgery in pregnant patients (acute appendicitis is more prevalent).[47] Acute cholecystitis in pregnancy presents a challenging clinical scenario, which has been the cause of some debate regarding surgical management in this patient population. The surgical dogma advocated by many surgeons in the past has been to pursue nonoperative management of pregnant patients until after delivery, when a cholecystectomy can be performed without risk to the fetus. This treatment algorithm has been challenged in recent years, because laparoscopic cholecystectomy has proved to be a safe operation, which is tolerated well in most patient populations.

Pregnant patients are at increased risk of developing gallstones, because of increased levels of estrogen and progesterone. Estrogen increases cholesterol secretion and progesterone decreases bile acid secretion as well as decreasing gallbladder contractility caused by smooth muscle inhibition.[48] Gallstones have been reported in as many as 1% to 3% of pregnant patients and biliary sludge in as many as 30%, although acute cholecystitis is not more common in pregnancy. About 0.1% of pregnant patients develop acute cholecystitis.[48]

There are no prospective randomized trials comparing nonoperative management and cholecystectomy in pregnant women with acute cholecystitis. A comprehensive literature search that evaluated a total of 277 laparoscopic cholecystectomies performed during pregnancy showed a fetal demise rate of 2.2%. Of the 6 reported cases of fetal demise, 4 of the cases involved gallstone pancreatitis.[49] The reported fetal death rates after nonoperative management are varied and range from 0% to 12%. One report indicated a 12% fetal death rate after nonoperative management of biliary colic and acute cholecystitis and an increase to 60% if gallstone pancreatitis developed.[50] An additional factor to consider aside from fetal death rates is the added morbidity of recurrent episodes of biliary colic and cholecystitis in those women treated nonoperatively. Individual reports indicate a wide variability in relapse rate. One study reported recurrence rates of 92%, 64%, and 44% in the first, second, and third trimesters, respectively.[51] Another study reported lower rates of 20%, 45%, and 35% in the first, second, and third trimesters, respectively.[47] In this series, the rates of premature contractions, labor induction for treatment, and preterm delivery were all higher in the nonoperative group compared with the cholecystectomy group.

SUMMARY

It is estimated that up to 15% of the American population have gallstones, and disorders of the gallbladder are the most common diseases confronting general surgeons. It is important for general surgeons to be aware that EC for acute cholecystitis has been shown to decrease overall hospital days without leading to increased complications, mortality, or conversion to open procedures. Although cholecystitis is one of the most common general surgical diseases, variations in cause, clinical presentation, and severity require that surgeons fully understand the disease process and treatment approaches.

REFERENCES

1. Stinton LM, Myers RP, Shaffer EA. Epidemiology of gallstones. Gastroenterol Clin North Am 2010;39(2):157–69, vii.
2. Shaffer EA. Gallstone disease: epidemiology of gallbladder stone disease. Best Pract Res Clin Gastroenterol 2006;20(6):981–96.
3. Halldestam I, Enell EL, Kullman E, et al. Development of symptoms and complications in individuals with asymptomatic gallstones. Br J Surg 2004;91(6):734–8.
4. McSherry CK, Ferstenberg H, Calhoun WF, et al. The natural history of diagnosed gallstone disease in symptomatic and asymptomatic patients. Ann Surg 1985;202(1):59–63.

5. Ransohoff DF, Gracie WA, Wolfenson LB, et al. Prophylactic cholecystectomy or expectant management for silent gallstones. A decision analysis to assess survival. Ann Intern Med 1983;99(2):199–204.

6. Riall TS, Zhang D, Townsend CM Jr, et al. Failure to perform cholecystectomy for acute cholecystitis in elderly patients is associated with increased morbidity, mortality, and cost. J Am Coll Surg 2010;210(5):668–77, 677–9.

7. Bates T, Harrison M, Lowe D, et al. Longitudinal study of gall stone prevalence at necropsy. Gut 1992;33(1):103–7.

8. Venneman NG, van Erpecum KJ. Pathogenesis of gallstones. Gastroenterol Clin North Am 2010;39(2):171–83, vii.

9. Steiner CA, Bass EB, Talamini MA, et al. Surgical rates and operative mortality for open and laparoscopic cholecystectomy in Maryland. N Engl J Med 1994; 330(6):403–8.

10. Orlando R 3rd, Russell JC, Lynch J, et al. Laparoscopic cholecystectomy. A statewide experience. The Connecticut Laparoscopic Cholecystectomy Registry. Arch Surg 1993;128(5):494–8 [discussion: 498–9].

11. Pulvirenti E, Toro A, Gagner M, et al. Increased rate of cholecystectomies performed with doubtful or no indications after laparoscopy introduction: a single center experience. BMC Surg 2013;13:17.

12. Petersen JM, Knight TT. Gunshot cholecystitis. J Clin Gastroenterol 1995;21(4): 320–2.

13. Raine PA, Gunn AA. Acute cholecystitis. Br J Surg 1975;62(9):697–700.

14. Hafif A, Gutman M, Kaplan O, et al. The management of acute cholecystitis in elderly patients. Am Surg 1991;57(10):648–52.

15. Gruber PJ, Silverman RA, Gottesfeld S, et al. Presence of fever and leukocytosis in acute cholecystitis. Ann Emerg Med 1996;28(3):273–7.

16. Kiewiet JJ, Leeuwenburgh MM, Bipat S, et al. A systematic review and meta-analysis of diagnostic performance of imaging in acute cholecystitis. Radiology 2012;264(3):708–20.

17. Kalimi R, Gecelter GR, Caplin D, et al. Diagnosis of acute cholecystitis: sensitivity of sonography, cholescintigraphy, and combined sonography-cholescintigraphy. J Am Coll Surg 2001;193(6):609–13.

18. Chatziioannou SN, Moore WH, Ford PV, et al. Hepatobiliary scintigraphy is superior to abdominal ultrasonography in suspected acute cholecystitis. Surgery 2000;127(6):609–13.

19. Gill PT, Dillon E, Leahy AL, et al. Ultrasonography, HIDA scintigraphy or both in the diagnosis of acute cholecystitis? Br J Surg 1985;72(4):267–8.

20. Hardy KJ. Carl Langenbuch and the Lazarus Hospital: events and circumstances surrounding the first cholecystectomy. Aust N Z J Surg 1993;63(1): 56–64.

21. Soper NJ, Stockmann PT, Dunnegan DL, et al. Laparoscopic cholecystectomy. The new 'gold standard'? Arch Surg 1992;127(8):917–21 [discussion: 921–3].

22. Beal JM. Historical perspective of gallstone disease. Surg Gynecol Obstet 1984; 158(2):181–9.

23. Lo CM, Liu CL, Fan ST, et al. Prospective randomized study of early versus delayed laparoscopic cholecystectomy for acute cholecystitis. Ann Surg 1998; 227(4):461–7.

24. Johansson M, Thune A, Blomqvist A, et al. Management of acute cholecystitis in the laparoscopic era: results of a prospective, randomized clinical trial. J Gastrointest Surg 2003;7(5):642–5.

25. Lai PB, Kwong KH, Leung KL, et al. Randomized trial of early versus delayed laparoscopic cholecystectomy for acute cholecystitis. Br J Surg 1998;85(6): 764–7.
26. Kolla SB, Aggarwal S, Kumar A, et al. Early versus delayed laparoscopic cholecystectomy for acute cholecystitis: a prospective randomized trial. Surg Endosc 2004;18(9):1323–7.
27. Skouras C, Jarral O, Deshpande R, et al. Is early laparoscopic cholecystectomy for acute cholecystitis preferable to delayed surgery?: Best evidence topic (BET). Int J Surg 2012;10(5):250–8.
28. Gurusamy K, Samraj K, Gluud C, et al. Meta-analysis of randomized controlled trials on the safety and effectiveness of early versus delayed laparoscopic cholecystectomy for acute cholecystitis. Br J Surg 2010;97(2):141–50.
29. Sato N, Yabuki K, Shibao K, et al. Risk factors for a prolonged operative time in a single-incision laparoscopic cholecystectomy. HPB (Oxford) 2014;16(2):177–82.
30. Antoniou SA, Pointner R, Granderath FA. Single-incision laparoscopic cholecystectomy: a systematic review. Surg Endosc 2011;25(2):367–77.
31. Leung D, Yetasook AK, Carbray J, et al. Single-incision surgery has higher cost with equivalent pain and quality-of-life scores compared with multiple-incision laparoscopic cholecystectomy: a prospective randomized blinded comparison. J Am Coll Surg 2012;215(5):702–8.
32. Pisanu A, Reccia I, Porceddu G, et al. Meta-analysis of prospective randomized studies comparing single-incision laparoscopic cholecystectomy (SILC) and conventional multiport laparoscopic cholecystectomy (CMLC). J Gastrointest Surg 2012;16(9):1790–801.
33. Z'Graggen K, Wehrli H, Metzger A, et al. Complications of laparoscopic cholecystectomy in Switzerland. A prospective 3-year study of 10,174 patients. Swiss Association of Laparoscopic and Thoracoscopic Surgery. Surg Endosc 1998; 12(11):1303–10.
34. Nuzzo G, Giuliante F, Giovannini I, et al. Bile duct injury during laparoscopic cholecystectomy: results of an Italian national survey on 56 591 cholecystectomies. Arch Surg 2005;140(10):986–92.
35. Fletcher DR, Hobbs MS, Tan P, et al. Complications of cholecystectomy: risks of the laparoscopic approach and protective effects of operative cholangiography: a population-based study. Ann Surg 1999;229(4):449–57.
36. Lillemoe KD, Lin JW, Talamini MA, et al. Laparoscopic cholecystectomy as a "true" outpatient procedure: initial experience in 130 consecutive patients. J Gastrointest Surg 1999;3(1):44–9.
37. Wu JS, Dunnegan DL, Luttmann DR, et al. The evolution and maturation of laparoscopic cholecystectomy in an academic practice. J Am Coll Surg 1998; 186(5):554–60 [discussion: 560–1].
38. Lau H, Brooks DC. Transitions in laparoscopic cholecystectomy: the impact of ambulatory surgery. Surg Endosc 2002;16(2):323–6.
39. Metcalfe MS, Ong T, Bruening MH, et al. Is laparoscopic intraoperative cholangiogram a matter of routine? Am J Surg 2004;187(4):475–81.
40. Khan OA, Balaji S, Branagan G, et al. Randomized clinical trial of routine on-table cholangiography during laparoscopic cholecystectomy. Br J Surg 2011; 98(3):362–7.
41. Ryu JK, Ryu KH, Kim KH. Clinical features of acute acalculous cholecystitis. J Clin Gastroenterol 2003;36(2):166–9.
42. Kalliafas S, Ziegler DW, Flancbaum L, et al. Acute acalculous cholecystitis: incidence, risk factors, diagnosis, and outcome. Am Surg 1998;64(5):471–5.

43. Melloul E, Denys A, Demartines N, et al. Percutaneous drainage versus emergency cholecystectomy for the treatment of acute cholecystitis in critically ill patients: does it matter? World J Surg 2011;35(4):826–33.

44. Abi-Haidar Y, Sanchez V, Williams SA, et al. Revisiting percutaneous cholecystostomy for acute cholecystitis based on a 10-year experience. Arch Surg 2012; 147(5):416–22.

45. Anderson JE, Chang DC, Talamini MA. A nationwide examination of outcomes of percutaneous cholecystostomy compared with cholecystectomy for acute cholecystitis, 1998-2010. Surg Endosc 2013;27(9):3406–11.

46. Mulholland MW, Lillemoe K, Doherty GM, et al. Greenfield's surgery: scientific principles and practice. 4th edition. Philadelphia: Lippincott Williams & Wilkins; 2006. p. 2277.

47. Lu EJ, Curet MJ, El-Sayed YY, et al. Medical versus surgical management of biliary tract disease in pregnancy. Am J Surg 2004;188(6):755–9.

48. Gilo NB, Amini D, Landy HJ. Appendicitis and cholecystitis in pregnancy. Clin Obstet Gynecol 2009;52(4):586–96.

49. Jelin EB, Smink DS, Vernon AH, et al. Management of biliary tract disease during pregnancy: a decision analysis. Surg Endosc 2008;22(1):54–60.

50. Muench J, Albrink M, Serafini F, et al. Delay in treatment of biliary disease during pregnancy increases morbidity and can be avoided with safe laparoscopic cholecystectomy. Am Surg 2001;67(6):539–42 [discussion: 542–3].

51. Swisher SG, Schmit PJ, Hunt KK, et al. Biliary disease during pregnancy. Am J Surg 1994;168(6):576–9 [discussion: 580–1].

Postscript

The following article is an addition to Acute Care Surgery, the February 2014 issue of *Surgical Clinics of North America* (Volume 94, number 1).

Small Bowel and Colon Perforation

Carlos V.R. Brown, MD

KEYWORDS

- Small bowel • Large bowel • Colon • Intestine • Perforation • Peritonitis
- Pneumoperitoneum

KEY POINTS

- For patients with small bowel and colonic perforations, a definitive diagnosis of the cause of perforation is not necessary before operation.
- Bowel obstruction and inflammatory bowel disease are the most common causes of non-traumatic intestinal perforations in industrialized countries, whereas infectious causes of intestinal perforations are more common in developing countries.
- Treatment of small bowel and colonic perforations generally includes intravenous antibiotics and fluid resuscitation, but the specific management of the bowel depends on the underlying cause of the perforation.

INTRODUCTION

Nontraumatic perforations of the small bowel and colon are relatively uncommon. The clinical presentation and diagnosis of intestinal perforation are fairly consistent and straightforward. However, causes of nontraumatic intestinal perforation are quite varied. Management typically involves intravenous antibiotics, resuscitation, and either primary repair or resection and reanastomosis, depending on the underlying cause of the perforation. The following section describes the common causes and treatment options for various types of nontraumatic small bowel and colonic perforations.

CLINICAL PRESENTATION/EXAMINATION

Regardless of the cause, clinical presentation for small and large bowel perforation should be relatively consistent. Patients will typically present with the acute onset of abdominal pain that is persistent, progressive, and unremitting. Severity of the pain will depend on the type and amount of intestinal contents released into the peritoneal cavity. Patients may have associated symptoms including fever, nausea, and vomiting. On physical examination, a patient with intestinal perforation will typically manifest diffuse tenderness to palpation and peritonitis.

University Medical Center Brackenridge, 601 East 15th Street, Austin, TX 78701, USA
E-mail address: CVRBrown@seton.org

Surg Clin N Am 94 (2014) 471–475
http://dx.doi.org/10.1016/j.suc.2014.01.010   **surgical.theclinics.com**

DIAGNOSTIC PROCEDURES

Most patients with intestinal perforation will present with diffuse peritonitis and little if any diagnostic evaluation is necessary. Laboratory tests, including complete blood count, serum chemistries, and arterial blood gas, are nonspecific but may be helpful in guiding preoperative resuscitation. If the diagnosis is in question, an acute abdominal series may show pneumoperitoneum, confirming diagnosis of intestinal perforation. If there is still a diagnostic dilemma, computed tomography can be obtained as a confirmatory study. However, in the setting of intestinal perforation, a definitive diagnosis of the cause of perforation is not necessary before operation.

CAUSES AND TREATMENT
Mechanical Obstruction

In industrialized countries bowel obstruction is a leading cause of intestinal perforation. Small bowel obstruction is typically caused by adhesive disease, hernia, or intraluminal mass, whereas colonic obstruction is caused by a mass, volvulus, or stricture.[1,2] In the context of intestinal perforation, an untreated small bowel obstruction will lead to proximal bowel dilation, venous outflow obstruction, and eventually bowel wall ischemia and perforation. This process may be accelerated in the setting of a closed loop obstruction of the small bowel, as in the case of an incarcerated hernia. Treatment of perforation as a result of small bowel obstruction will usually require a small bowel resection and primary anastomosis, as the perforated segment will be dilated and relatively ischemic. In addition, the cause of obstruction (adhesion, hernia, mass) should be addressed at the same operation. Colonic obstruction follows a similar pathophysiology but in a more consistent fashion. As the proximal colon dilates, the mural tension across the bowel increases as radius increases, according to Laplace's law. Because the cecum has the largest radius, it is the most likely part of the colon to become dilated and ischemic and subsequently perforate. Colonic perforation due to distal obstruction will usually require resection of the colonic segment proximal to the obstruction. Colonic perforation as a result of a rectosigmoid obstruction due to mass or stricture will most often require a subtotal colectomy as the proximal colon will be thin, friable, and not amenable to primary repair. Decisions regarding primary anastomosis versus end ileostomy depend on the condition of the patient and the integrity of the two ends of bowel.

Inflammatory Bowel Disease

Inflammatory bowel disease, both Crohn's disease and ulcerative colitis, may lead to small and large bowel perforation. Crohn's disease of the small and large bowel is typically a chronic disease involving transmural inflammation of the bowel wall. Intestinal perforation as a result of Crohn's disease usually results during an acute exacerbation and will most commonly occur just proximal to a strictured segment of bowel.[3] Although intestinal perforation as a result of Crohn's disease is uncommon, perforation remains a continued cause for acute surgical intervention in patients with inflammatory bowel disease. Perforation of the small or large bowel secondary to Crohn's disease requires resection and primary anastomosis, making sure to resect the grossly diseased segment of bowel. The most extreme form of acute exacerbation of colonic inflammatory bowel disease comes in the form of toxic colitis or toxic megacolon. Toxic megacolon is typically caused by ulcerative colitis but may result from Crohn's disease as well. Similar to obstructive disease of the colon, perforation in the setting of toxic megacolon will usually occur in the cecum. Toxic megacolon with perforation should be treated with subtotal colectomy with end ileostomy.

Diverticular Disease

Diverticulitis is the most common cause of colonic perforation.[4] Sigmoid diverticulitis occurs as a result of diverticular obstruction, inflammation, microperforation, and infection. Although most cases of sigmoid diverticulitis are mild and can be managed without an operation, the most severe forms of the disease may result in free perforation that requires prompt surgical intervention. Colonic perforation as a result of diverticulitis can be managed with sigmoid resection, oversewing of the rectal stump, and end descending colostomy or with resection and primary anastomosis. Although there are proponents for both approaches until there are randomized trials, the treatment of perforated sigmoid diverticulitis will need to be based on clinical judgment, taking into account patient age, physiologic status, comorbidities, and an understanding that a "temporary" colostomy may actually be permanent in a significant percentage of patients. Laparoscopic irrigation and drainage has recently developed as a treatment option for patients with acute perforated diverticulitis, although only a small number of studies have been published to date.[5] Perforation as a result of diverticular disease of the small bowel is much less common, but a Meckel's diverticulum may be complicated by acute inflammation and perforation.[6] Diverticulectomy can be performed if the Meckel's perforates at its tip, whereas segmental bowel resection with primary anastomosis should be performed if the perforation occurs at the base of the diverticulum or the bowel wall proper. In addition, segmental bowel resection should be performed if there is ectopic mucosa associated with the diverticulum.

Ischemia

Primary visceral ischemia is a relatively uncommon disease and an uncommon cause of bowel perforation. Acute mesenteric ischemia may be caused by arterial embolism, arterial thrombosis, venous thrombosis, or nonocclusive ischemic disease. Patients with acute mesenteric ischemia will typically present with severe abdominal pain long before perforation ensues, but a delay in presentation or diagnosis may lead to transmural bowel wall ischemia and perforation.[7] Treatment of perforation due to acute mesenteric ischemia involves segmental resection of diseased segment of bowel and definitive management of underlying vascular cause if treatable. A primary anastomosis may be performed if the remaining bowel is healthy and viable. However, if the remaining bowel is questionable, it may be left in discontinuity. Either way, a second-look operation should be considered to assess the viability of the remaining bowel.

Radiation Enteritis

Radiation therapy for pelvic malignancy (prostate, cervical, endometrial, bladder, rectum) is common. Virtually all patients who receive pelvic radiation will sustain some form of radiation injury to the bowel, typically the ileum and rectum.[8] However, the subsequent radiation enteritis either is asymptomatic or can be controlled with medical therapy. Although radiation enteritis is rarely associated with intestinal perforation (usually involving the distal ileum), management of patients with perforation as a result of radiation injury can present a challenge because much of the bowel surrounding the perforation may have sustained radiation injury as well. Treatment of perforation in the context of radiation enteritis involves resection of the perforated segment and in most situations a primary anastomosis. If the remaining bowel is too diseased for anastomosis, exteriorizing the two ends of bowel may be considered.

Foreign Body

Intestinal perforation secondary to intraluminal foreign body is relatively uncommon, because most foreign bodies will transit the gastrointestinal tract without sequelae.[9] Foreign bodies prone to cause intestinal perforation are typically long, hard, and sharp and may include toothpicks, or fish or chicken bones. If the foreign body perforation is small and the edges are clean, the bowel may be repaired primarily. Otherwise a segmental resection and primary anastomosis should be performed.

Infectious

Infectious causes of intestinal perforation are far more common in developing countries[10–12] and immunocompromised patients. Infectious diseases such as typhoid and tuberculosis are the most common cause of intestinal perforation in developing countries, whereas viral enteritis (particularly cytomegalovirus) is a potential cause of intestinal perforation in the immunocompromised patient.[13] Intestinal perforations caused by infection usually occur in the terminal ileum but viral enteritis may cause right-sided colonic perforations as well. Perforations caused by an infectious cause should be treated with segmental resection of the diseased segment of bowel. Most situations will allow a primary anastomosis but, depending on patient condition, degree of contamination, and integrity of the remaining bowel, exteriorization of the remaining bowel may be considered.

SUMMARY

Nontraumatic perforations of the small intestine and colon are uncommon. Mechanical obstruction and inflammatory bowel disease are the leading causes in industrialized

Table 1
Nontraumatic causes of small and large bowel perforation and respective treatment options

Cause	Treatment Options

Obstruction	• Small bowel
	  ○ Resection and primary anastomosis
	  ○ Alleviate cause of obstruction
	• Large bowel
	  ○ Resection and primary anastomosis
	  ○ Subtotal colectomy
	  ○ Alleviate cause of obstruction

Inflammatory bowel disease	• Resection of grossly involved bowel and primary anastomosis • Toxic megacolon—subtotal colectomy with end ileostomy

Diverticular disease	• Sigmoid diverticulitis
	  ○ Resection and end colostomy
	  ○ Resection and primary anastomosis
	  ○ Laparoscopic washout and drainage
	• Meckel's diverticulum
	  ○ Diverticulectomy
	  ○ Segmental bowel resection and primary anastomosis

Ischemia	• Resection and primary anastomosis or leave bowel in discontinuity • Management of underlying vascular pathologic abnormality • Second-look laparotomy
Radiation enteritis	• Resection and primary anastomosis or exteriorization
Foreign body	• Primary repair • Resection and primary anastomosis
Infectious	• Resection and primary anastomosis or exteriorization

nations, whereas infectious causes are more common in developing countries. Patients typically present with peritonitis and definitive diagnosis is made at the time of laparotomy. General treatment includes intravenous antibiotics and fluid resuscitation, whereas operative management depends on the underlying cause of perforation. **Table 1** summarizes the most common causes and treatment options for perforations of the small intestine and colon.

REFERENCES

1. Zielinski MD, Bannon MP. Current management of small bowel obstruction. Adv Surg 2011;45:1–29.
2. Cappell MS, Batke M. Mechanical obstruction of the small bowel and colon. Med Clin North Am 2008;92:575–97.
3. Gardiner KR, Dasari BV. Operative management of small bowel Crohn's disease. Surg Clin North Am 2007;87:587–610.
4. Lopez DE, Brown CV. Diverticulitis: the most common colon emergency for the acute care surgeon. Scand J Surg 2010;99:86–9.
5. Alamili M, Gogenur I, Rosenberg J. Acute complicated diverticulitis managed by laparoscopic lavage. Dis Colon Rectum 2009;52:1345–9.
6. Sharma RK, Jain VK. Emergency surgery of Meckel's diverticulum. World J Emerg Surg 2008;3:27.
7. Bobadilla JL. Mesenteric ischemia. Surg Clin North Am 2013;93(4):925–40, ix.
8. Ruiz-Tovar J, Morales V, Hervas A, et al. Late gastrointestinal complications after pelvic radiotherapy: radiation enteritis. Clin Transl Oncol 2009;11:539–43.
9. Hines J, Rosenblat J, Duncan DR, et al. Perforation of the mesenteric small bowel: etiologies and CT findings. Emerg Radiol 2013;20:155–61.
10. Eid HO, Hefny AF, Joshi S, et al. Non-traumatic perforation of the small bowel. Afr Health Sci 2008;8:36–9.
11. Jain BK, Arora H, Srivastava UK, et al. Insight into the management of non-trauamtic perforations of the small intestine. J Infect Dev Ctries 2010;4:650–4.
12. Wani RA, Parray FQ, Bhat NA, et al. Nontraumatic terminal ileal perforation. World J Emerg Surg 2006;1:7.
13. Michalopoulos N, Triantafillopoulou K, Beretouli E, et al. Small bowel perforation due to CMV enteritis infection in an HIV-positive patient. BMC Res Notes 2013; 6:45.

Index

Note: Page numbers of article titles are in **boldface** type.

A

Ampulla, adenoma of, endoscopic retrograde cholangiopancreatography in, 401–403
   anatomy and physiology of, 214–215

B

Bariatric population, biliary imaging in, 415
   biliary issues in, **413–425**
Bariatric surgery, 413–414
   cholelithiasis and, 414–415
Bile duct, common, endoscopy of, laparoscopic, 287–291
      open, 291–292
      laparoscopic exploration of, in gallstone pancreatitis, 269–270
   evaluation and exploration of, technical aspects of, **281–296**
   evaluation of, resident training implications in, 293
   fluoroscopic cholangiography of, 285–287
   injuries of, biliary reconstruction in, timing of, 306
      class I, 305
      class IV, 305–306
      classification of, Bismuth and Strasberg, 298, 299
         Stewart-Way, 298–301
      complete cholangiography in, 303
      identification of, 298–301
      intraoperative, 301–302
      management of, 304–306
      postoperative, 303–304
      specific, 305–306
      vascular injury associated with, 303–304
   intraoperative cholangiography of, 283–287
   postsurgical leaks of, endoscopic retrograde cholangiopancreatography in, 401
   preoperative cholangiography in, 282
      indications for, 282
      types of, 282–283
   ultrasound cholangiography of, 285
Bile duct stones, endoscopic retrograde cholangiopancreatography in, 399
Bile metabolism, 361–363
   and lithogenesis, **361–375**
   bile acid synthesis and, 362–363
   bile acids in, 362
   bile composition and, 362
   enterohepatic circulation and, 363–365
   farnesoid X receptor and, 364–365
   interorgan transport and, 363

Surg Clin N Am 94 (2014) 477–483
http://dx.doi.org/10.1016/S0039-6109(14)00022-X
0039-6109/14/$ – see front matter © 2014 Elsevier Inc. All rights reserved.

Moving?

Make sure your subscription moves with you!

To notify us of your new address, find your **Clinics Account Number** (located on your mailing label above your name), and contact customer service at:

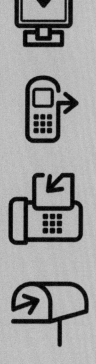

Email: journalscustomerservice-usa@elsevier.com

800-654-2452 (subscribers in the U.S. & Canada)
314-447-8871 (subscribers outside of the U.S. & Canada)

Fax number: 314-447-8029

Elsevier Health Sciences Division
Subscription Customer Service
3251 Riverport Lane
Maryland Heights, MO 63043

*To ensure uninterrupted delivery of your subscription, please notify us at least 4 weeks in advance of move.

Printed and bound by CPI Group (UK) Ltd, Croydon, CR0 4YY

07/10/2024

01040498-0012